Minor oral surgery

Minor Oral Surgery

Geoffrey L. Howe
TD MDS(Dunelm) MRCS(Eng) LRCP(Lond)
FDS RCS(Eng) FFD RCS(Irel)

*Formerly Professor of Oral Surgery and Oral
Medicine, University of Hong Kong and Professor of
Oral Surgery in the Universities of London, Durham
and Newcastle upon Tyne*

With a Chapter by

Ross J. Bastiaan
MDSc(Melb) LDS(Vic) MSc(Lond) FRACDS

*Periodontist, Clinical Consultant to the Royal Dental
Hospital of Melbourne and Senior Demonstrator,
Department of Dental Medicine and Surgery,
University of Melbourne*

With a Foreword by

the late Professor **F. C. Wilkinson**
CBE LLD MD DDSc MSc FRCS FDS RCS

THIRD EDITION

WRIGHT
Bristol
1985

Published by
John Wright & Sons Ltd, Techno House, Redcliffe Way, Bristol BS1 6NX, England

BY THE SAME AUTHOR
The Extraction of Teeth
(Bristol: John Wright & Sons Ltd)

With F. Ivor Whitehead
Local Anaesthesia in Dentistry
(Bristol: John Wright & Sons Ltd)

First edition, 1966
Second edition, 1971
Reprinted, 1973
Reprinted, 1976
Reprinted, 1977
Reprinted, 1978
Reprinted, 1980
Reprinted, 1983
Third edition, 1985

British Library Cataloguing in Publication Data

Howe, Geoffrey L.
    Minor oral surgery. – 3rd ed.
    1. Mouth – Surgery   2. Surgery, Minor
    I. Title   II. Bastiaan, R. J.
    617′.522   RK529

ISBN 0 7236 0823 7

Typesetting by
BC Typesetting
51 School Road, Oldland Common, Bristol BS15 6PJ

Printed in Great Britain by
John Wright & Sons (Printing) Ltd at The Stonebridge Press, Bristol BS4 5NU

Preface to the Third Edition

This book has been reprinted six times since the second edition was published fourteen years ago. Thus it would appear that it still fulfils the purpose for which it was designed.

Nevertheless, knowledge of all aspects of oral surgery continues to expand and so this third edition has been prepared. The opportunity has been taken to further clarify the text and to include both new material and suggestions for further reading. However the size, scope and design of the book remain virtually the same.

I am grateful to Dr Ross Bastiaan for completely rewriting chapter 14 and to Dr T. M. Moles for his help in updating the sections dealing with collapse, cardiac and respiratory arrest and obstruction of the airway. Many new illustrations have been included. Mr P. Darton of the University of Hong Kong has drawn *Figs*. 3.19, 5.45, 6.25, 6.49, 10.32, 10.35, 10.37, 11.11, 14.5, 14.6, 14.11, 15.1, 15.2*a*, 15.3, 15.4, 15.5, 15.6, 15.7, 15.8, 15.9 and 15.10. Ms Georgina Au of the Chinese University of Hong Kong drew *Figs*. 3.14, 3.37, 8.10, 8.14, 9.2, 9.3, 9.6, 9.7 and 10.15, whilst *Figs*. 14.3, 14.4, 14.8, 14.9, 14.10 and 14.13 are the work of Ms Anne Pottage of the University of Melbourne and *Fig*. 10.33 that of Ms J. A. Middleton. Dr L. M. Brocklebank provided *Figs*. 4.10, 6.14, 6.15, 6.33, 6.34, 7.3 and 7.5. The vast majority of the photographic work was undertaken most efficiently by Mr Raymond Leung of the University of Hong Kong but *Figs*. 14.2, 14.7, 14.12 and 14.16 are the work of Mr T. Dobrostanski of the University of Melbourne. The forthright detailed and constructive criticisms of Mr F. G. Hardman have been most helpful to me. My secretary Mrs Winnie Chiu has cheerfully typed and retyped much of the text and my wife has once again been a tower of strength to me during proof reading. I am deeply indebted to them all and greatly appreciate their assistance.

GLH

From the Preface to the First Edition

The amount and type of oral surgery performed in general dental practice are governed by many factors, the most important of which are the surgical experience, ability, and skill of the particular dental practitioner concerned. This facility can only be acquired by practice which is best obtained by holding worthwhile junior hospital appointments after qualification. The location and type of general practice may also influence the amount of surgical work undertaken by those engaged in it. If an oral surgery centre providing a first-class service is nearby the necessity to undertake this type of work within the practice is less compelling, whereas the dentist practising in a remote area may find it necessary to perform a considerable amount of surgery.

As a general rule it is usually inadvisable for the general dental practitioner to undertake any surgical procedure which, in his estimation, cannot be completed in thirty minutes under local anaesthesia. This time allowance can on occasions be increased by dental surgeons who have received postgraduate training in oral surgery and have access to either hospital or nursing-home facilities which permit the use of endotracheal anaesthesia.

Most patients who present with conditions remediable by means of oral surgery are seen in the first instance by a general dental practitioner, and it thus becomes obligatory for every dentist to have a good working knowledge of basic oral surgical principles and practice if he is to be an efficient dental surgeon.

Whilst there are excellent textbooks on oral diagnosis well suited to the needs of practising dental surgeons and large tomes which cover every aspect of oral surgery, there appears to be a need for a concise manual of practical oral surgery suitable for use by senior dental students and general dental practitioners. This work is designed solely to meet this need and for this reason major procedures, which are best performed by specialist oral surgeons working in hospitals, and interesting but rare clinical entities are deliberately excluded from it.

If it had not been for the ready and freely given assistance of many colleagues and friends this work would never have been completed. It is a pleasure to record my gratitude to Messrs P. Bradnum, L. W. Kay, and R. Sutton Taylor who read the complete text and suggested many improvements, to Mr D. P. Hammersley whose excellent line drawings do so much to clarify the text, and to Mr J. Davies and Mr B. Hill of the Photographic Department of the Newcastle Dental Hospital who have undertaken most of the photographic work. I am particularly indebted to my secretary, Mrs V. G. Dyer, who has typed and retyped the manuscript on innumerable occasions.

The knowledge and skill of every dental surgeon are compounded from personal experience, extensive and prolonged study, and the wisdom and guidance of his clinical teachers. Like every other professional man, I am for ever a debtor to those colleagues who taught me, not least of whom is that doyen of academic oral surgery, Professor F. C. Wilkinson, to whom I gratefully dedicate this book.

GLH

Contents

Foreword

by the late Professor F. C. WILKINSON,
CBE LLD MD DDSc MSc FRCS FDS RCS

Before the inception of the National Health Service in 1947 there were relatively few dental surgeons in Great Britain who either considered oral surgery to be the most important part of their daily work or who limited their practice to the speciality alone. Under the provisions of the Act a hospital service was set up, consultant dental surgeons were appointed to the staffs of general hospitals, and dental departments were established for the treatment of patients referred by general practitioners practising in the area served by the hospital.

Today, dental schools and many general hospitals have oral surgery departments, fully equipped with all the facilities necessary for the treatment of the various oral conditions which require surgical intervention and of accidental injuries to the jaws, and these units are staffed by well-qualified and experienced dental surgeons. With such excellent teaching and training centres to hand it is unfortunate that the time that can be allotted to the study of oral surgery, in the present over-crowded undergraduate curriculum, is too short for the dental student to avail himself of the opportunities afforded by such institutions and so he graduates with only a very superficial knowledge of the subject.

This book will therefore particularly appeal to the general dental practitioner who will find it a mine of information, and will appreciate the value and clarity of the advice it contains concerning the management of all types of patients requiring surgical treatment who are liable to seek his aid. The work is based upon the long experience that the author has had in teaching both undergraduate and post-graduate students. The close contact he has enjoyed with general practitioners in his capacity as a consultant has enabled him to appreciate and understand their problems. A full description is given of the methods employed in making a differential diagnosis, and I was pleased to note the repeated emphasis upon the fundamental importance of preoperative assessment and treatment planning in all cases. Complications which might arise during or following each operation are fully discussed. Intelligent anticipation is undoubtedly the best insurance against accidents.

The advice given on how to distinguish between the difficult case that looks simple, which is best referred to a consultant, and the simple case which looks difficult but can be treated in the surgery, should prove very valuable. The book is written in such a way as to arouse interest and I am sure that many readers will seek postgraduate training as a result of reading it. Although the work deals with minor oral surgery alone I would recommend it to candidates preparing for higher qualifications who will find the exposition of basic principles of considerable value, for they form a sound basis on which to extend one's knowledge.

Chapter 1

Diagnosis in oral surgery

The experienced clinician quickly recognizes many diseases due to his familiarity with the signs and symptoms which characterize them. Whilst such 'spot diagnosis' may facilitate diagnosis and treatment in many patients, there is no doubt that the method is also the underlying cause of many errors in the practice of medicine, surgery, and dental surgery. Therefore it is important that every clinician, however experienced he may be, uses 'spot diagnosis' with discretion and employs a methodical system of diagnosis whenever he is called upon to deal with a condition the nature of which is not immediately apparent to him.

The traditional system of diagnosis in all branches of medicine and surgery is detailed in *Table* 1.1 and comprises:

1. *History-taking*: during which the clinician listens to the patient's story and lists the *symptoms* in order of severity. A *symptom* may be defined as any change in the body, or its functions, which is perceptible to the patient and may indicate disease. In other words, symptoms are what the patient complains of.

2. *Clinical examination*: during history-taking the dental surgeon observes his patient and notes his demeanour and any obvious abnormality. These observations are then supplemented by a careful and thorough clinical examination of those areas and systems indicated by the patient's history. A *sign* may be defined as any change in the body or its functions which is perceptible to a trained observer and may indicate disease. The clinician elicits signs during his examination. Some lesions such as a lump may present as both a symptom and a sign.

After performing the first two stages of diagnosis it is often possible to make a provisional or presumptive diagnosis.

3. *Special methods of examination* (e.g., radiography, examination of the blood, or biopsy) are then employed either to confirm or to exclude diagnostic possibilities, thus enabling a definitive diagnosis to be made, and a treatment plan formulated which copes with operative difficulties and avoids possible complications.

Although in a busy dental practice it is all too easy to neglect the importance of diagnostic method, it is absolutely vital that the dental surgeon, confronted with any oral surgical problem, should proceed in an orderly, unhurried, and systematic fashion if embarrassing mistakes are not to occur. A common error is the failure to give a patient time to describe the pain of which he complains, before a mirror and probe examination of the teeth is performed. In these circumstances, it is possible to incriminate an impacted mandibular third molar as a cause of a pain which in fact is pulpal in origin and due to caries elsewhere. *Fig*. 1.1 is the radiograph of the right lower molar region of such a patient. This young man attended his general

Table 1.1. A Method of Diagnosis

---

1. History

    a. Personal Details—name, address, telephone number, sex, age, racial or ethnic group, occupation, marital status, habits.
    b. History of Present Complaint
    c. Past Medical History
    d. Drug History
    e. Family History
    f. Past Dental History
    g. Social History

2. Clinical Examination

    Inspection
    Palpation—extra-orally and intra-orally
    Percussion
    Auscultation

3. Provisional or Presumptive Diagnosis

4. Special Methods of Examination, including:

    Radiographic Examination
    Haematological Examination
    Biochemical Examination
    Histological Examination
    Bacteriological Examination
    Special Tests

5. Definitive Diagnosis

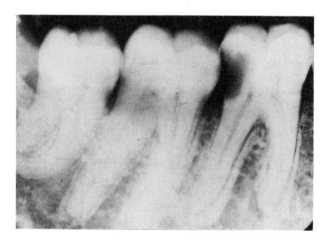

Fig. 1.1. Radiograph showing gross distal caries in a right mandibular first permanent molar.

dental practitioner complaining of 'toothache' in the right side of his mandible. Without further inquiry he was examined by his dentist, who noted the presence of a mandibular third molar, attributed the symptoms to this tooth, and referred the patient to hospital for specialist treatment. After putting the patient at ease the oral surgeon asked him to describe the pain that he was experiencing. The patient stated that at first the pain was precipitated by taking hot, cold and sweet things, but later came on at intervals without any obvious precipitating cause and kept him awake at night. Thus a pulpal cause of pain was immediately suspected and examination revealed the presence of a carious exposure of the pulp of the first permanent mandibular molar. Extraction of this tooth by the referring dentist relieved the patient of his symptoms but not his doubts regarding the abilities and competence of the practitioner concerned.

Every dental surgeon evolves a personal method of diagnosis from his experience, but the beginner is obliged to use a standard system and modify it to suit the needs of the individual patient.

Detailed notes should be made of the patient's history and all relevant examination findings. The need for good records cannot be overemphasized. The practice of maintaining carefully compiled clinical records is designed to further the interests of patients, but there have been numerous occasions on which they have been of great value to the clinician concerned either when retrospective studies are undertaken or when litigation ensues. All too many surgeons think that they remember everything about their patients when in fact they do not. Even if they did so, it must never be forgotten that case records are not only of value to the person who makes them, but also to other clinicians who may be called upon to treat the patient at a later date.

History-taking

The main components of a history are listed in *Table* 1.1 and each part may be of especial importance in the management of an individual patient.

Care should be taken to record accurately the *personal details* of the patient. The surname may indicate that he or she is a member of a family known to be afflicted with an hereditary disease or in which such anomalies as mandibular prognathism or dentinogenesis imperfecta occur. Poor access to medical and dental aid may influence a treatment plan and so both the *address and telephone number* should be recorded. As the patterns of disease vary between both the *sexes and racial and ethnic groups* a note should be made of these details. Some diseases are age-related and so the patient's *date of birth* should be recorded. Others, like silicosis in coalminers, are related to *occupations* whilst sailors and jet-setting businessmen may find difficulty in either obtaining treatment or keeping follow-up appointments. Pregnancy and family ties may also be important in this context and so the *marital status* of the patient should be noted.

A note should invariably be made of the *reason for the patient's attendance* at his or her first visit even when the patient is symptom-free and merely requests a dental check-up.

Many patients attend regularly for dental care and so usually have no complaints when first seen by a different dentist. The *past medical and dental histories* as well as details of any *drug therapy* that the patient either is, or has recently been receiving, may be of great significance in both diagnosis and treatment planning. All patients should be asked as a routine whether they have ever been afflicted with rheumatic fever, St Vitus' dance (chorea), heart, chest or lung disease or have any known allergies. Details of previous hospital admissions and operations should be sought together with particulars of any difficulties experienced with previous dental extractions or any history of post-extraction haemorrhage, abnormal bleeding or bruising. The *social history* may include such important details as a recent bereavement, stress either at work or at home, cigarette smoking and either alcohol or drug abuse.

During history-taking the dentist should encourage the patient to describe his symptoms in his own words, interrupting his story only to clarify a point or stop a lengthy digression.

Many patients are very anxious to help their dental surgeon and so he must take particular care to phrase every question so that an answer is not suggested. For example, the question, 'Does the pain come on when you take hot, cold, or sweet things into the mouth?' invites an affirmative answer and is therefore called a 'leading question'. A more accurate answer would probably be obtained if the question was reworded and the patient was asked, 'Is there anything that brings on the pain?'

During the early stages of his clinical career the student will find that history-taking can be, and often is, a time-consuming process. He will also note that his teachers elicit the relevant points of a case history in a fraction of the time he has taken. Speed in history-taking comes only with practice and must never be achieved at the price of either accuracy or completeness. The experienced clinician is able to facilitate the process by concentrating upon those features which practice has taught him to be of importance in the particular type of case being investigated.

A clear and concise summary of the patient's complaints should be recorded in the case notes, the symptoms being listed in order of importance. It is a useful practice to distinguish between those facts which the patient volunteers and those which are elicited as a result of direct questioning. Any relevant negative answer to a direct question should also be noted.

Clinical examination

Careful history-taking should be followed by a thorough clinical examination. Indeed the experienced clinician notes many features about his patient whilst he is taking the case history. He notes such details as the age and demeanour of the patient, whether the patient looks well or ill, or is pale or flushed, in addition to observing the presence of any local lesion which may exist.

Clinical examination should begin with extra-oral examination. It is often helpful to compare the condition of the similar organ or area on the other side in cases of difficulty. The size, shape, attachments and consistency of any swellings present should be noted. Swellings around the jaws may be tender or non-tender, soft, firm, or brawny, fluctuant or oedematous, or red and hot. The technique of eliciting fluctuation is illustrated in *Figs.* 1.2 and 1.3, and the best way of detecting a local rise in temperature is shown in *Fig.* 1.4. The facial, sublingual, submandibular and cervical lymph nodes should be palpated, and any enlargement or tenderness of the nodes noted (*see Fig.* 9.7). These lymph nodes can be felt more easily if, whilst the patient relaxes with his neck flexed, the soft tissues of

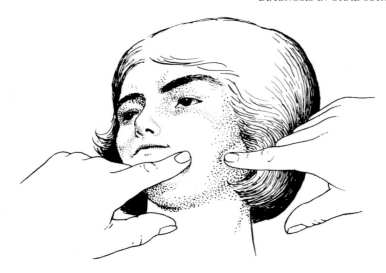

Fig. 1.2. Fluctuation may be elicited by placing the tips of two fingers on the lesion being examined. Pressure is applied with the tip of the 'examining finger' whilst the 'watching finger' is kept still. The presence of an impulse or fluid 'thrill' can be readily detected by the 'watching finger'.

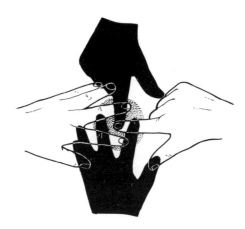

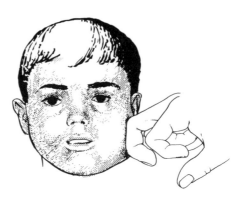

Fig. 1.3. When examining small lesions for fluctuation the 'examining finger' is applied between two 'watching fingers'. Fluctuation should always be elicited in two planes at right-angles to each other, as it is possible to elicit fluctuation in one plane in normal tissues such as large muscle masses.

Fig. 1.4. The dorsal surface of the middle phalanx of the fingers should be used to detect local rises in temperature, for it is the site of optimum thermotactile sensation.

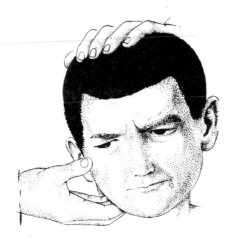

Fig. 1.5. Technique of palpating sub-mandibular lymph nodes.

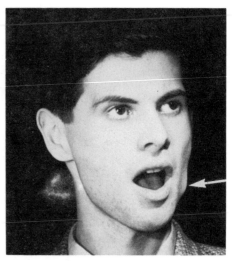

Fig. 1.6. This patient presented with a tender enlargement of the left facial lymph node 10 weeks after the removal of an impacted lower third molar (*see Fig.* 9.15).

the region being examined are firmly palpated with the finger-tips and rolled over a bony surface, such as the transverse processes of the vertebrae in the case of cervical nodes or the lower border of the mandible in the case of submandibular lymph nodes (*Fig.* 1.5).

The facial group of lymph nodes is situated just in front of the border of the lower attachment of the masseter muscle. In younger patients particularly, they sometimes become enlarged and tender as a result of a dental infection (*Fig.* 1.6). When such involvement occurs, these nodes may become tethered to either the overlying skin or the periosteum adjacent to them. This fact, and the tendency of these nodes to break down and form an abscess of the cheek, may be the cause of considerable diagnostic difficulty.

Firm pressure in the infra-orbital region may elicit tenderness in the presence of acute maxillary sinusitis. Any limitation of mouth opening, or deviation of the midline of the mandible during it, should be noted. Palpable clicking during movements of the temporomandibular joints is best felt if the examiner inserts his forefingers with the pulps forward in the patient's external auditory meatuses (*Fig.* 1.7). Whenever infection is present, the patient's temperature, pulse and respiration rates should be recorded.

Intra-oral examination should include inspection of the buccal and labial sulci, the tongue, palate, pharynx, and the floor of the mouth. When indicated, the ducts of the salivary glands should be palpated bimanually for the presence of calculi and saliva expressed from them (*Fig.* 1.8). The teeth present on clinical examination should be noted and any tooth absent from the arch accounted for (*Fig.* 1.9). Caries, abnormal mobility, faceting and the periodontal condition of the standing teeth should be recorded. The teeth should be lightly percussed and any abnormality of percussion note or tenderness noted. The presence of either dental plaque or food packing should also be recorded. Any edentulous area of gum should be dried and carefully examined for the presence of sinuses. If a sinus is detected, a fine probe should be carefully passed along it. Retained roots or unerupted teeth can often be felt in this way, thus enabling their precise location to be ascertained with some degree of accuracy. When it is possible to express pus from a sinus, a description of the pus should be recorded.

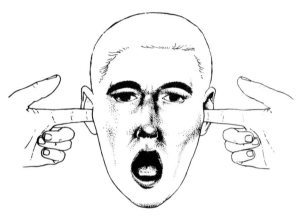

Fig. 1.7. Intra-aural palpation of temporomandibular joints. Dentists with broad index fingers should use the little fingers for this purpose.

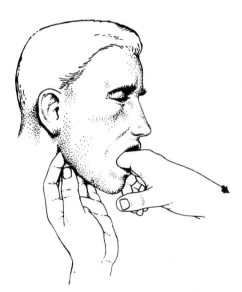

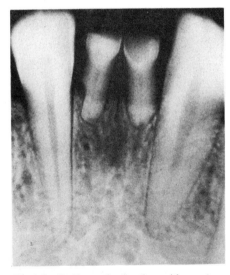

Fig. 1.8. Bimanual palpation of the sub-maxillary ducts.

Fig. 1.9. Radiograph of patient with congenital absence of lower permanent central incisors and retention of the deciduous predecessors.

Special methods of examination

Radiography is the special method of examination which is most frequently employed in the practice of oral surgery. The number of radiographic illustrations in this book serves both to emphasize the importance of this form of examination and to illustrate some of the ways in which it can be of value in the practice of oral surgery.

'Vitality' testing of the pulps of standing teeth is another useful aid to diagnosis, and both thermal and electrical methods are employed for this purpose. However, it must not be forgotten that they only test the integrity of the pulpal nerve supply whilst the vitality of the pulp is dependent upon its blood supply. Nerves appear to be more easily damaged than blood vessels. All methods of testing in clinical use are dependent upon the same unknown variables, namely the co-operation and response of the patient.

The teeth being examined should be isolated and dried before either a piece of hot gutta-percha, or a pledget of cotton-wool soaked in ethyl chloride, is applied to the crown of the tooth. Care should also be taken to avoid contact with the gingival tissues if 'false positive' responses are to be avoided. Despite this precaution being taken experience reveals that heat applied to a pulpless tooth may give a 'false positive' response on occasions. This finding is sometimes attributed to gaseous expansion within the closed pulp canal. Electrical pulp testing is a more sophisticated method of determining the vitality of tooth pulps (*Fig.* 1.10). Occasionally, a 'false positive' response is obtained when a pulpless tooth is tested in this way or with hot gutta-percha. This finding is usually associated with the presence of pus in the pulp chamber and canal of such a tooth. Whenever the results of pulp testing conflict with the overall clinical picture it is sound practice to suspect their accuracy. On occasions burring into the amelocemental junction to test pulp vitality may be justified. It should never be forgotten that the most common cause of facial pain is the presence of a dental lesion.

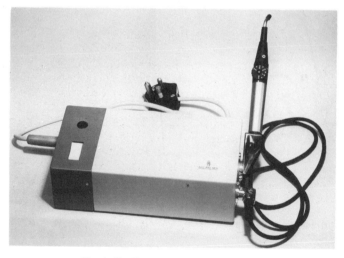

Fig. 1.10. Siemens' electric pulp tester.

Diagnostic method

A systematic technique of diagnosis is best illustrated by means of examples.

1. The diagnosis of 'toothache'

The commonest symptom which causes patients to seek dental aid is 'toothache', a term used by the laity to describe a variety of types of pain which may be due to many causes some of which are local and others systemic. Careful history-taking is essential if diagnostic errors are to be avoided. In the vast majority of cases, the patient's description of his symptoms makes diagnosis of the likely cause easy, and the experienced dentist knows what kind of lesion he is likely to find when he examines his patient.

The characteristic features of 'toothache' due to some common local causes are listed in *Table* 1.2, and in most cases diagnosis is a brief, obvious and satisfying procedure. In those relatively rare cases where difficulty or doubt is experienced, a very detailed history of the pain should be taken, and particular attention paid to the following points.

a. The Site of the Pain. The patient should be asked to point to the place where the pain is felt, using only one finger for the purpose.

b. The Onset and Duration of the Pain, and whether any incident, which might have played some part in the aetiology of the symptom, preceded its appearance (e.g., a blow on the jaw, recent dental treatment, etc.).

c. Any Radiation of the Pain. If the pain radiates, the patient should be asked to demonstrate its course with the tip of one finger. On other occasions pain may be felt in a site other than that of the causative lesion and is then described as 'referred pain'. Pain is never referred across the midline.

d. The Precise Characteristics of the Pain. Facial pain may be either continuous or intermittent, with or without exacerbations, which may or may not be precipitated. Episodes of pain may alternate with periods in which the patient is free from pain. The number, length and frequency of such episodes, together with the duration of the periods of freedom from pain, may prove to be of diagnostic significance.

e. The Severity of the Pain, and whether it is either increasing or decreasing, or is persisting at a uniform level. The degree to which the pain interferes with either the patient's activities or sleep may provide an indication of its severity.

f. The Timing of the Pain. Some pains are characteristically worse at particular times in the 24 hours, e.g., pulpal pain often wakens the patient at night and tends to keep him awake.

g. Any Factors which Precipitate the Pain. Thus pulpal pain is often precipitated by thermal and osmotic stimuli, antral pain by both stooping and jolting, and anginal pain by exercise. Periodontal pain is often precipitated by biting and chewing, although in the earliest stages of acute periodontitis many patients obtain relief by biting upon the affected tooth. Pain may also be precipitated by biting upon a cracked tooth or cusp.

h. Any Factors or Drugs which Relieve the Pain. The nature and duration of relief afforded by mild analgesics may aid the diagnostician in his attempts to assess the severity of the pain.

Table 1.2. Clinical Features of Some Important

Pain due to	Character of pain	Site of pain	Radiates into	Precipitating factors
Pulpal causes	Sharp and severe at first. Later sharp, severe, and continuous	Affected tooth and/ or referred to another tooth or edentulous area in either jaw on same side of face	Ear (lower teeth) and cheek, eye, and temple (upper teeth)	Intra-oral thermal and osmotic changes at first. Later, nil
Cracked tooth syndrome	Sudden, lancinating pain or discomfort of short duration occasionally accompanied by a dull pain	In one segment of the dentition	—	Chewing in one segment of dentition. Sometimes intra-oral thermal and osmotic changes
Acute periodontitis	Dull at first. Later dull with acute exacerbations when tooth bitten upon	Affected tooth	—	At first nil but later biting on tooth
Acute dental abscess	Dull, throbbing, and severe, with sharp exacerbations when involved tooth bitten upon or touched	Affected tooth	Ear (lower tooth), and cheek, eye, and temple (upper tooth)	Biting upon or touching involved tooth
Acute pericoronitis	Dull and continuous. Closure of jaws increases pain if impinging tooth is present	Affected area. Lower third molar regions are the most common site	To the ear on occasions	Impinging upper molars. Inability to clean area efficiently. Upper respiratory infection
Dry socket	Dull, throbbing, continuous ache	Site of an extraction performed 2–4 days previously	To the ear when lesion in lower jaw	Touching affected area

Local Conditions Causing Facial Pain

Relieving factors	Timing	Other symptoms and signs	Progress if untreated
Withdrawal of stimulus (Stage 1). Mild analgesics at first but analgesics gradually lose effect	Occurs only whilst stimulus applied (Stage 1). Lasts 20–30 min after stimulus withdrawn (Stage 2). Usually lasts longer than 30 min (Stage 3)	Caries of crown of tooth. New restoration. Fracture of or crack in enamel	May progress to acute periodontitis and abscess formation
Stopping chewing	Occurs only during chewing	Fractured or cracked cusp which is painful when either percussed or loaded and bitten upon	Good once cracked cusp is located and either removed or supported
Biting on affected tooth in early stages only. Analgesics	Continuous but worse at mealtimes	Redness of overlying gum. Affected tooth 'high' to bite and periodontitic	May progress to abscess formation
Heat in early stages. Analgesics	Continuous. Worse at night and mealtimes. Prevents sleep	When swelling appears after few hours pain is less intense although involved tooth is still acutely tender to touch. Enlarged tender lymph nodes. Fluctuation and/or pitting oedema. Involved tooth may respond to pulp testing if abscess is periodontal in origin	Pus bursts into soft tissues and pain diminishes. Pus may discharge and lesion may become chronic.
Local applications of heat. Analgesics	Continous. Worse at meal-times. Seldom prevents sleep	Pyrexia. Swelling. Trismus. Unpleasant taste. Foetor, dysphagia (rare). Tender enlarged lymph nodes	Infection may either resolve or spread, or become chronic
Local applications of heat. Analgesics	Continuous. Worse at meal-times. May prevent sleep	Foetor oris. Involved bone is tender to touch. Socket either empty or contains only broken-down blood clot	May resolve in about 2 weeks or progress to sequestration

Table 1.2. (*cont.*)

Pain due to	Character of pain	Site of pain	Radiates into	Precipitating factors
Acute maxillary sinusitis	Dull, throbbing, and continuous	Infra-orbital part of cheek and related upper teeth. Rarely occurs bilaterally	Eye and temple on the affected side	Jolting and bending forwards
Acute ulcerative gingivitis	Dull, continuous pain. Touching lesions causes severe pain	Affected areas of mouth	May cross midline if affected areas do	Patient generally run down. Poor oral hygiene

i. The Presence of Other Symptoms. Intermittent swelling may characterize obstructions to the flow of saliva, whilst the discharge of pus intra-orally may cause the patient to complain of either a sweet or an unpleasant taste. Clicking, crunching and inability to open the mouth may occur in disorders of the temporomandibular joint.

j.   Relevant Past Medical History. Patients with facial pain of vascular origin may have either a personal or family history of allergic disease (i.e., migraine, bronchial asthma, hay fever, eczema, or urticaria). A history of previous 'nervous breakdowns' is often obtained from patients afflicted with pain of psychosomatic origin or who possess a low pain threshold. 'Angina of effort' may be felt in the mandible.

k. The Views of the Patient concerning the cause of the Pain may provide valuable clues to the correct diagnosis.

Careful history-taking should be followed by a thorough and systematic clinical examination, as previously described. Special attention should be paid to certain other features when a patient complaining of obscure facial pain is being investigated. For example, the presence of herpes scars in the skin supplied by the ophthalmic or first division of the fifth cranial nerve may indicate that a diagnosis of post-herpetic neuralgia must be considered (*Fig.* 1.11). Inequality of the size of the pupils, or their reaction to light and accommodation, may emphasize the need for a thorough examination of the cranial nerves. No patient complaining of pain in or about the face should be labelled a neurotic by a dentist whose essential role is to eliminate any possible oral cause for the pain of which the patient complains, and he should never attempt to exceed that duty. The patient's physician should be provided with a report detailing the dentist's findings and his opinion as to whether any dental condition is playing any part in the aetiology of the pain.

Relieving factors	Timing	Other symptoms and signs	Progress if untreated
Decongestant nose drops. Analgesics	Continuous and may prevent sleep	Previous 'cold in head'. Pyrexia. Feeling of fullness in affected cheek. Nostril blocked on affected side. Related teeth tender to percussion. Tender on infra-orbital pressure. May complain of post-nasal discharge. Enlarged tender lymph nodes	May become chronic and cause chronic discharge
Analgesics	Continuous but seldom prevents sleep	Mild pyrexia occasionally marked. Characteristic foetor oris. Gums bleed readily. Unpleasant taste. Enlarged tender lymph nodes. Trismus rare. Malaise	Becomes chronic and destroys supporting tissues of teeth

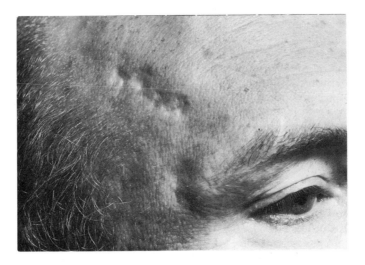

Fig. 1.11. Herpes scars on the forehead.

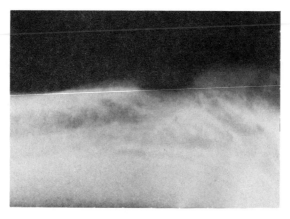

Fig. 1.12. Radiograph of premolar region of an atrophic mandible in which the mental foramen is situated on the crest of the ridge.

An isolated deep infected periodontal pocket may cause severe pain, and its presence can easily be missed unless particular care is taken to examine the depth of all the gingival crevices with a blunt probe. Interdental food packing is another cause of periodontal pain which may occur on both sides of the mouth concurrently. In edentulous patients, atrophy of the alveolar bone may result in the mental foramen being situated on the crest of the ridge (*Fig.* 1.12). In these circumstances, pressure from a denture may cause severe pain which radiates into the lower lip and may be accompanied by impairment of labial sensation. Palpation on the buccal side of the edentulous ridge in the premolar region reveals the presence of the thickened trunk of the mental nerve. If the denture is carefully eased in this site these unpleasant symptoms usually disappear and surgical repositioning of the nerve is seldom required.

No dental examination in a case of facial pain is complete unless good radiographs of both upper and lower jaws, and all the teeth on the affected side, have been taken and carefully examined. In some cases an obvious dental cause will be seen in the radiographs, whilst in other cases the absence of such a lesion will support a clinical impression that no dental cause for the pain exists. It is possible to interrupt sensation temporarily in localized areas by means of either periodontal, supraperiosteal or regional block injections of a local anaesthetic solution. The knowledge that such a diagnostic procedure alleviates the pain may aid localization of the lesion causing the pain and it is a great pity that this simple yet valuable diagnostic test is not employed more frequently.

When diagnosis is complete, any possible dental or oral cause of pain should be remedied as soon as possible. In most instances this results in complete relief of pain. Any patient in whom such a cause for facial pain cannot be detected or in whom the elimination of all possible dental and oral causes for the pain fails to produce relief, must be referred promptly either to her general medical practitioner or to a specialist oral surgeon for investigation. The dental surgeon should send a letter detailing his investigations, findings, treatment, and opinion to the physician concerned (*see* Chapter 16).

2. The investigation and management of a patient who requires multiple extractions and gives a history of post-extraction haemorrhage

Such a patient should be investigated by means of the classic method of diagnosis already described, and it will suffice for purposes of illustration if comment is limited to some points of special relevance in this particular kind of case. The importance of obtaining a detailed history from such patients cannot be over-emphasized for it often provides an indication as to whether or not an underlying coagulation defect is present.

Personal details may be of great assistance. Thus the patient's surname may indicate that he belongs to a family known to be afflicted with a haemorrhagic diathesis. The treatment plan may have to be altered if he lives a long way from medical and dental aid. Patients who possess a telephone can obtain medical and dental advice, and assistance, more readily if they bleed than those who are compelled to use public call boxes. Certain states which predispose to haemorrhage are commoner in one sex than the other and occur more frequently in certain ethnic groups. As age advances, it appears that some haemorrhagic diatheses (e.g., haemophilia) may become less severe in some cases. Nevertheless the dentist must remember that the mere fact that a patient has reached adult life without having been the subject of haematological investigations is not a reason for assuming that he is normal in this respect. The patient's occupation or compelling family commitments may affect the ease with which he or she can obtain treatment and attend for follow-up, whilst the marital status of women may reflect compelling family commitments.

A family history must be taken in every case, for some haemorrhagic diatheses have a familial background. Thus haemophilia occurs in males but is transmitted through females. Any tendency to abnormal bleeding in the male relatives of a male patient's mother is, therefore, of especial relevance. Congenital, as well as hereditary, abnormalities may be of importance in this context. Thus patients with hereditary haemorrhagic telangiectasia or Sturge–Weber syndrome (encephalo-trigeminal angiomatosis) may have angiomatous lesions in the oral cavity (*Figs.* 1.13, 1.14). Past dental history may help the dental surgeon to estimate the patient's interest in, and appreciation of, dental care in addition to indicating whether difficulty has been experienced with previous dental extractions. The patient should be carefully questioned about previous haemorrhagic episodes. It is important to discover how long ago the incident occurred, what precipitated it, and whether any teeth have been extracted without complications occurring since the episode in question. In this context the patient who bleeds after each and every dental extraction and who gives a history of having to return repeatedly for the treatment of haemorrhage from a single socket must be regarded as the one likely to have an underlying coagulation disorder. Such a patient should be referred to a haematologist for investigation prior to surgery being undertaken. Some idea of the severity of the bleeding can be obtained by thoughtfully worded questions concerning the methods which had to be employed to control the haemorrhage, their efficacy, and whether medical and dental aid was enlisted or admission to hospital necessitated. If it can be decided whether the bleeding was primary, reactionary, or secondary in nature, some light may be shed on the aetiology of the condition.

Past medical history may reveal a cause for abnormal bleeding. Some patients bleed excessively or bruise very easily in response to a trivial injury (*Fig.* 1.15). Others may be receiving either heavy doses of aspirin or anticoagulant therapy (*see* p. 26). A knowledge of both the general condition and domestic circumstances of the patient is required if a good dental treatment plan is to be formulated (*see* Chapter 2).

Care should be taken to ascertain whether the patient is in severe pain, for this may make it essential to expedite surgery.

Particular attention should be paid during clinical examination to the presence of pallor of the mucous membranes, bruising, or such lesions as angiomata.

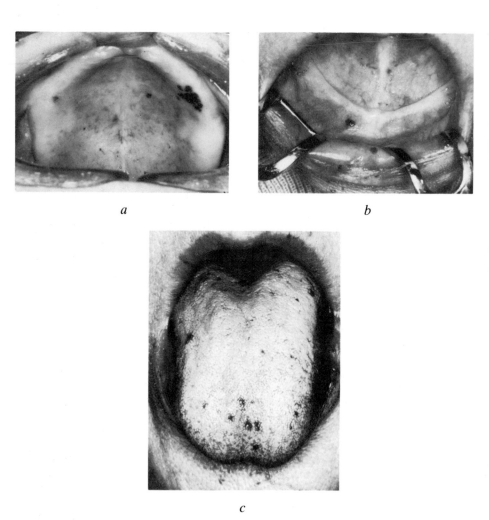

a   *b*

c

Fig. 1.13. Haemorrhagic telangiectasia. Lesions present on, *a*, palate, *b*, lower ridge and lip, and *c*, tongue.

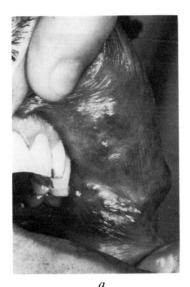

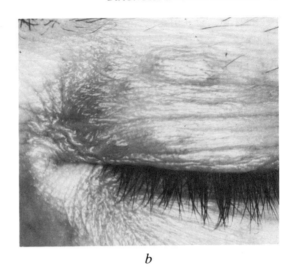

b

a

Fig. 1.14. Sturge–Weber syndrome. Lesions on, *a*, lip, and *b*, eyelid.

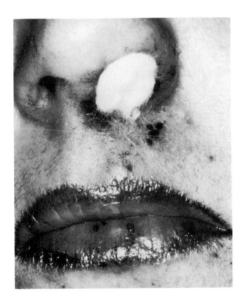

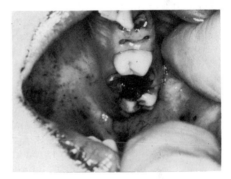

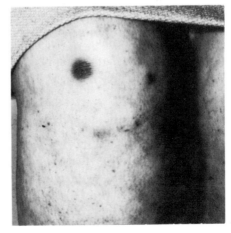

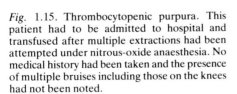

Fig. 1.15. Thrombocytopenic purpura. This patient had to be admitted to hospital and transfused after multiple extractions had been attempted under nitrous-oxide anaesthesia. No medical history had been taken and the presence of multiple bruises including those on the knees had not been noted.

The amount and character of previous dental treatment, the presence of local sepsis or calculus, are also of special importance in such a case. The number of teeth to be extracted should be decided on and note taken whether they are situated in several different quadrants of the mouth. An assessment of any difficulty which may be experienced in extracting the teeth should be made after taking a detailed history and performing a thorough clinical examination, supplemented by a careful study of pre-extraction radiographs (*Figs.* 1.16, 1.17). Other special methods of examination which may be performed by the dental surgeon are the estimation of the bleeding and clotting times and the tourniquet test (Hess's test) for capillary fragility.

The determination of the bleeding and clotting times are purely empirical tests, the results of which vary according to the particular technique employed. As the bleeding and clotting times are only prolonged in the presence of severe coagulation defects it is generally agreed that when the results fall within the range of normal, a tendency to abnormal post-extraction bleeding cannot be excluded. Prolongation of the bleeding and clotting time is, however, an indication for seeking the assistance of a haematologist. These tests are certainly no substitute for careful history-taking as a screening procedure and never suffice on their own as the haematological investigation of a patient in whom a coagulation defect is suspected.

A number of techniques are available for the determination of the clotting time. A convenient method is to collect blood from a needle stab wound of the lobe of the ear in a capillary tube containing a lead shot. The tube, which is about 2 cm long and about 1 mm in internal diameter, is inverted at intervals of 5 sec until the formation of blood clot prevents the movement of the lead shot within the tube. At room temperature this occurs in between 5 and 10 min in normal people. The bleeding time can be determined by timing the period taken for a freely bleeding stab wound of the lobe of the ear to stop bleeding. Excess blood is removed by very gentle application of the torn edge of a filter paper to the wound at 20-sec intervals. Excess blood is absorbed in this way without pressure being exerted on the bleeding point. In normal persons the bleeding is arrested in between 2 and 4 min.

The tourniquet test is performed in the following way. A sphygmomanometer cuff is applied to the upper arm, inflated to a pressure midway between the systolic and diastolic blood pressure, and kept at this level for 5 min. The cuff is then deflated and the arm raised for 1 min. The skin of the antecubital fossa is examined and in the normal patient not more than two or three tiny haemorrhagic spots are to be seen. The presence of more than eight petechiae in a circle 6 cm in diameter suggests that the capillaries are unusually fragile. A positive result may also be obtained if the platelets are deficient as in thrombocytopenic purpura.

The dental surgeon now has sufficient information to enable him to make a decision whether he can safely treat the patient in his own practice or whether he should refer the patient to a hospital with full haematological facilities. When he decides to undertake the treatment of the patient himself he should proceed in a systematic manner. Prior to performing an extraction he should clean up the mouth by means of pre-extraction scaling of the teeth which should be completed at least 1 week before extractions are commenced. A trial extraction of either the painful tooth alone or a single-rooted tooth, or other easy extraction, should be performed, care being taken to avoid tears in the soft tissues and fractures of the bony socket wall. If required a mucoperiosteal flap should be raised and the tooth

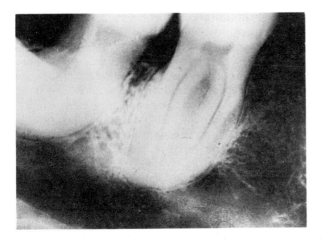

Fig. 1.16. Pre-extraction radiograph showing hypercementosis of tooth roots.

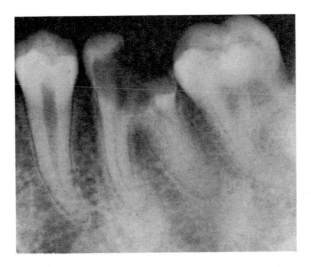

Fig. 1.17. This broken-down pulpless lower first molar has widely spread roots set in dense sclerotic bone and will be difficult to remove.

dissected from its attachments. The socket should be compressed between the operator's finger and thumb, and a gauze pressure pack inserted and bitten upon by the patient for a few minutes. If at the end of this time there is any sign of oozing, a horizontal mattress suture should be inserted to secure haemostasis (*see Fig.* 3.36). A suture should always be inserted whenever the patient has an established history of post-extraction haemorrhage or when any doubt exists as to whether the bleeding is under control.

Before the patient is discharged he should be asked either to walk around or go up and down some stairs in order to determine whether exercise causes the haemorrhage to recommence. Should this occur, pressure should be applied to the gum margins until the socket is filled with a firm clot. An effective method of exerting such pressure is by means of a block of composition, moulded so as to cover the bleeding tissues and to permit pressure to be applied to them when the patient closes his teeth together (*see Fig.* 15.11). The patient should then be discharged with instructions to avoid violent exercise, and to abstain from taking alcohol, very hot drinks, or using hot saline mouth baths for 24 hours. In case bleeding recurs, he should be instructed how to apply pressure to the bleeding point by means of either a clean folded handkerchief or the specially moulded composition block, and told to return should these simple measures fail to control the haemorrhage.

At a follow-up visit, 2–7 days after extraction, the patient should be questioned about his postoperative progress before the remainder of the treatment is planned. The results of the trial extraction are of great assistance in determining both the number of teeth to be extracted at one sitting and the measures likely to be required to secure haemostasis.

Accurate preoperative diagnosis and careful detailed treatment planning are the basis of the successful practice of oral surgery. In the succeeding chapters particular attention will be paid to those features which are of especial importance during such a preoperative assessment of individual cases.

SUGGESTED READING

Allen F. J. (1967) Post-extraction haemorrhage. *Br. Dent. J.* **122**, 139–43.
Blau J. N. (1982) How to take a history of head or facial pain. *Br. Med. J.* **285**, 1249–1251.
Fisher F. J. (1982) Toothache and cracked cusps. *Br. Dent. J.* **153**, 298–300.
Gillbe G. V. and Fellingham F. R. (1968) Repeated post-extraction haemorrhage. *Br. Dent. J.* **125**, 385–8.
Grundy J. R. (1957) History taking for cases of toothache. *Br. Dent. J.* **102**, 100–2.
Halpern I. L. (1975) Patient's medical status—A factor in dental treatment. *Oral Surg.* **39**, 216–26.
Haskell R. (1975) Drug treatments affecting the management of dental patients. *Br. Dent. J.* **139**, 249–51.
Hurwitz L. J. (1968) Facial pain of non-dental origin. *Br. Dent. J.* **124**, 167–71.
Hussar D. A. (1973) Interactions involving drugs used in dental practice. *J. Am. Dent. Assoc.* **87**, 349–58.
Joseph E. K. (1963) Dental and facial pain. *Dent. Pract.* **13**, 273–80.
Little J. W. (1976) Detection and management of the potential bleeder in dental practice. *J. Oral Med.* **31**, 11–18.
MacFarlane R. G. and Biggs I. R. (1955) *The Diagnosis and Treatment of Haemophilia*, MRC Memorandum No. 32.
Naylor M. N. and Moore J. R. (1962) Post extraction haemorrhage. *Br. Dent. J.* **112**, 349–53.
Orr J. A. and Douglas A. S. (1957) Dental extraction in haemophilia and Christmas disease. *Br. Med. J.* **1**, 1035–9.

Rosen H. (1982) Cracked tooth syndrome. *J. Prosthet. Dent.* **47**, 36–43.

Sutton R. B. O. (1982) The problem of obscure facial pain. *Dent. Update* **9**, 159–64.

Trieger N. and Goldblatt L. (1978) The art of history taking. *J. Oral Surg.* **36**, 118–24.

Walker D. G. (1969) Outline of a method for the detection of coagulation disorders. *J. Oral Surg.* **27**, 670.

Chapter 2

The importance of the general condition of the patient in oral surgery

The dental surgeon must always remember that he treats patients and not just their teeth. Every treatment plan must be based upon a careful assessment of the general condition of the patient in addition to his dental state. Many conditions may make it necessary to modify an otherwise ideal dental treatment plan in the best interests of the patient. For this reason it is necessary to make detailed inquiries concerning the past and present medical condition of all dental patients. At his first attendance the new patient should be asked a series of questions designed to obtain information concerning those conditions and treatments which have a direct bearing on dental treatment (*see* p. 50). A patient returning for treatment at a later date should be asked whether there has been any change in either his health or any medication he is receiving since the previous history was recorded. Parents must be carefully questioned concerning the medical histories of child patients.

Whenever the dental surgeon finds himself confronted with such a medical problem he should seek the advice, opinion and aid of the patient's physician. The patient is bound to benefit if there is mutual respect, informed understanding, and close co-operation between his medical and dental advisers.

For purposes of discussion it is convenient to divide such general medical problems into several ill-defined arbitrary groups.

CONDITIONS WITH A POOR PROGNOSIS

When patients are afflicted with diseases which have a poor prognosis, dental treatment should be limited in amount and of the simplest nature possible. There is little purpose in submitting them to prolonged, involved and expensive courses of treatment when a systemic factor exists which is likely to preclude the patient from enjoying the benefits of such treatment. Patients with such conditions as incurable cancer, untreatable uraemia, or those in terminal cardiac failure should only have dental treatment performed for the relief of pain which cannot be controlled by conservative measures and the use of analgesics. In most instances, extraction of the offending tooth under local anaesthesia brings relief, but in cases of leukaemia or agranulocytosis surgery must be avoided if possible.

Oral surgery in senile patients should only be undertaken when it is absolutely essential. Buried and semi-erupted teeth should be left in situ unless symptoms supervene which cannot be controlled by such conservative methods as antibiotic therapy and the prescription of analgesics. It is best to avoid the clearance of a number of remaining natural teeth in elderly patients who do not master dentures so readily as younger folk. When surgical treatment is obligatory, it should be performed under local anaesthesia rather than general anaesthesia whenever possible. If practicable, individual sessions of dental treatment should be planned so as not to exceed 15 min in duration in such cases.

CONDITIONS RESULTING IN LACK OF CO-OPERATION

Dental treatment may be both difficult and time-consuming when the patient has any condition which results in a lack of co-operation with the dentist. Thus dental treatment plans have to be modified when the patient is either insane or mentally deficient. The constant involuntary movements seen in paralysis agitans and the spasticity of cerebral palsy make the dental care of patients severely afflicted with these diseases very difficult unless endotracheal anaesthesia is employed. Young children below the age of reason are often unable to distinguish between pain and pressure, and in such cases an oral surgical procedure may have to be performed under general anaesthesia, although local anaesthesia would be the method of choice in an older patient. On occasions the combination of relative analgesia and local anaesthesia is a preferable alternative. Young children lose interest and patience quickly and should not be subjected to prolonged sessions of treatment.

Most patients afflicted with *epilepsy* are well controlled by medical treatment and usually present no problem in the practice of oral surgery, provided that they have not omitted to take the anticonvulsant drugs prescribed for them prior to attending for treatment. It is good practice to ask an epileptic patient to remove any denture he may be wearing before commencing dental treatment, and to limit the amount of dental apparatus inserted into his mouth as much as possible. Whilst he is actually receiving dental treatment he should be asked to bite upon a small mouth prop to which is attached a chain which hangs out of the mouth, thus providing a means of control over the prop. Should an attack of 'grand mal' occur during dental treatment, the dentist should remove all loose debris and dental apparatus from the patient's mouth as quickly as possible and lay the patient on the floor in the left lateral position in a clear area where he cannot harm himself during the convulsions. Alternatively, if the design of the dental chair permits it should be placed in the 10° head down position. A clear airway must be maintained at all costs and if the patient is wearing a tight collar it should be loosened. If the prop is left in position blood and secretions can be sucked out more easily. Oxygen should be administered by a face mask at a rate of 5–10 litres/min. Lorazepam 4 mg may be given by intramuscular injection to control the convulsions if required. Recovery is not usually long delayed and in some cases the dental treatment may be completed if in the opinion of the operator circumstances warrant this course of action. Although some patients feel a little drowsy after recovering from a seizure they are usually fit to travel home accompanied by a relative or friend. If recovery takes much more than a few minutes, medical aid should be obtained.

Epilepsy is usually treated by the administration of both long-acting barbiturates and anticonvulsant drugs. One of the latter group of drugs, phenytoin sodium (Epanutin, Dilantin sodium), may produce a hyperplastic gingivitis which is said to be characterized by the presence of vertical clefts (*Fig.* 2.1). Not all patients taking the drug are affected and the dosage does not seem to influence the degree

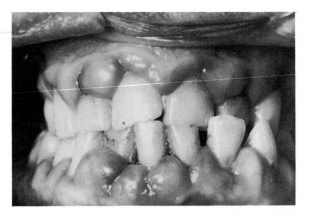

Fig. 2.1. Gingival hyperplasia due to phenytoin sodium.

of involvement. Although the presence of such local irritant factors as dental plaque, calculus or the overhanging margins of restorations play some part in the development of hyperplasia, this is not always the case. These hyperplastic masses recur after gingivectomy has been performed (p. 365) unless the administration of phenytoin is discontinued. Before periodontal surgery is undertaken in such a case, the patient's physician should be consulted and asked if it is practicable to prescribe an alternative anticonvulsant drug such as primidone (Mysoline) or methoin (Mesontoin), neither of which has been found to cause hyperplastic gingivitis. As both phenobarbitone and primidone tend to be hypnotic they are seldom prescribed together. Phenytoin sodium has little or no sedative effect.

No opportunity should be neglected to encourage epileptic patients to maintain a high standard of oral hygiene and receive regular dental care in an attempt to control plaque and preserve the natural dentition and so avoid the need for dentures. Unfortunately many of these patients have poorly cared-for mouths, a finding which may in part be related to the degree of long-term sedation required to keep them free of fits.

When general anaesthesia is required it must not be forgotten that methohexitone (Brietal sodium) is itself a convulsant. For this reason this barbiturate should not be employed when a patient has a history of epileptic convulsions because its use may predispose to status epilepticus under anaesthesia.

CONDITIONS PREDISPOSING TO EXCESSIVE HAEMORRHAGE

Most patients suffering from conditions which predispose to excessive haemorrhage are best treated in a hospital in which full haematological and blood transfusion facilities exist. The general dental practitioner should refer any patient whom he believes to be suffering from any of the haemorrhagic diatheses (e.g., haemophilia, Von Willebrand's disease, purpura, or Christmas disease) to such an institution for investigation and treatment (*Fig.* 2.2). Patients who have liver disease of such a degree as to affect blood coagulation are usually already under the care of a physician when they seek dental treatment. The advice and assistance of the

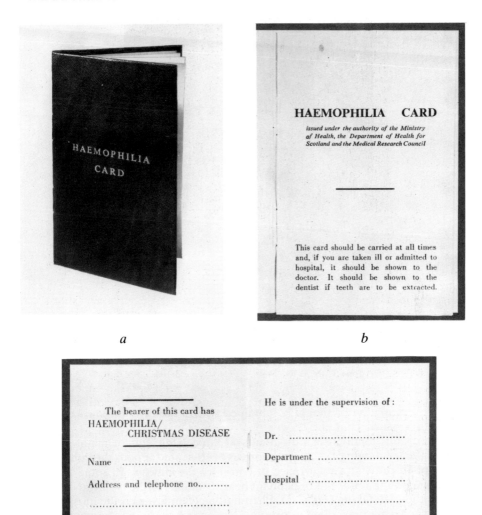

Fig. 2.2. Official card (10·6 × 7·6 cm (4·2 × 2·6 in), 8 pp.) issued to haemophiliacs. The card has, *a*, dark-green stiff covers, *b*, clear instructions on the title page, and, *c*, contains a great deal of useful information.

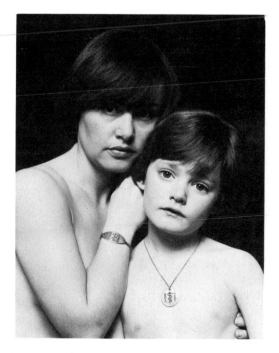

Fig. 2.3. 'Medic-Alert' wrist bracelet and pendant. (*By courtesy of Medic-Alert Foundation.*)

patient's medical adviser should be obtained before the dental treatment plan is formulated for such a patient.

An increasing number of outpatients are receiving anticoagulant therapy, either for the treatment of such conditions as deep-seated venous thrombosis or in an attempt to prevent a recurrence of coronary thrombosis. In some instances such patients wear a bracelet or pendant bearing details of the type and dosage of the drugs they are taking (*Fig.* 2.3). Phenindione (Dindevan) is the most popular anticoagulant drug prescribed at present, although heparin and coumarin drugs are also in use. There is good reason to believe that the likelihood of coronary thrombosis occurring is higher in patients in whom anticoagulant therapy has been temporarily suspended than in those patients who have never been treated with these drugs. When dental extractions are to be performed on such a patient, the advice and assistance of the physician responsible for the anticoagulant therapy should be obtained. In many cases the prothrombin level will be such as not to necessitate any alteration in dosage, whilst in others it may be wise to gradually reduce the dosage until the prothrombin time is maintained at one and a half to two times the regular control level. In practice, difficulties are seldom experienced when a limited number of teeth are extracted from an outpatient who is taking his usual dose of anticoagulants, provided that the pre-extraction prothrombin ratio is within the therapeutic range, especial care is taken to minimize damage to the supporting structures and the sockets are sutured immediately, using mattress sutures.

Pressure is applied to the socket margins by means of either a previously constructed removable appliance, or a moulded block of composition impression material, which is bitten upon by the patient. In most instances these measures arrest the haemorrhage, but occasionally it is necessary to sew a pack of either Whitehead's varnish or thrombin on ribbon gauze over the socket. On the rare occasions when these local measures fail to stop the bleeding, phytomenadione (Konakion) 10–20 mg may be given either by mouth or intramuscularly. In cases of emergency this substance can be slowly injected intravenously (1 mg/min) and the patient should be transferred to a hospital.

The dental surgeon must be guided by the physician when deciding whether to treat each individual patient in his practice, or whether to refer him to a centre in which facilities for blood transfusion are readily available.

If the patient is treated in a dental practice or as an outpatient he must be given clear instructions how and where he can obtain the assistance of trained personnel if required during the postoperative period.

Anaemia may be accompanied by a tendency to either postoperative haemorrhage or delayed healing, and all patients who appear upon clinical examination to be anaemic should be referred for a haemoglobin estimation prior to surgery. When this test confirms the clinical impression the dental surgeon should enlist the aid of the patient's physician in the management of the case. Whilst preoperative correction of anaemia is always desirable it is of particular importance in patients afflicted with cardiac disease. Surgical treatment should be deferred until the anaemia is controlled whenever it is possible to do so, for blood loss during and after the operation aggravates the condition. When surgery cannot be postponed the patient should be treated in hospital and general anaesthesia should be avoided if possible, for any episode of oxygen deprivation may cause either myocardial or cerebral damage due to ischaemia. General anaesthesia is also contra-indicated in patients afflicted with sickle-cell disease, a condition mainly confined to Negroes, in which oxygen deprivation may precipitate a severe sickling crisis in which the erythrocytes become distorted and disintegrate. Whilst the 'Sickledex' test is a convenient and quick method of screening patients for the presence of either sickle-cell anaemia or the sickle-cell trait, it occasionally gives false positive results. Furthermore it cannot distinguish the relatively common sickle-cell carrier from the uncommon patient with a sickle-cell disease who may react badly to anaesthesia. Such patients may have no history of previous ill health. When it is positive the patient should either be treated under local anaesthesia or referred to a colleague who has the facilities and expertise to perform further haematological tests including electrophoresis and to deal effectively with any complication which may occur.

CONDITIONS AFFECTING THE CHOICE OF ANAESTHESIA

A number of general conditions affect the choice of the form of anaesthesia to be employed for an oral surgical procedure. Oral surgery may be performed under either local or general anaesthesia, and the dental surgeon must assess the indications and contra-indications of both before deciding which to use in a particular case. On many occasions either method will suffice, and in these circumstances the patient may be allowed to choose between them. However, if there is a positive contra-indication to the method of anaesthesia for which the patient has a preference, the dental surgeon should not be persuaded to use a technique which is not in the best interests of his patient, but should follow the dictates of his trained opinion.

Hurry is the enemy of good oral surgery and an ill-chosen form of anaesthesia is a common cause of hurry. The dental surgeon must learn to estimate with accuracy the time required to complete each operation, for this enables him to choose a form of anaesthesia which provides adequate operating time for the completion of his task.

Modern anaesthesia is such that specialist anaesthetists with full hospital facilities seldom, if ever, refuse to give a general anaesthetic to an inpatient, however unfit he may be, provided that such an anaesthetic is administered for an essential procedure. Conversely, the use of general anaesthesia for oral surgical procedures performed upon outpatients has many limitations. A good dental anaesthetist can usually provide 5–10 min operating time under a general anaesthetic of inhalational type in the dental chair without the risk of anoxia or other complications. Although some exceptionally experienced and skilled anaesthetists are able to double this operating time, as a general rule the dental surgeon should not choose this form of anaesthesia for any operation which may last for more than 5 min. Local anaesthesia may be used for any dental operation of 30–45 min duration, but any surgical procedure requiring longer than this is an indication for the use of either sedation or relative analgesia or for admission to hospital and the administration of an endotracheal general anaesthetic.

Both general and local factors govern the choice of anaesthesia for oral surgery, and the operator must be fully conversant with them if he is to make a correct choice.

GENERAL FACTORS GOVERNING THE CHOICE OF ANAESTHESIA

Very large or very obese patients are often unsuitable subjects for a general anaesthetic in the dental chair, especially if they have any tendency towards alcoholism. The co-operation of the patient is not only essential when local anaesthesia is being employed, but it can be used to great advantage to facilitate the operation. Some patients are incapable of this co-operation for such reasons as fear, apprehension, extreme nervousness, hysteria, mental deficiency, or insanity. Young children below the age of reason find it impossible to distinguish between pressure and pain and so are liable to prove uncooperative if local anaesthesia is used. In some instances the judicious use of premedication may make the employment of local anaesthesia possible, but in most cases oral surgery upon such patients is easier if general anaesthesia is used. The induction of general anaesthesia in these circumstances may be difficult and may tax to the full both the skill and patience of the most experienced anaesthetist. Epileptics are usually good subjects for either local or general anaesthesia provided that they have not omitted to take the anticonvulsant drugs to which they are accustomed, and anoxia and the use of methohexitone are avoided.

Systemic disease may be the deciding factor which influences the choice of anaesthesia. Any condition which impairs either respiratory efficiency or the patency of the airway is a contra-indication to general anaesthesia in the dental chair. Chronic bronchitis, emphysema, bronchiectasis, asthma, tuberculosis and excessive smoking interfere with respiratory exchanges, whilst nasal obstruction, paralysis of the vocal cords and space-occupying lesions of the neck may interfere with the patency of the airway. Any acute infection of the respiratory tract is an absolute contra-indication to general anaesthesia in the dental chair, and in these cases local anaesthesia should be employed if the surgery cannot be postponed. Acute infection in the floor of the mouth is a contra-indication to any form of anaesthesia as an outpatient. Oedema of the glottis and laryngeal obstruction may complicate general anaesthesia in such circumstances, whilst local anaesthesia is impracticable. These patients should be admitted to hospital and any necessary surgery performed under endotracheal anaesthesia.

Whilst patients with rheumatic heart disease usually tolerate both surgery and anaesthesia better than the middle-aged or elderly patient with either hypertensive or ischaemic heart disease, most patients with any form of cardiovascular disease do not withstand anoxia or hypotension well, however temporary it may be. The use of hypotensive agents to treat patients with high blood pressure may cause problems when general anaesthesia is employed (see p. 46). For this reason it is better to employ local anaesthesia in these cases whenever it is practicable to do so. Whilst some authorities advise the omission of adrenaline from the local anaesthetic solutions administered to patients suffering from cardiovascular disease, it is widely believed that the small amounts of adrenaline administered for dental purposes are, in fact, beneficial, because they ensure a more certain, prolonged and profound anaesthesia and thus decrease the amount of adrenaline secreted by the patient himself in response to pain or fear. Other authorities prefer to use an alternative agent such as a 3% solution of prilocaine (Citanest) containing the vasoconstrictor, felypressin, when treating such patients. The patient's tolerance to exercise is the best guide to his ability to withstand both anaesthesia and surgery. In severe heart disease the patient should be admitted to hospital for any form of oral surgery whatever type of anaesthesia is to be used (see p. 40).

Many anaesthetists prefer not to administer a general anaesthetic in the dental chair to a woman in the first or last 3 months of pregnancy, as they fear that any anoxic episode during the anaesthetic may damage the foetus. Pregnancy is not a contra-indication to the use of local anaesthesia, which, however, should not be used in certain rare haemorrhagic diseases such as haemophilia, Christmas disease, or Von Willebrand's disease, due to the risk of bleeding at the injection site. Whilst it has been claimed that conservative treatment may be performed under intraligamentary anaesthesia the dangers associated with dental extractions in these patients are such as to make admission to hospital and full haematological cover imperative. In general, the patient classified as a poor anaesthetic risk should be treated as an in-patient under either local anaesthesia or endotracheal anaesthesia.

Until comparatively recent times most local anaesthetic agents available for use in dental surgery contained the p-aminobenzoic acid ring. This molecular structure is also found in certain other drugs (e.g., sulphonamides) and some patients acquire a sensitivity to it. The administration of any substance which contains this ring in its molecule (e.g., procaine and benzocaine) is contra-indicated in sensitized subjects (Fig. 2.4). Fortunately, the introduction of lignocaine (lidocaine, xylocaine), a local anaesthetic agent with a completely

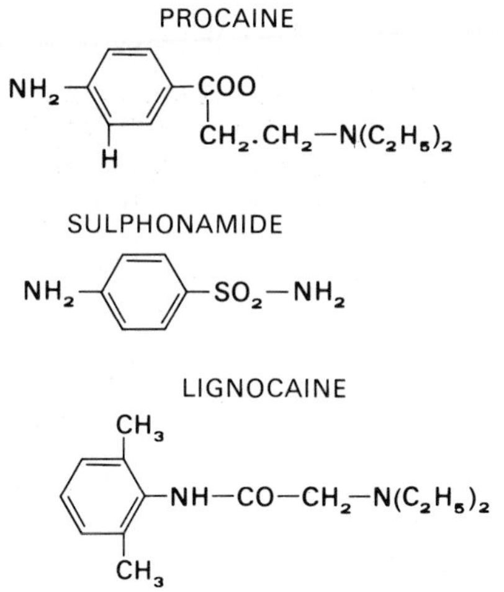

PROCAINE

SULPHONAMIDE

LIGNOCAINE

Fig. 2.4. Although chemically related to procaine and sulphonamide, lignocaine does not contain the *p*-amino group which seems to be responsible for inducing allergic sensitivity.

different chemical structure, has made it possible to utilize an alternative agent when the patient either gives a history of or exhibits sensitivity to a particular drug. Whilst it is conceivable that in very rare instances patients can react to both ester-linked local anaesthetics (e.g., procaine) and their amide link successors (e.g., lignocaine) such a possibility has yet to be confirmed.

Certain practical considerations may govern the choice of anaesthesia when undertaking oral surgery. The techniques of local anaesthesia are easily mastered, and the equipment required is limited in amount, economical and easily transportable. No preoperative preparation of the patient is required for local anaesthesia, and the patients can leave the surgery unescorted and often return to work after a local anaesthetic has been used.

LOCAL FACTORS GOVERNING THE CHOICE OF ANAESTHESIA

The most important contra-indication to local anaesthesia is the presence of acute infection at the site of operation. Injections of local anaesthetic solution into acutely inflamed areas spread the infection and seldom produce anaesthesia. It is sometimes possible to use regional anaesthesia to obtain the desired effect, but no attempt should be made to use an inferior dental block in patients with infections in either the floor of the mouth or retromolar area. The vasoconstrictor contained in most local anaesthetic solutions assists haemostasis, thus providing a drier field of operation, and this materially assists the surgeon. If there is a tendency to bleed due to the presence of a local abnormality, such as a haemangioma, local anaesthesia should be avoided and the operation undertaken only in a hospital with full haematological facilities (*Fig.* 2.5). The blood supply of any bone which has received therapeutic irradiation is impaired and the use of local anaesthesia

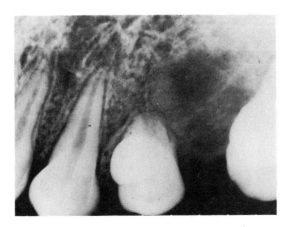

Fig. 2.5. Periapical radiograph showing an intra-osseous cavernous haemangioma.

with its contained vasoconstrictor is contra-indicated for oral surgery in these cases due to the risk of osteoradionecrosis supervening (*see* p. 33).

Of necessity the many contra-indications, advantages, and disadvantages of local and general anaesthesia in the dental chair have been emphasized. It is very important to remember that both methods have been in widespread use for a long time and that the morbidity is infinitesimal if care is taken in the selection of the appropriate method. The dental surgeon should make careful inquiries into the general medical history of any patient consulting him about an oral surgical problem, and in cases of difficulty he should confer with the patient's physician before selecting the form of anaesthesia to be employed.

CONDITIONS DICTATING THE DEFERMENT OF DENTAL TREATMENT

Deferment of all but urgent and essential dental treatment is dictated by the presence of such general conditions as shock, thyrotoxicosis, acute poliomyelitis, acute pulmonary tuberculosis, acute viral hepatitis and the exanthematous fevers. If such a patient has severe pain which cannot be controlled by conservative methods of treatment, minimal surgery can sometimes be performed under local anaesthesia, provided that full medical cover is available. Clinically, the incidence of dental decay in patients suffering from active pulmonary tuberculosis appears to be increased and severe pain may result from this and necessitate surgical treatment. The use of para-aminosalicylic acid (PAS) or its derivatives and of isonicotinic hydrazine (INH) or its derivatives, for the treatment of tuberculosis prior to dental and oral surgical procedures, is believed to predispose to haemorrhage. Dental treatment undertaken for patients receiving one or more of these drugs may be complicated by slow but persistent bleeding. The onset of these haemorrhages may occur several days after oral surgical interventions, but the bleeding can usually be arrested by pressure. It is occasionally necessary to use either a suture or a haemostatic agent to secure haemostasis. It has been claimed

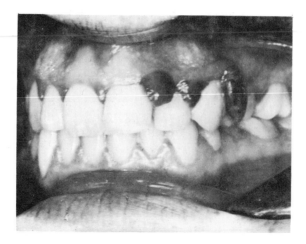

Fig. 2.6. Pregnancy gingivitis with 'tumour' formation interdentally.

that patients receiving INH have a greater chance of developing a 'dry socket' after tooth extraction, and the use of antibiotic cover has been advocated in such cases (*see* p. 392). The patient's physician should be consulted if it is proposed to employ such cover under these circumstances.

As drugs may cross the placental barrier and produce adverse effects upon the fetus it is wise to limit medication in pregnant women as far as is practicable. When general anaesthesia must be employed anoxia, however transient, must be avoided. Pregnancy gingivitis and 'tumours' (*Fig.* 2.6) are usually seen during the last 6 months of pregnancy, and when these conditions merit surgical treatment, local anaesthesia with or without premedication should be employed. A pregnancy 'tumour' is often related to some local source of irritation, e.g., calculus, an overhanging margin of a filling, or the sharp margin of a carious cavity, and it is important to eliminate any such predisposing factor, when excising the lesion, if recurrence is to be avoided. The haemorrhage which accompanies the removal of a 'pregnancy epulis' can often be controlled by the insertion of an interdental pack of zinc oxide and oil of cloves paste on cotton-wool to cover and compress the site from which the haemorrhage originates.

CONDITIONS ASSOCIATED WITH DENTAL OR ALVEOLAR ABNORMALITIES

General conditions associated with dental or alveolar abnormalities are fortunately rare. Cleidocranial dysostosis is often accompanied by failure of eruption of some teeth. Supernumeraries may be present and the unerupted teeth are often of bizarre form and have hooked roots (*Fig.* 2.7). Surgical exposure of such teeth does not facilitate their eruption. In addition to the bony abnormalities which often affect the jaws in osteitis deformans (Paget's disease of bone) the teeth may be either hypercementosed or ankylosed (*Fig.* 2.8). The deformed alveolar bone can be cut easily with either a hand gouge or chisel, but tends to bleed readily during the operation and heal slowly after it. A chronic bony infection with sequestration may follow quite simple surgery in a bone affected by the disease.

The jaws fracture readily in patients suffering from fragilitas ossium who may also be afflicted with odontogenesis imperfecta (*Fig.* 2.9). In the rare disease known as osteopetrosis (marble bone disease) great difficulty may be experienced in cutting the sclerotic bone which heals badly, chronic osteomyelitis often complicating minor surgery in these patients. Patients afflicted with this disease are usually anaemic due to the obliteration of the marrow cavities in their bones and have enlarged spleens in which active haemopoietic tissue is demonstrable. Fibrous dysplasia may affect the jaws and cause deformity (*Fig.* 2.10). Any surgery designed to deal with such a lesion and improve the patient's appearance should only be undertaken by a specialist oral surgeon and must be deferred until the disease has 'burned itself out', if recurrence of the deformity is to be avoided.

CONDITIONS ASSOCIATED WITH DELAYED HEALING AND LOWERED RESISTANCE

Therapeutic irradiation has proved to be a weapon of great value in the management of malignant disease. Therefore it is unfortunate that its use may be complicated by side-effects, the incidence of which has not decreased with the introduction of megavoltage therapy. Fibrosis in irradiated salivary glands leads to a diminution in the flow of saliva and dryness of the mouth (xerostomia). This is often associated with poor oral hygiene, rampant caries and advanced periodontal disease. The blood supply of the jaws is impaired by endarteritis obliterans and the healing potential of the bone is reduced. In these circumstances either a trivial injury or the extraction of a tooth may be complicated by osteoradionecrosis, a painful and debilitating condition. For this reason many radiotherapists insist upon the patient having a dental clearance of the area to be irradiated prior to the treatment of an oral malignant lesion. Although ideally 6 weeks should elapse between the completion of the dental extractions and the start of a course of radiotherapy, such a delay is seldom either practicable or clinically justifiable, and so the irradiated sockets often heal slowly. When teeth are extracted prior to irradiation it is usual to delay therapy for 3 days if the healing socket is in an area which is not scheduled to receive heavy irradiation, and for between 7 and 10 days if the socket is to receive intensive therapy. Even when healing is complete the patient may experience difficulty in wearing dentures due to xerostomia and denture trauma may cause a breakdown of the irradiated soft tissues leading to osteoradionecrosis. For this reason some authorities feel that the provision of prostheses is contra-indicated. Sometimes patients require either a dental extraction or some other oral surgical procedure in an irradiated area. This should only be undertaken after consultation with the radiotherapist concerned, and precautions should be taken in an endeavour to reduce the likelihood of osteoradionecrosis occurring. The number of extractions should be limited to two or three at a time and be performed under general anaesthesia and antibiotic cover. The delivery of the teeth should be followed by careful trimming of the alveolus, debridement and suturing to obtain primary closure of the extraction wounds. A good standard of oral hygiene must be maintained throughout the healing period.

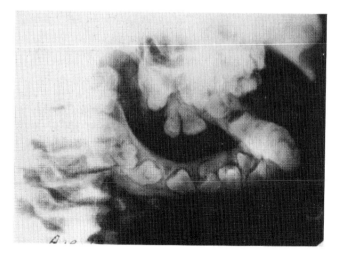

a

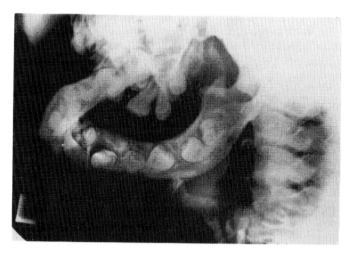

b

Fig. 2.7. Cleidocranial dysostosis. *a*, Right, *b*, left lateral oblique, and *c*, occlusal radio-graphs. All the permanent teeth are present but most of them are unerupted and misplaced. A number of supernumerary teeth are present.

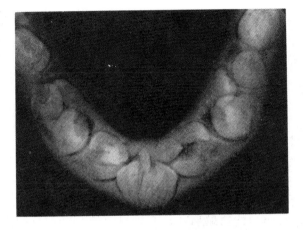

c

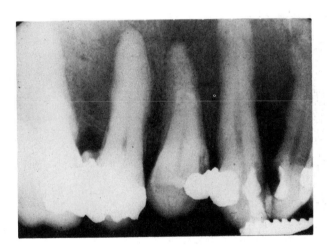

Fig. 2.8. Periapical radiograph of patient with osteitis deformans.

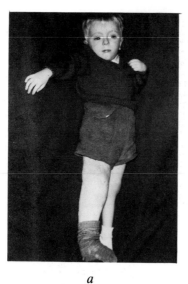

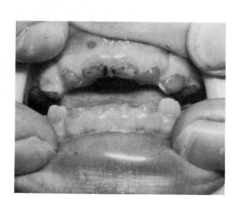

a *b*

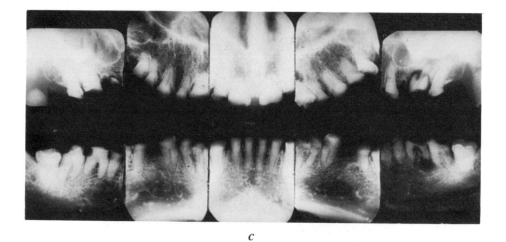

c

Fig. 2.9. Dentinogenesis imperfecta. *a*, Patient with fragilitas ossium who, *b*, exhibits odontogenesis imperfecta. *c*, Typical radiographic appearances of odontogenesis imperfecta in an adult patient. Note the poor quality of enamel with marked attrition, obliteration of pulp canals, short roots, and apical rarefaction. This patient did not have an osteodystrophy.

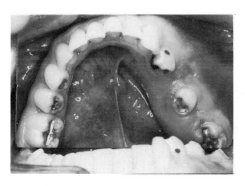

a

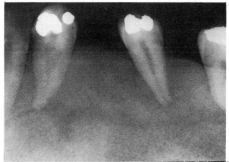

b

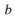

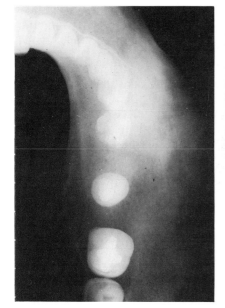

c

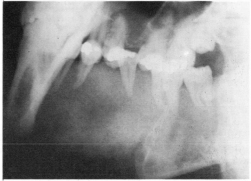

d

Fig. 2.10. Monostotic fibrous dysplasia of the mandible. *a*, Mirror picture of the clinical appearance. *b* and *c*, Radiographic appearances in intra-oral films. *d*, Radiographic appearance in extra-oral film.

Any debilitating diseases, such as chronic nephritis, cirrhosis of the liver, or diabetes mellitus, may be associated with poor healing of the tissues and a lowered resistance to infection.

Uncontrolled *diabetes mellitus* may be accompanied by severe periodontal disease and acute infections. Well-controlled diabetics stand surgery and anaesthesia well if their general condition is carefully supervised by a competent physician before, during, and after surgery.

Diabetes varies in its severity and is usually treated by dietary measures alone, or diet combined with either an oral antidiabetic agent such as chlorpropamide (Diabenese) or injections of insulin.

Diabetics whose condition is controlled by either diet alone or diet combined with an oral antidiabetic agent seldom present any problems in dental practice provided that they adhere to their usual therapeutic régime. The timing of dental treatment is not critical in such cases.

If the patient is receiving insulin, minor oral surgery should be performed under local anaesthesia if this is practicable, and it is not usually necessary to alter the dosage of insulin. It is wise to arrange dental appointments in the morning about 1 or 2 hours after breakfast and after the usual dose of insulin has been administered, for control of the condition is likely to be better at this time than later in the day.

The administration of a general anaesthetic to a diabetic whose condition is controlled by insulin is best undertaken in the morning. If the surgery can be performed just prior to the midday meal the normal diet and insulin dosage can be taken, and the timing provides the required period of abstinence from food in preparation for the anaesthesia without upsetting the patient's routine. If the normal dose of insulin were taken and the patient was denied breakfast, hypo-glycaemia could occur. For this reason some physicians reduce the normal morning dose of insulin by half in these circumstances, and then take steps to ensure a normal postoperative dietary intake to counteract the effects of missing the morning meal. Any diabetic patient receiving a total of more than 60 units of insulin daily, or whose condition is unstable, should be admitted to hospital for dental treatment. Acute infection increases the need for insulin and may cause the condition of even a well-controlled diabetic to become unstable. The amount and severity of surgery required may also be an indication for referring the patient to a specialist (*see* Chapter 16). These patients are best admitted to a medical ward in which the staff are familiar with the clinical problems presented by such cases, rather than to a dental unit.

If a diabetic who has taken his normal dose of insulin misses a meal he may have too little glucose in his blood, a condition called 'hypoglycaemia'. When he either misses a dose of insulin or has an increased requirement due to either stress or acute infection, he will have too little circulating insulin and diabetic ketosis may supervene. Both states can result in a loss of consciousness and it is important to distinguish between them. The clinical features of these conditions are shown in *Table* 2.1. Hypoglycaemia is characterized by the rapid onset of signs and symptoms and is more commonly seen in dental practice. If there is any doubt about the diagnosis the administration of a glucose drink, a few lumps of sugar, or some boiled sweets normally rectifies the condition fairly rapidly. A hypoglycaemic attack requires urgent treatment, and if the patient is either unconscious or unable to swallow, intravenous glucose must be administered. Ampoules of 50% dextrose solution are available, and 20–100 ml should be given intravenously (*see* p. 342).

Table 2.1. The Clinical Features of Hypoglycaemia and Diabetic Ketosis

	Condition	
	Hypoglycaemia	Ketosis
Cause	An excess of insulin/lack of food	A lack of insulin
Symptoms	Weakness Hunger	Weakness Excessive thirst

Signs	Anxiety
	Sweating
		Deep laboured respirations
		Dry skin and mucous membranes
		  (dehydration)
		Sweet breath
		  (said to smell like acetone)

	BP normal or elevated Pulse full and rapid Coma	Decreased BP Pulse weak and rapid Coma

Medical assistance should be obtained, especially if the administration of glucose has proved ineffective.

On rare occasions the dental surgeon may be working in a situation where medical aid is not readily available and be consulted by a diabetic patient who complains of severe pain which can be relieved by surgery of a minor nature. In these circumstances the necessary treatment can be safely undertaken if a system of pre- and postoperative care based upon 6-hourly urine testing is employed. In practice the following system has been found to work well when *local* anaesthesia is used.

One 'acetest' tablet is laid on a clean white surface and one drop of urine is placed on it. Thirty seconds later the test is read. If the tablet remains white or turns cream in colour the test is negative. In the presence of ketones in the urine a mauve colour appears, which should be compared with the 'acetest' colour scale in order to assess the degree of ketosis. Oral surgery should not be undertaken in the presence of ketosis and medical aid must be sought.

Provided that ketosis is absent 5 drops of urine are then placed in a test-tube. After rinsing, the dropper is used to add 10 drops of water to the urine. A 'clinitest' tablet is then dropped into the test-tube and the reaction carefully watched. Fifteen seconds after bubbling stops, the tube is gently shaken and compared with the 'clinitest' colour scale. If the solution turns orange or dark greenish-brown (+ + + +) the patient is given 24 units of soluble insulin, if burnt sienna (+ + +) 20 units, if light greenish-brown (+ +) 16 units, and if green (+) 12 units. If the solution is dark blue the test is negative and no insulin is required. At the time of surgery 50 g of glucose are given by mouth.

The nature of *cardiovascular disease* is such that there is often a progressive decline in the patient's ability to withstand stress. Therefore any dental disease present should be eliminated and such preventative measures as are practicable are instituted as soon as possible. Periodic re-examination is required, for piecemeal dentistry is contra-indicated. A complete dental treatment plan should be formulated, account being taken of the patient's general and dental condition. If the mouth is neglected it is often better to perform a dental clearance under hospital conditions and antibiotic cover (*see* p. 256). Whenever possible dental procedures should be performed using local anaesthesia.

Patients who are able to take strenuous exercise, such as walking rapidly upstairs without any discomfort of cardiovascular origin, usually tolerate dental treatment, including surgery, well. In all other cases the dental treatment plan must be formulated in co-operation with the patient's physician. The extent of surgery undertaken on each occasion should be decided after consideration of all relevant factors, but it is essential to keep dental treatment within the patient's range of tolerance. Patients who complain of chest pain, breathlessness, or exhibit pallor or lapses in consciousness are best treated under hospital conditions.

Dental treatment should be postponed for at least 3 months after a patient has had a cardiac infarction. Should a dental emergency occur during this period the patient should be referred to hospital (*see* Chapter 15).

Most patients suffering from debilitating diseases stand local anaesthesia well and antibiotic cover should be given when surgery is undertaken in these cases.

CONDITIONS PREDISPOSING TO COMPLICATIONS OF DENTAL TREATMENT

Whilst many general conditions predispose to complications of dental treatment some conditions are of especial importance in dental surgery. It has been demonstrated that both the extraction of teeth and the removal of dental calculus by means of scaling are accompanied by a transient bacteraemia. Indeed it is now known that the brushing of clinically healthy gingivae or the use of an oral irrigation device can cause such a bacteraemia. In persons in normal health the organisms are speedily removed from the bloodstream by natural defensive mechanisms. If, however, the patient has either *rheumatic* or *congenital valvular heart disease*, or has had either a *synthetic vascular graft or prosthesis or a cardiac pacemaker* implanted or who has suffered a *coronary thrombosis*, colonies of the circulating organisms may settle on the abnormal or scarred endothelium or the appliance to form the vegetations which characterize the condition known as subacute bacterial endocarditis. This disease has a high mortality and morbidity, and it is the duty of the dental surgeon to make every endeavour to prevent its occurrence by planning his dental treatment in such a way as to minimize the risk of bacteraemia whenever he is dealing with any patient who has a history of rheumatic fever, chorea, valvular heart disease, cardiac surgery or infarction. In these cases, only teeth with vital pulps should be conserved and all scaling and extractions must be performed under adequate antibiotic cover (p. 256). The demonstration that instrumentation confined to the root canal does not provoke a bacteraemia has led some authorities to claim that endodontics is not contra-indicated absolutely in such patients provided that proper precautions are taken and a skilled technique is employed. However, involvement of the periapical tissues provokes a bacteraemia, albeit a small and transient one, whilst surgery in the region causes a larger bacteraemia which lasts longer. Though endodontics and even apical surgery may be justified on occasions repeated attempts to salvage pulpless teeth under deteriorating conditions are to be condemned. Especial care should be taken to minimize trauma when teeth are removed and to ensure that no dental remnants remain in the jaws. The presence of periodontitis predisposes to bacteraemia during scaling, the incidence and severity of which can be reduced by the local use of germicidal drugs. After isolating the affected area with cotton rolls 10 ml of a 1% (v/v) aqueous solution of either chlorhexidine or povidone-iodine is instilled into the periodontal pockets via a blunt-tipped needle attached to a plastic disposable syringe. The patient should be asked to retain the solution in the mouth for 2 min before rinsing out. Scaling or extractions can then be commenced. This procedure must only be used as an additional precaution to antibiotic cover and not regarded as a substitute for it.

The risk of transient bacteraemias occurring is related to the amount of dental disease, especially periodontal disease, present in the patient concerned. Thus, preventive measures designed to maintain the oral health of patients likely to be susceptible to infective endocarditis should be utilized to the full.

It would appear that infective endocarditis can also develop in patients with a previously normal heart when their resistance to infection is lowered as a result of either immunosuppressive treatment, chronic alcoholism or drug addiction. Thus the total prevention of dentally-associated infective endocarditis is an impossibility. Nevertheless the dentist has a moral obligation to do everything possible to try to prevent such a lethal complication of dental treatment. Cardiac patients in whom certain older types of artificial pacemakers have been implanted may be adversely affected by ultrasonic cleaning or scaling equipment.

Prosthetic replacements of major joints, such as the hip joint, may become infected by haematogenous spread in the presence of active dental infections. Thus dental infections afflicting patients with major joint replacements must be treated with speed and effectiveness in an endeavour to prevent haematogenous spread to the replacement site. Whilst some orthopaedic surgeons advocate that all dental procedures performed on such patients must be undertaken under antibiotic cover there is little scientific evidence to support such a practice. Antibiotic prophylaxis is not necessary when dental treatment is undertaken on patients who have undergone minor joint replacement or in whom pins or screws have been inserted during the treatment of bone fractures.

Steroid therapy may cause problems when oral surgical treatment is undertaken. The adrenal cortex is under the control of the anterior pituitary gland which stimulates its growth and secretory activity by means of adrenocorticotrophic hormone (ACTH). The production of ACTH is itself suppressed by increased quantities of hormones from the adrenal cortex and the level of balance is regulated by the hypothalamus. This beautiful self-regulating mechanism is illustrated diagrammatically in *Fig.* 2.11. A large variety of stimuli, both physical and psychological, which can be referred to collectively as 'stress', cause increased adrenocortical activity by stimulating the hypothalamic centre, and in many cases this increased activity is essential to preserve life. This is the so-called 'fight, fright, or flight' mechanism described by physiologists.

If hydrocortisone or an allied substance is given either parenterally or by mouth, the concentration of hydrocortisone (cortisol) in the blood passing through the hypothalamus rises. This results in a decreased output of ACTH and hence there is decreased function and atrophy of the adrenal cortex (*Fig.* 2.12). Under these circumstances a rapid withdrawal of the hydrocortisone will result in the adrenal cortex secreting little, if anything, for a period of varying duration. If during this period of lowered adrenocortical activity the patient has an infection,

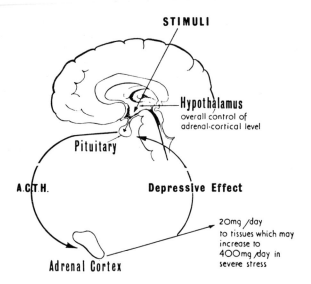

Fig. 2.11. Normal adrenal cortical cycle.

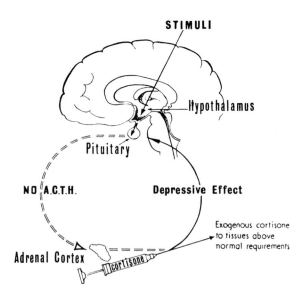

Fig. 2.12. Adrenal atrophy following steroid therapy.

an accident, or an operation, he may pass into a form of profound shock, the so-called 'adrenal crisis', which may prove fatal.

If hydrocortisone has been given for a prolonged period it may take a considerable time before adrenocortical function returns to normal. Whilst the level of secretion may have become sufficient for ordinary everyday activity, the adrenal cortex may be unable to secrete the greatly increased amounts of cortisol necessary to cope with conditions of stress. Dental infections or operations, whether performed under either local or general anaesthesia, may have disastrous consequences in such circumstances.

The commonest conditions for which steroids are administered are chronic degenerative or autoimmune diseases such as arthritis and status asthmaticus. The high incidence of these diseases and the increasing use of steroids in treating them combine to ensure that most dental surgeons are called upon to treat such patients in practice. Direct questioning should be used to determine whether the patient has taken steroids during the 2 years preceding his attendance for dental treatment. Nowadays most patients are warned of the dangers inherent in the therapy and are either issued with a card of the type illustrated in *Fig.* 2.13, with instructions to produce it whenever they attend for medical or dental treatment or wear a 'Medic-Alert' wrist bracelet (*Fig.* 2.3).

Injection of steroids into joints or applications to the skin are not important in this context unless they are extensive enough to affect the blood levels of hydrocortisone. Any patient requiring surgery and/or general anaesthesia and who either is, or recently has been, receiving systemic steroid therapy should be treated as an inpatient under the care of a physician. If the patient is taking corticosteroids at the time of admission it is usual to supplement the dose during the period of stress, and if the patient has stopped taking steroids during the preceding 18 months steroid therapy is reinstituted. Whilst many physicians have differing views, it is a common practice to give such patients 100 mg of hydrocortisone sodium succinate intramuscularly 1 hour preoperatively.

During the postoperative period 100–200 mg of cortisone are given daily by mouth if the patient is not vomiting, and by intramuscular injection if he is, and the dose is gradually reduced during the following week. A widely-used alternative

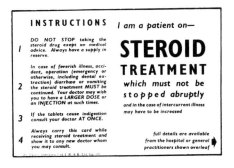

a   *b*

Fig. 2.13. Official card issued to patients on steroid therapy. The card is blue in colour and is usually folded down the centre. *a*, Outside; *b*, Inside.

régime is to double the daily oral dose on the day before and the day of surgery and follow this by gradually reducing the dosage until the maintenance level is reached during the 48 hours after operation.

The patient's blood pressure should be carefully checked during surgery and the postoperative period, and if it falls hydrocortisone hemisuccinate, 100 mg in 2 ml should be given intravenously. If the blood pressure does not rise in 20 min the dose should be repeated. If a patient has an 'adrenal crisis' in the dental surgery the dentist should give the emergency treatment outlined above and summon medical aid.

Examination of *Figs.* 2.11 and 2.12 would seem to indicate that atrophy of the adrenal cortex could be either prevented or minimized by giving ACTH at the same time as hydrocortisone or allied substances. Unfortunately ACTH has to be given by injection and most medical practitioners dislike treating chronic conditions by means of injections if this can be avoided. There is also some evidence that the parenteral administration of ACTH reduces the output of ACTH by the anterior pituitary gland. The possibility that long-term steroid therapy may inhibit the inflammatory response to such a degree that infections of dental origin can assume an unusually dangerous character is an indication for the early institution of antibiotic therapy in a substantial dosage (*see* p. 255).

As every doctor is only too well aware, new drugs are constantly being developed and introduced into medical practice. Some of these remedies create problems in dental practice and the incidence of undesirable side-effects and unwanted drug reactions is undoubtedly increasing. For this reason a 'drug history' should be taken from every patient attending for dental treatment. When questions are framed it is important to remember that in the lay mind such substances as aspirin, contraceptive pills, or other remedies taken without medical advice are seldom regarded as drugs. The patient should be asked whether he has suffered from any illness in the past for which 'drugs, medicines, pills, or tablets' were given, and whether he reacts adversely to any substance. It is also wise to ask for details of medication, with or without medical supervision, which he either is or has been taking in the previous 2 years. As patients often forget to produce warning cards unless they are reminded to do so, they should be asked whether one has been issued to them (*Figs.* 2.2, 2.13).

In recent years the treatment of depressive illness has been revolutionized by the introduction of the *monoamine oxidase inhibitor* and *tricyclic drugs*. When the former (*Table* 2.2) were first introduced it was thought that they would potentiate the action of adrenaline or noradrenaline to provoke a dangerous rise in blood pressure. In the light of experience it is now accepted that the small amounts of amine vasoconstrictors contained in local anaesthetic solutions used in dentistry do not constitute any danger to patients taking this type of drug. However such patients may experience hypertension with headache and risk a cerebral haemorrhage if they take amine-containing foods. For this reason they should be warned to avoid the ingestion of cheese, Marmite, Bovril, broad beans, yoghurt, pickled herrings, chicken livers, strong wines and beers. Severe drug reactions have complicated the administration of pethidine to patients who have been taking these drugs due to potentiation of the analgesic agent. This phenomenon is of little importance in dental practice where pethidine is seldom used. But potentiation is also stated to occur with numerous other drugs, including morphine and its derivatives, amphetamine, adrenaline and other pressor agents, barbiturates, and alcohol. The potentiating effect of a monoamine oxidase inhibitor may last for 2–3 weeks after the drug itself has been discontinued. Greater caution must be exercised if local anaesthesia is required for patients taking any of the tricyclic group of antidepressive drugs (*Table* 2.3) which are also used to treat nocturnal enuresis in children. It has been demonstrated that the effects of noradrenaline are potentiated significantly by drugs of the tricyclic group and the effects of adrenaline to a lesser extent. These vasoconstrictors should not be injected in patients taking tricyclic antidepressive drugs because of

Table 2.2. Some Monoamine Oxidase Inhibitors and Drugs Potentiated by them

Monoamine oxidase inhibitors	*Drugs*

Used to treat anxiety states and depression:
  Phenelzine (Nardil)
  Isocarboxazid (Marplan)
  Nialamide (Niamid)
  Tranylcypromine (Parnate)
  Tranylcypromine and trifluoperazine (Parstelin)
  Pargyline (Eutonyl)*
  Mebanazine (Actomol)
  Phenoxypropazine (Drazine)
  Pheniprazine (Cavodil)
 	
Used to treat angina pectoris:
  Iproniazid (Marsalid)
  Pivhydrazine (Tersavid)
 	
* Occasionally used to treat hypertension
	Pethidine
	Morphine and its derivatives
	Amphetamine
	Adrenaline and other pressor agents
	Barbiturates and alcohol
	Hypotensive agents

Potentiation may last for up to 3 weeks after the withdrawal of the monoamine oxidase inhibitor.

Treatment: Either acidify urine by intravenous sodium acid phosphate, or lysine, or arginine hydrochloride,
  or treat hypotension with hydrocortisone hemisuccinate, 100 mg intravenously,
  and hypertension with an intravenous injection of phentolamine methane sulphonate (Rogitine) 5 mg (an adrenergic-blocking agent).

Table 2.3. Some Tricyclic Antidepressive Drugs

Official name	*Proprietary names*
Amitriptyline	Amizol, Domical, Larozyl (Sweden), Limbitrol (also contains chlordiazepoxide), Saroten, Triptafen, and Tryptizol
Clomipramine	Anafranil
Desipramine	Pertofran
Imipramine	Berkomine, Tofranil, Praminil, Norpramine, Impril (Canada), Imiprin (Australia), Iramil
Nortriptyline	Allegron, Aventyl; Motipress and Motival are compound preparations of nortriptyline and fluphenazine
Opipramol	Insidon
Protriptyline	Concordin
Trimipramine	Surmontil

the risk of producing hypertension or cardiac arrhythmia. Either local anaesthetic solutions that do not contain adrenaline or noradrenaline, or a prilocaine preparation containing felypressin, a non-amine vasoconstrictor (Citanest with Octapressin), should be used under these circumstances.

The profound hypertensive reaction which occurs is characterized by the sudden onset of a severe headache. Whilst this phenomenon is usually transient, it may be complicated by either intracranial haemorrhage or acute heart failure. These complications may be avoided by the intramuscular or intravenous injection of 5 mg phentolamine (Rogitine), but as such treatment may produce a labile blood pressure it is best carried out by experts with the aid of electronic monitoring equipment. For this reason any patient exhibiting such a reaction should be transferred to hospital without delay.

Although no mishaps due to the use of antidepressant drugs have been reported in the dental literature to date, the possibility cannot be excluded, for many of the drugs said to be potentiated are in daily use. For this reason the use of pre-medication, analgesics, and general anaesthesia should be avoided as far as is possible, and a 3% prilocaine (Citanest) solution containing felypressin should be used whenever local anaesthesia is required during the treatment of such a patient.

Occasionally a dentist performing surgery under general anaesthesia may wish to use a solution containing a vasoconstrictor in order to reduce the vascularity of the operative site. If so, he should always consult the anaesthetist prior to the induction of anaesthesia, for adrenaline or noradrenaline may provoke cardiac arrhythmia when used in conjunction with such agents as *halothane, ethyl chloride, trichlorethylene* and *cyclopropane*. There is no evidence that felypressin produces a similar complication, so that prilocaine with felypressin may be used safely under these circumstances. However, it is a less effective vasoconstrictor.

An increasing number of patients afflicted with high blood pressure are taking potent *hypotensive drugs*. Most of them are receiving adrenergic neurone-blocking drugs such as guanethidine (Ismelin) or methyldopa (Aldomet), for the use of such ganglion-blocking agents as pentolinium (Ansolysen), mecamylamine (Inversine), and pempidine (Perolysen, Tenormal) tends to be reserved for the treatment of such severe complications as hypertensive encephalopathy. Both types of drug may cause postural hypotension, and so patients taking them may feel either giddy or even faint when rising from the dental chair especially following treatment in the supine position. The administration of barbiturates including methohexitone or such general anaesthetic agents as halothane (Fluothane) to such a patient may potentiate the hypotensive effects and so produce a dangerous fall in blood pressure. Local anaesthesia may be used on an outpatient basis, but if general anaesthesia is required the services of a highly skilled anaesthetist must be enlisted and the patient is best treated under hospital conditions.

CONDITIONS WHICH POSE A THREAT TO THE HEALTH OF THE DENTIST

During the practice of his profession the dentist is at risk from droplet infection, the inhalation of anaesthetic vapours, mercury intoxication and radiation. He should take sensible precautions, such as wearing a face mask when indicated, ensuring that his X-ray apparatus is regularly serviced and checked, adhering strictly to sound radiographic practices, and arranging for waste anaesthetic gases to be scavenged in an endeavour to minimize the effect of such health hazards. It is also a wise precaution to wear rubber gloves when treating patients especially those who have or have recently had acute herpetogingivostomatitis or recurrent herpes labialis.

In recent years there has been increasing concern amongst dentists regarding the transmission of *hepatitis* in dental practice.

It is now known that the majority of infections with the viruses that cause hepatitis are asymptomatic and are not characterized by jaundice. Whilst hepatitis A virus causes infectious hepatitis, a most unpleasant acute illness, infection with hepatitis B virus causes 'serum hepatitis', a much more sinister malady.

Hepatitis B

The hepatitis B virus, or Dane particle (HBV), is described as being spherical in shape and 42 μm in diameter. Its outer coat is composed of the hepatitis B surface antigen (HBsAg), whilst the inner coat or 'core' contains DNA polymerase and double-stranded DNA. Hepatitis e antigen (HBeAg) is thought to be a component of the core.

As far as is known, the HBV replicates only in live cells and is released from there into the bloodstream. This process may continue for a variable period after infection in some cases. When this period exceeds 6 months the individual is regarded as a carrier, a state which may persist for many years or even be life-long.

Primary carcinoma of the liver is much more common in carriers than in health controls. Males are more likely to become carriers than females.

HBV may be present in the blood of carriers and those in the incubation period and suffering overt disease. Excess outer coat, the hepatitis B surface antigen is found in the tissues and in the blood as 20 μm spheres and tubules 22 μm in diameter and 100 μm long and is known as 'Australian antigen'. All carriers have HBsAg in their blood and are thus described as being 'Australian antigen positive', but fail to produce an antibody to HBsAg. Anti-HBc, the antibody to the core of the Dane particle, is present in high titre in all carriers but affords no protection against infection with HBV. Determination of the level of anti-HBc is useful in the diagnosis of carriers. In some carriers HBeAg persists in the blood and its presence indicates continuing infection of the liver and a carrier of a highly infectious kind. Conversely, carriers with anti-HBe in their sera constitute a very low risk but it would be a mistake to regard them as being non-infectious.

The presence of HBsAg means that the individual is a carrier and has some circulating HBV: if anti-HBe is also demonstrable then HBV is likely to be scarce and only a large volume of blood (e.g. blood transfusion) would be likely to transmit the infection. However, if HBeAg is present then HBV is in high concentration and even tiny quantities of blood may prove infectious. As little as 0·0001 ml of infected blood is sufficient to transmit the disease by injection and about ten thousand times this amount is infectious by mouth. Whilst in developed countries only one or two persons in a thousand are carriers the incidence is much higher in the developing countries of Africa and Asia. For example, in Hong Kong 9·6% of the population are carriers of HBsAg and the presence of anti-HBs can be detected in one-third of the population as a whole and in 68·5% of those aged 50 years or more. It is estimated that 5% of the population of the world (some 200 million persons) are carriers. Medical and dental personnel have a slightly higher carrier rate and amongst dentists, oral surgeons have a higher carrier rate than general practitioners.

Hepatitis B is spread predominantly by the parenteral route (needle pricks, injections and transfusions) and the whole virus, the Dane particle, is the infectious agent. Although infection is accompanied by the production of a vast excess of HBsAg this antigen is not infectious. Blood-sucking arthropods may serve as vectors whilst saliva, like semen, is probably infectious. Intra-family spread by means of close contact, kissing, the sharing of utensils and sexual contact is a well-recognized feature of the condition. A carrier mother may also transmit the disease to her baby either during or shortly after birth.

HBsAg is not secreted into the saliva but gains access by leakage of blood into the mouth mainly via the gingival crevice. Thus saliva can be regarded as highly diluted blood and a case of transmission of hepatitis B by 'human bite' is on record. If exposure to saliva meant greater exposure to the disease then dentists would be especially at risk. In fact the prevalence of the disease among dentists is only slightly higher than the population in general and infection is clearly related to blood and not saliva.

The course of the disease

A variety of non-specific symptoms, especially gastrointestinal symptoms, usually precede the onset of jaundice. Severe anorexia, nausea, vomiting and right upper quadrant abdominal pain are commonly found and may be accompanied by constipation, diarrhoea, headache, low-grade fever and coryza. The onset of a hepatitis B infection is more insidious than that of a hepatitis A infection.

Deepening in colour of the urine heralds the onset of clinically detectable jaundice. The stools become clay-coloured and pruritus may be experienced. The icteric phase usually lasts from 1 to 4 weeks and tender enlargement of the liver, spleen and cervical lymph nodes may occur. On occasions cholestatic jaundice may last for as long as 6 months. In such cases a predominantly conjugated hyperbilirubinaemia and a raised alkaline phosphatase level are usually present.

With the subsidence of jaundice the patient's general condition improves although he or she becomes easily fatigued for some time. The serum transaminase level may be doubled or trebled for up to 6 months but is compatible with complete recovery. In some patients convalescence is protracted and symptoms of ill-health persist disproportionate to the biochemical disturbance. This post-hepatic syndrome usually affects intelligent patients, often those with a medical background and reassurance regarding prognosis should be given.

In a small minority of cases several episodes of remission and relapse can occur and may continue for several years. Alcohol excess and premature strenuous physical activity may be predisposing factors. In some cases death can occur within 4 weeks of onset. Of those patients who suffer acute type B hepatitis 5–10% subsequently develop chronic liver disease, a complication which is commonest in males, the very young, the very old and immunosuppressed.

There is no specific treatment for the disease.

Bed rest with toilet privileges is the classic treatment, a gradual increase in physical activity being permitted during convalescence when the serum bilirubin is less than 26 μmol/l. A low fat, high carbohydrate diet is usually advocated although a high protein, high calorie diet may hasten recovery if the patient can take it. As most studies report increased mortality and morbidity with the use of steroids they are seldom prescribed now.

Prevention

Every endeavour should be made to *prevent* the spread of the disease. Thus good sanitation and the provision and the use of proper facilities for personal hygiene should prevent the occurrence of epidemics. The use of sensitive methods to detect the presence of HBsAg in blood and blood products should eliminate most post-transfusion infections. Intra-family spread may be decreased by not sharing the use of utensils. Direct transmission and sexual transmission may be prevented by the use of hepatitis B immunoglobulin and the hepatitis B vaccine where indicated.

It is essential that all medical, dental and nursing personnel are trained to handle correctly patients known to be Australian antigen-positive. In practically all cases the dentist will not know that he is treating a carrier. It would be neither sensible nor practicable to test all dental patients for the presence of HBsAg and so a commonsense approach must be employed and an endeavour should be made to recognize those patients in whom there is a high risk that they will be Australian antigen-positive. These include hospitalized and institutionalized patients as a whole, those involved in drug addiction programmes, patients who receive blood transfusions frequently, such as those with cancer or haemophilia, and those on haemodialysis, epileptics, patients afflicted with cerebral palsy, male homosexuals and female prostitutes.

When treating a patient who is either known or thought to be Australian antigen-positive the potentially infective nature of blood must never be forgotten. Both the operator and his assistant should wear disposable rubber gloves when treating such patients, especially if there is the slightest danger of their hands becoming bloodstained. Protective glasses and disposable masks should be worn to protect mucosal surfaces especially when high-speed rotary instruments are being used. Disposable gowns, overshoes, needles and scalpel handles and blades should be used and the patient's clothing could be protected by a disposable barrier sheet secured with tape. All waste should be placed in a strong double thickness bag or container clearly labelled 'Infectious material' and incinerated without delay.

Extreme care should be exercised during the handling and sterilization of instruments. A tangled 'hedgehog' of instruments should never be picked up in one handful. Instruments should be picked up separately and placed in receptacles for washing and sterilization. Heavy duty gloves should be worn when collecting instruments which should either be cleansed by the use of ultrasound and detergents or scrubbed whilst submerged in hot water to prevent splashing and aerosol formation. HBV in bloodstains, either on cloth or on other surfaces, can be destroyed by applying a solution containing sodium hypochlorite solution (10 000 parts per million available chloride) using a squeeze bottle, heavy duty gloves and disposable paper tissues. A viricidal agent, such as 5% Printol, should be used routinely and regularly to disinfect working surfaces, sinks, spittoons, and aspirators and their traps.

Dental handpieces readily become contaminated and so either a handpiece of sterilizable type must be employed or conventional handpieces must be sterilized by the use of ethylene oxide.

If sensible precautions are taken infection of the operator or his assistant is only likely to occur if there is a 'needle stick' kind of accident when handling blood-stained sharp instruments. Should this occur, or some other form of contamination be suspected, then hepatitis B immunoglobulin (HBIG) should be given in a dose of 0·05–0·07 ml/kg of body weight within 24–48 hours of injury or contamination, as it is effective in either preventing or reducing the severity of infection. A second dose is given one month later.

Hepatitis B vaccine

Although HBsAg is not infectious the antibody response to it (anti-HBs) protects the individual against subsequent infections. Antibodies to other components of the virus do not confer immunity and it is the production of anti-HBs in a susceptible individual alone which provides protection against hepatitis B infection.

Vaccines prepared after HBsAg particles have been extracted from serum, concentrated and purified are now available and dentists, oral surgeons and dental hygienists are amongst the high-risk groups for whom vaccination has been recommended.

Before the vaccine is given it is necessary to test for susceptability to hepatitis B by testing a blood sample from the potential recipient for the presence of anti-HBs and HBsAg. The vast majority of subjects are shown by these tests not to have been previously infected with HBV and so are suitable for vaccination.

Three doses of the vaccine are given intramuscularly, the two initial doses being given a month apart whilst the booster dose is administered 6 months after the first dose. Specific antibody develops in 75–90% of healthy adults after the first two doses and in 85–95% after the third dose. Vaccine-induced antibodies have persisted for at least 3 years, but it has been estimated that a booster dose may be required after 5 years. Present vaccines provide protection in about 95% of those receiving them and no serious immediate or long-term adverse reactions have been reported to date.

Research continues and vaccines prepared by the use of purified polypeptides, obtained by breaking down virus particles, as the immunogen are now being tested.

The importance of the general condition of any patient receiving dental treatment is such that inquiries about his past and present medical condition should be an unalterable routine. Special emphasis should be directed towards obtaining a history of any diseases of the respiratory and cardiovascular systems, including rheumatic fever, chorea, or severe 'growing pains', or any episode of abnormal bleeding or bruising. Every patient should also be asked for details of previous hospital admissions or steroid therapy, in addition to any medical condition present, or drugs which are being taken, or to which he is sensitive, at the time he attends for dental treatment. Only when the dental surgeon has all relevant data at his disposal can he formulate a proper dental treatment plan in the best interests of his patient.

SUGGESTED READING

Bailey B. M. W. and Fordyce A. M. (1983) Complications of dental extractions in patients receiving warfarin anticoagulant therapy. *Br. Dent. J.* **155**, 308–10.

Biggs R., Matthews J. M., Rush B. M. et al. (1965) Further experience in use of human antihaemophilic globulin (HAHG) for the control of bleeding after dental extraction in haemophilic patients. *Lancet* **1**, 969–74.

Cawson R. A. (1966) The problem of the newer drugs in dentistry. The role of Medindex. *Br. Dent. J.* **120**, 109–10.

Cooke B. E. D. (1957) Benign fibro-osseous enlargement of the jaws. *Br. Dent. J.* **102**, 1–14, 49–59.

Cooley R. L. and Lubow R. M. (1982) Hepatitis B vaccine: implications for dental personnel. *J. Am. Dent. Assoc.* **105**, 47–9.

Dormer A. E. (1958) Bacterial endocarditis. Survey of patients treated between 1945 and 1956. *Br. Med. J.* **1**, 63–9.

Duperon D. F. and Dobbs T. M. (1976) Dental care for patients with congenital haemorrhagic disorders. *J. Canadian Dent. Assoc.* **42**, 269–73.

Garrod L. P. and Waterworth P. M. (1962) The risks of dental extraction during penicillin treatment. *Br. Heart J.* **24**, 39–46.

Holbrook W. P., Willey R. F. and Shaw T. R. D. (1981) Dental health in patients susceptible to infective endocarditis. *Br. Med. J.* **283**, 371–2.

Lindemann R. A. and Henson J. L. (1982) The dental management of patients with vascular grafts placed in the treatment of arterial occlusive disease. *J. Am. Dent. Assoc.* **104**, 625–8.

MacFarlane T. W., Ferguson M. M. and Mulgrew C. J. (1984) Post extraction bacteraemia: role of antiseptics and antibiotics. *Br. Dent. J.* **156**, 179–81.

MacFarlane T. W. and Follett E. A. C. (1983) Hepatitis B vaccine. *Br. Dent. J.* **154**, 39–41.

McGowan D. A. (1982) Endodontics and infective endocarditis in hospital dentistry. *Int. Endodont. J.* **15**, 127–31.

McIntyre H. (1960) Dental extractions in patients with heart disease. *Br. Med. J.* **1**, 1778–81.

McIntyre H. and Wilkinson J. F. (1964) Dental treatment in the haemophilia syndrome. *Lancet* **1**, 584–5.

Martin C. M. (1983) Hepatitis B vaccine—What to expect. *Oral Surg.* **56**, 455–59.

Mason D. A. (1970) Steroid therapy and dental infection. *Br. Dent. J.* **128**, 271–4.

Masterton J. B. (1965) Restorative dentistry for haemophiliacs. *Br. Dent. J.* **119**, 148–52.

Millard H. D. and Tupper C. J. (1960) Subacute bacterial endocarditis: a clinical study. *J. Oral Surg.* **18**, 224–9.

Ministry of Health (1967) *Emergencies in Dental Practice.* London, HMSO.

Okell C. C. and Elliott S. D. (1935) Bacteriaemia and oral sepsis: with special reference to the aetiology of subacute endocarditis. *Lancet* **2**, 869–72.

Parnell A. G. (1964) Adrenal crisis and the dental surgeon. *Br. Dent. J.* **116**, 294–8.

Peterson M. S. and Goldberg A. F. (1981) Hepatitis—the risk in hospital dentistry. *Spec. Care Dent.* **1**, 256–8.

Shira R. B., Hall R. J. and Guernsey L. H. (1962) Minor oral surgery during prolonged anticoagulant therapy. *J. Oral Surg.* **20**, 93–99.

Sims W. (1981) Serum hepatitis and the dental hygienist. *Dental Health* **20**, 5–8.

Stones H. H. (1951) Oral manifestations in systemic diseases: hypovitaminoses and blood dyscrasias. *Ann. R. Coll. Surg.* **9**, 234–44.

Thom A. R. and Howe G. L. (1972). The dental status of cardiac patients. *Br. Heart J.* **34**, 1302–7.

Thornton J. B. and Alves J. C. M. (1981) Bacterial endocarditis. *Oral Surg.* **52**, 379–83.

Walker R. O. and Rose M. (1965) Oral manifestations of haematological disorders. *Br. Dent. J.* **118**, 286–9.

Walton J. G. and Thompson J. W. (1969) Systemic disease in dental practice. *Br. Dent. J.* **127**, 227–30, 281–7, 333–7.

Walton J. G. and Thompson J. W. (1969) Unwanted effects due to drugs. *Br. Dent. J.* **127**, 134–8, 177–82, 379–86, 421–3.

Watkinson A. C. (1982) Primary herpes simplex in a dentist. *Br. Dent. J.* **153**, 190–1.

Whitehead F. I. (1962) The significance of anticoagulant therapy and steroid therapy to the dental practitioner. *Dent. Pract.* **13**, 139–41.

Chapter 3

Basic principles upon which the successful practice of oral surgery is dependent

Once a definitive diagnosis has been made in a particular case, the dental surgeon must endeavour to select the appropriate method of treatment to be employed. In broad terms only three types of treatment are available for use in dental practice.

1. *Expectant treatment or treatment by observation*: This is often combined with reassurance and may be used to treat patients afflicted with conditions such as non-erosive lichen planus, benign hyperkeratosis, or those in whom such lesions as an aphthous ulcer or a haematoma are resolving.

2. *Conservative treatment*, such as the insertion of a sedative dressing into a carious cavity or an infected socket, the removal of dental calculus, or an alteration in denture design or the technique of toothbrushing employed by the patient.

3. *Radical treatment by means of surgery*, the technique with which this book is concerned.

In many instances the dentist will employ a combination of techniques during the treatment of a particular patient. Thus he may excise a dental cyst, apicect and root-fill a pulpless tooth related to it, and carefully observe the patient post-operatively to ensure that bone regeneration occurs and that healing progresses in a satisfactory manner. Such postoperative treatment by observation may involve the use of radiography to supplement clinical examination. The dental surgeon may advise a patient who has a white lesion of the oral mucosa to give up smoking, either fill or extract any sharp tooth related to the lesion, biopsy the affected mucosa, and, after recording precise details of the site, consistency and size of the lesion, review the patient's condition at regular intervals.

TREATMENT PLANNING

Every treatment plan must be designed to suit the particular dental, medical, social and economic needs of the individual patient, and the dentist should never fall into the error of forgetting that he treats people and not isolated carious cavities, periodontal pockets, or mouths. He must endeavour to restore his patient to oral health as soon as is practicable by the use of those methods of treatment which his professional training leads him to believe are the most suitable in the particular circumstances.

Successful treatment planning must be based upon a thorough preoperative assessment of any difficulties which may be encountered, any possible complications which might occur, and both the advantages and disadvantages of the various methods of treatment available for use. Accurate and thorough preoperative assessment enables the dentist to prepare and implement a treatment plan designed to cope with anticipated difficulties and to avoid possible complications. Certain factors are of especial importance during treatment planning and these must now be discussed.

Before embarking upon any surgical procedure the dentist should ask himself whether he has sufficient knowledge of, and proficiency in, the surgical techniques involved to serve the best interests of his patient. Such proficiency is best acquired by practical experience gained under the supervision of a colleague skilled in these techniques, and is based upon a sound knowledge of surgical and radiographic anatomy, pathology, physiology, and pharmacology, If any doubt exists on these points the advice and assistance of a more experienced colleague should be sought (*see* Chapter 16). The dentist must also ensure that not only are efficient sterilization facilities and an adequate armamentarium available for his use, but that his arrangements are such as will permit him to perform the procedure in a systematic and unhurried manner under optimum conditions. This last requirement can only be met if the illumination of the site of operation is adequate, any skilled assistance required is available, and the choice of the form of anaesthesia to be employed is correct.

Thus the use of general anaesthesia in the dental chair limits both the operating time and surgical access, and so in general dental practice it is usually wiser to perform oral surgical procedures under local anaesthesia either with or without the use of premedication. The oral premedication of a really nervous patient should begin at least 2 and preferably 3 days before the dental appointment.

Although barbiturates have been used fairly extensively in the past it is now recognized that they may have severe limitations in producing tranquil sleep and actually lower the pain threshold. For these reasons they are not favoured by the author for premedication of patients prior to the use of local anaesthesia.

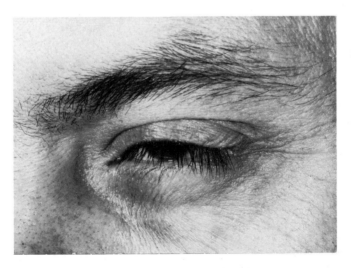

Fig. 3.1. Verril's sign: the upper eyelid has drooped to a position half-way across the pupil of the eye.

Preoperative apprehension may be controlled by the oral administration of a tranquillizer, for example, diazepam (Valium) 5–10 mg before retiring on the 3 nights preceding the visit to the dentist and about 1 hour prior to the surgery.

Immediate sedation may be achieved in the dental surgery by the intravenous administration of a tranquillizing drug. However as syncope has complicated the parenteral use of such substances in elderly and debilitated patients it is a wise precaution to place the patient in a supine position when this route of administration is employed. When given intravenously a 5 mg/ml solution is utilized and 2·5 mg of diazepam are given every 30 sec until either ⅓ mg/kg bodyweight (2 mg/stone bodyweight) has been given or ptosis, with the margin of the upper eyelid at least half-way across the pupil, has occurred (Verril's sign) (*Fig.* 3.1). The local anaesthetic should be given immediately sedation is achieved because the amnesic effect of diazepam is greatest at this time. There is some evidence that depression of the laryngeal reflex occurs, which is maximal during the first 5 min of sedation but has disappeared completely within 20 min. Therefore adequate mouth packs must be used and suction apparatus utilized whenever this technique is employed.

Non-barbiturates and other tranquillizers may be used to sedate dental patients (*Table* 3.1). They are particularly suitable for children because they are available in the form of elixirs.

Table 3.1. Sedative Drugs available for Oral Administration which are included in the *Dental Practitioners' Formulary*

Proprietary name	Approved name	Average adult dose
Non-barbiturates		
Welldorm	Dichloralphenazone	1300 mg (2 tablets)
Tricloryl	Triclofos	1000 mg (2 tablets)
Tranquillizers		
Librium	Chlordiazepoxide	} 5–10 mg (1–2 tablets)
Valium	Diazepam	
Equanil }	Meprobamate	400 mg (1 tablet)
Miltown		

The sedation of a really nervous child should ensure a good sleep for 2 or 3 nights prior to the surgery. The drug of choice is diazepam elixir (Valium) in a dose of 2·5–5 mg about half an hour before retiring to bed and a similar amount about 1 hour before the dental appointment. The intravenous administration of diazepam may also be used immediately prior to treatment but the effects in children under 12 years of age are somewhat unpredictable. For this reason the technique should only be employed by experts.

Sedation may also be achieved by using a hypnotic such as Chloral Elixir Paediatric BPC which contains 200 mg chloral hydrate in 5 ml. The dose recommended for a child aged between 1 and 5 years is 5–7·5 ml (1–1½ British standard spoonfuls). An alternative preparation is triclofos elixir BPC (Tricloryl Syrup) which contains 500 mg triclofos sodium in 5 ml, and which is given to children aged 1–5 years in a dosage of 2·5–5 ml (½–1 British standard spoonful).

The regimen of administration should be similar to that recommended for diazepam elixir but with only half of the initial dose given 1 hour before surgery.

Whenever premedication is prescribed the patient should be warned of the possibility of preoperative drowsiness or ataxia, and must be escorted to the surgery. No premedicated patient should be allowed to leave the surgery unaccompanied or to drive a motor-vehicle for at least 4 hours, and preferably 24 hours postoperatively. He or she must be told not to take any other central nervous system depressant, such as alcohol or antihistamines, during this period.

As a general rule it is preferable to perform any oral surgical operation which is likely to take more than 30 min to complete under endotracheal anaesthesia in a hospital. A dental surgeon called upon to undertake such a prolonged procedure should enlist the aid of a colleague if he cannot obtain the use of the required facilities himself (*see* Chapter 16). The dentist must train himself to be able to estimate, with accuracy, the time required to complete any surgical procedure. Unless he can do this with facility he will be unable to make the correct decisions with regard to the type of anaesthesia to be employed or the need for hospital admission when planning any oral surgical procedure.

Except in the case of soft-tissue lesions unrelated to bone, such as mucous retention cysts of the lips, the careful preoperative interpretation of good radiographs is a necessary preliminary to surgery. A sound knowledge of surgical and radiographic anatomy is an essential prerequisite to the acquisition of surgical judgement and skill. Throughout this book it is assumed that the reader possesses such knowledge, for comment is limited to those anatomical and radiographic features which are considered to be of importance in the surgical treatment of the particular condition under discussion.

STERILIZATION

Many diseases are caused by infection with micro-organisms, and those micro-organisms which cause disease are described as being pathogenic. If pathogenic micro-organisms are introduced into an operation wound there is a serious risk that the wound will break down and healing will be delayed. The surgeon attempts to prevent the occurrence of this undesirable postoperative complication by using aseptic techniques and by sterilizing the instruments and materials used during the operation. *Sterilization* may be defined as the removal of all micro-organisms from a given object or their effective destruction, whilst *disinfection* is the destruction of pathogenic micro-organisms in the non-sporing or vegetative state. Sterilization rather than disinfection is mandatory wherever tissue is penetrated or there is contact with blood or serum.

The healthy mouth is always contaminated with micro-organisms of many types, some of which are potentially pathogenic. It is quite impossible to render the mouth sterile, although the number of micro-organisms present can be reduced considerably by attention to oral hygiene and scaling of the teeth a week or two prior to operation (*Fig.* 3.2). Despite every care being taken, it is still necessary to operate in a non-sterile field, and it is fortunate that the oral tissues appear to have especially efficient defensive mechanisms which usually deal with the contamination of the wound which inevitably occurs. Although coping successfully with autogenous infection, these defences are more vulnerable to micro-organisms

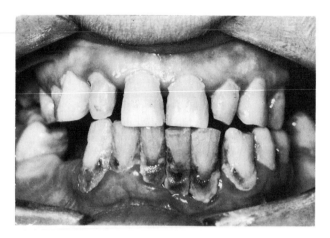

Fig. 3.2. Gross periodontal disease with calculus deposits. It is undesirable to perform oral surgery in the presence of such a condition.

introduced into the mouth from other sources at the time of operation, so that the operator should use an aseptic technique. *Asepsis* is a method of surgery which is designed to prevent the introduction of infection into a wound at the time of operation or when wounds are dressed.

The hands of the operator should be thoroughly cleansed and instruments sterilized before use. The operator should keep his finger-nails short and clean, and the hands should at least be scrubbed with soap and water and dried upon a clean towel immediately before performing a dental extraction or any other intra-oral surgery. Whenever it is practicable, more elaborate precautions should be taken by the operator, including a carefully timed 3-minute 'scrub-up' using either a hexachlorophane detergent cream or an iodophor such as povidone-iodine surgical scrub and the use of sterile rubber gloves (*see Fig.* 3.9 and p. 61).

In order to kill the most resistant micro-organisms, namely bacterial spores, it is necessary either to subject them to moist heat at 120° C for 10–12 min in an autoclave or steam-pressure sterilizer, or to dry heat at 160° C for 60 min in a hot-air oven. Water boils at 100° C at normal temperature and pressure, and bacterial spores may resist these conditions for 60 min and fungi and thread organisms for 20 min. Therefore, hot-water 'sterilization' cannot produce complete sterility, and as this form of disinfection is still widely employed in general dental practice it is fortunate that the majority of pathogenic bacteria which may be present are in the vegetative phase and are destroyed by immersion in boiling water for 5–10 min.

The limitations of the method make careful techniques essential if a breakdown of sterility is not to occur and render it unsuitable for use when syringes and needles are to be sterilized. The instruments must be thoroughly washed and all blood, pus and other debris removed from them. All the instruments should be completely submerged in boiling water so that their entire surface area is in contact with water. After boiling point has been regained the instruments should be boiled for a minimum of 5 min, and during this time no other instruments must

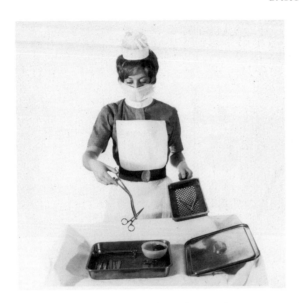

Fig. 3.3. Sterile instruments being transferred from the autoclave tray to a sterile dish. N.B. that the points of the Cheatle forceps are always kept pointing downwards and that the tray lid is laid down with its inner surface upwards.

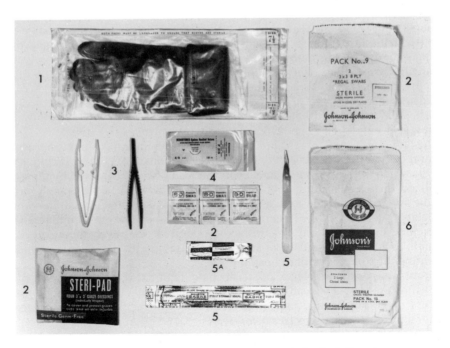

Fig. 3.4. Sterile disposable surgical equipment. 1, Gloves; 2, Swabs; 3, Dressing tweezers; 4, Sutures; 5, Scalpel; 5A, Blades; 6, Towels.

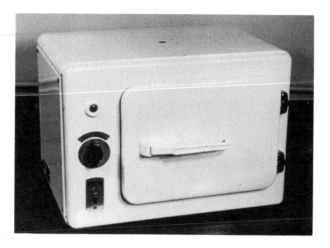

Fig. 3.5. Electrohelios hot-air oven.

be added to the load in the hot-water bath. When the period of boiling is complete, the instruments are transferred with sterile Cheatle forceps to trays containing a chemical sterilizing agent until required for use (*Fig.* 3.3). Most chemical sterilizing agents do not make an instrument completely sterile, but immersion in 70% ethyl alcohol with 0·075% chlorhexidine digluconate and 0·75% cetrimide BP for 30 min will kill vegetative micro-organisms, and these agents are useful for maintaining the cleanliness of instruments previously disinfected by boiling. They are also employed to disinfect the hands of the surgeon and the skin and mucous membrane of the patient as previously described. Metal and glass surfaces can also be prepared by wiping them down with alcoholic chlorhexidine solution (0·5% Hibitane gluconate 20 w/v in 70% alcohol). This technique is employed when laying up an operating trolley (*see* p. 60).

The general dental practitioner who intends to undertake any appreciable amount of oral surgery has a duty to maintain a standard of both sterilization and asepsis which is above the average level. This can often be achieved by the use of sterilized disposable equipment and dressings (*Fig.* 3.4), a reasonably priced hot-air oven (*Fig.* 3.5), and a completely automatic high-speed instrument autoclave, such as the type illustrated in *Fig.* 3.6. No endeavour should be spared to exclude extraneous bacteria from the operative site, even though it is not possible to achieve a standard of asepsis comparable with that maintained in the operating theatre of a modern hospital.

Monitoring of the efficiency of sterilizing equipment is an integral part of the sterilizing process. This can be achieved by the regular and systematic use of process or colour change indicators and biological monitors according to the manufacturers' instructions (*see below*).

Disposable equipment is sterilized by gamma-radiation and a high standard of packaging is required if contamination is not to occur. It is essential to ensure that the packaging of all presterilized articles is intact prior to using them.

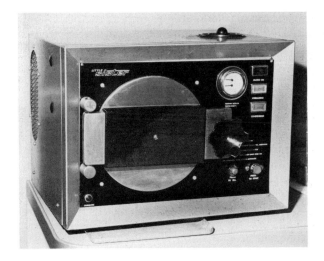

Fig. 3.6. 'Little Sister' high-speed automatic instrument autoclave.

Sharp instruments should be sterilized in a hot-air oven which, however, will destroy rubber, glassware, and dressings. The long duration of the sterilizing cycle is the main disadvantage of the method and makes it necessary for the dentist to have several sets of instruments available for use, as rapid sterilization is not possible (*see* Appendix A). Conventional handpieces but not air turbine handpieces can be sterilized in a hot-air oven provided that a silicone oil is used as a lubricant although some deleterious effects are seen over a period of time. After each use they should be dismantled and immersed in 100% xylene followed by 95% methylated spirits to remove contaminated oil prior to relubrication and sterilization. The handpiece, together with a selection of burs, is then loosely packed in a colour-coded aluminium container and placed in the hot-air oven. Other instruments are placed in heat-sealed paper envelopes which must be handled carefully to prevent puncture after sterilization. Strict adherence to correct timing is essential for successful sterilization regardless of whether a hot-air oven or an autoclave is used, and the dentist must stress this fact when instructing his staff. The efficacy of sterilization can be checked in autoclaves and hot-air ovens by the use of Browne's tubes (Types 1 and 3 respectively) which alter colour once the correct time and temperature have been reached. The use of autoclave tape (3M No. 1222) is a further safeguard.

Two main types of autoclave are currently in use, the high-vacuum type in which the air is evacuated from the chamber by a pump prior to the entry of the steam, and the downward-displacement type in which the air is displaced by the steam. The former type is so expensive that it is found only in hospitals and similar institutions, whilst most of the autoclaves found in dental practices work on the downward-displacement principle. In the latter kind of apparatus the contents can only be sterilized if unwrapped, and so these appliances are usually employed to sterilize instruments in trays. Corrosion of metal instruments occurs during autoclaving, and, except in the presence of dissimilar metals, can be overcome by the addition of a vapour-phase inhibitor, such as cyclohexylamine in a concentration of 0·1%, to the water in the autoclave. This substance is vaporized under the conditions found when the autoclave is working, and forms a protective coating on the instruments during cooling.

Preparation of materials and instruments for sterilization in an autoclave of the high-vacuum variety must be such that penetration by steam occurs easily. Airtight containers are unsuitable for this method of sterilization. Polyamides (nylons) have been shown to be ill-suited for this purpose, for although they are penetrated by steam to a limited extent, bursting may occur or pinholes or holes at the seams may develop. For small packs it is far better to seal the instruments or dressings in a double layer of suitable paper through which both air and steam diffuse readily. Only air turbines or conventional handpieces or air motors that can be autoclaved should be used for oral surgery unless ethylene oxide sterilization is available to the operator. They must be stripped, cleansed, lightly oiled and autoclaved before each use.

Once the instruments have been sterilized they must neither be handled nor laid down on a non-sterile surface. The top of an operating trolley is thoroughly cleaned by the application of alcoholic chlorhexidine solution and dried. Using two pairs of sterile Cheatle forceps this is covered first with a sterile waterproof disposable towel and then with a sterile disposable towel. The risk of contamination should a wet instrument be placed upon an ordinary disposable towel during surgery makes the use of a waterproof towel essential. The dry instruments are laid out with their handles pointing towards the operator in the order in which they will be used. The use of wet instruments should be avoided, especially when gloves are not being worn, because bacteria from the operator's hands may be carried in fluid which runs down the handles, on to the blades and into the wound.

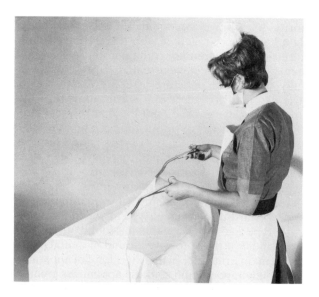

Fig. 3.7. Use of two pairs of Cheatle forceps to lay a sterile towel over a trolley top.

If there is to be a delay before the operation is commenced, the trolley top should be protected from contamination by covering it with a sterile towel applied with sterile Cheatle forceps (*Fig.* 3.7).

Unless gloves are worn the surgeon and his assistants must touch the handles of sterile instruments alone and avoid touching those parts which enter the wound. For this reason double-ended instruments should not be used and the surgeon should train himself to replace each instrument he discards in its correct place on the trolley top during the operation. Investigations have revealed that about

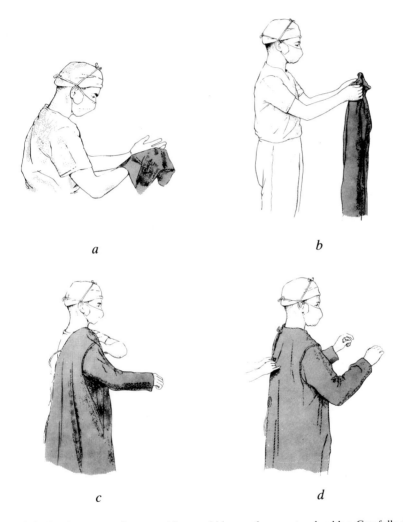

a *b*

c *d*

Fig. 3.8. Putting on a sterile gown. After scrubbing-up the operator should: *a*, Carefully dry his hands on a sterile towel; *b*, Pick up the gown by holding its inner surface; *c*, Insert his right arm into the sleeve without touching the outside of the gown; *d*, Insert his left arm and be tied up by an assistant who is not scrubbed-up.

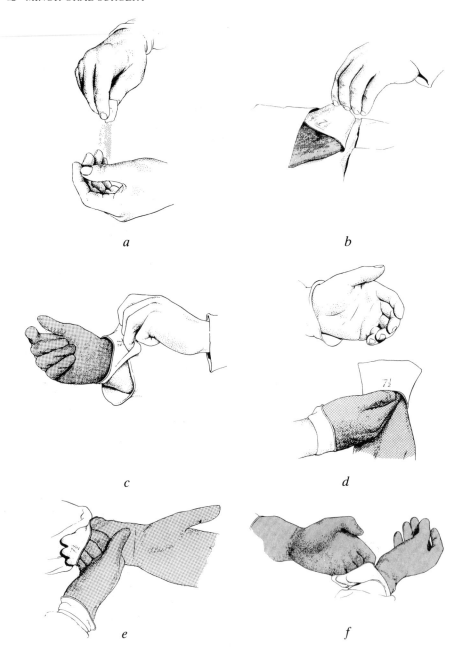

a   *b*

c   *d*

e   *f*

Fig. 3.9. Putting on sterile gloves. The operator should open the sterile glove pack and then: *a*, Powder his hands; *b*, Pick out the right glove by grasping its folded cuff with the left hand; *c*, Draw the right glove on to the hand without touching its outer surface; *d*, Pick up the left glove by inserting the gloved right hand under its folded cuff; *e*, Draw the left glove on to the hand, turning the cuff on to the sleeve of the gown; *f*, Turn the cuff of the right glove on to the sleeve of the gown.

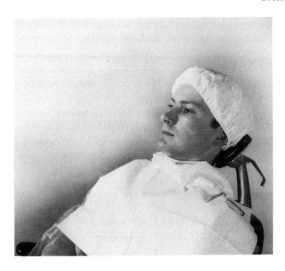

Fig. 3.10. Patient prepared for minor oral surgery under local anaesthesia (*see* text for explanation).

one-quarter of the rubber gloves used in oral surgery are perforated during use, and so it is obvious that the wearing of gloves does not diminish the importance of cleansing the hands. The operator should scrub up with bare forearms, having first removed rings, watches, and bracelets which may harbour infection. The hair and breath are sources of infection and caps and masks should be worn. Facemasks soon become contaminated in use and should be adjusted prior to hand washing and should not be touched again by the surgeon. The hands and forearms should be carefully, repeatedly, and thoroughly cleansed with a sterile brush for at least 3 minutes. The repeated use of 3% hexachlorophane in a detergent cream (pHisohex), in a liquid soap (Sterzac) or 4% chlorhexidine solution throughout the day produces a great reduction in resident bacterial flora of the skin. Dentists who are sensitive to hexachlorophane can use a povidone-iodine (Betadine) surgical scrub which is equally effective. The operator should then dry his hands on a sterile disposable towel and don a clean, or preferably sterile, operating gown in the manner illustrated in *Fig.* 3.8 and sterile rubber gloves as shown in *Fig.* 3.9.

The patient is also a potential source of infection. Just prior to operation he should clean his teeth thoroughly by using a tooth-brush and mouth rinsing. His outer garments should be left outside the surgery, the remainder of his clothing protected with a waterproof apron and his hair enclosed within a disposable cap. A sterile disposable towel is then placed around the patient's neck and held in place with towel clips (*Fig.* 3.10). The mucous membrane at both the site of injection and operation can be prepared by drying it with sterile cotton-wool and applying a solution of 0·5% chlorhexidine (Hibitane) in 70% alcohol.

Major items of dental equipment such as engines, lights, and chairs are inevitably a source of cross-infection and for this reason should be regularly cleaned with disinfectants containing 1% of available chlorine or a 2% glutaraldehyde solution. Despite these measures such equipment must always be regarded as being a source of infection and any necessary adjustments to it should be made, whenever possible, by an assistant who is not participating in the operation. Should circumstances preclude this, a sterile clothes-peg or a piece of sterile gauze should be used to prevent contamination when any alteration in the position of the operating light is required. Cable engine arms should be enclosed within a sterile tube of gauze throughout the operation.

For purposes of discussion it is convenient to separate minor oral surgical procedures into those operations which involve both hard and soft tissues and those which are performed upon the soft tissues alone. All such procedures are in essence a series of steps, each of which should be planned by the dental surgeon before he embarks upon surgery.

MINOR ORAL SURGICAL OPERATIONS ON BOTH HARD AND SOFT TISSUES

The successive stages of such an operation are: (1) the creation of a mucoperiosteal flap; (2) the removal of bone; (3) the delivery of the tooth, root, or other intra-bony lesion; (4) débridement; (5) wound closure and/or packing; (6) after-care; and each of these stages will now be discussed separately.

Mucoperiosteal flaps

Mucoperiosteal flaps are raised in order to render the operative site clearly visible and accessible to instrumentation, and they must be designed so as to provide the adequate visual and mechanical access for which they are created. Postoperative healing is facilitated by ensuring that the base of the flap is broader than its free end, and thus contains an unimpaired blood supply, and that accurate apposition of soft tissues is possible when the flap is replaced at the end of the operation. Whenever it is practicable, the incision should be designed so that at the end of the operation the suture line lies upon, and is supported by, bone which has not been cut on this particular occasion. Healing by first intention, which is always to be preferred to healing by granulation, cannot be obtained if the suture line, which must inevitably leak, rests upon a blood clot in which bacteria multiply. Mucoperiosteal flaps should be designed in such a way as to ensure that post-operative prosthetic difficulties are not created either by obliteration of the buccal sulcus or by the presence of residual tags of flabby mobile tissue.

The scalpel handle No. 3 fitted with a detachable disposable No. 15 blade is the most widely used scalpel in the practice of oral surgery (*Fig.* 3.11).

The incision should be made with firm pressure upon a sharp scalpel through both the mucous and periosteal layers of the gingiva down to the bone. The knife must be used as a pen and not as a plough (*Fig.* 3.12), and the soft tissues should be cut at right-angles to the surface of the underlying bone. It is best to make incisions of adequate length in one operation for extensions and 'second cuts' usually render the flap margin ragged and delay healing.

If the gingival margin of a standing tooth is involved in the flap it should be incised vertically, and not just levered away from the neck of the tooth (*Fig.* 3.13). If clean incisions are made and the tissues accurately replaced, the depth of the gingival pocket is not deepened when healing is complete.

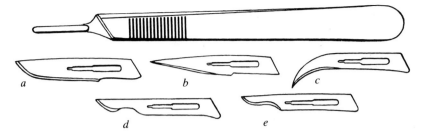

Fig. 3.11. Scalpel handle No. 3 with disposable blades: *a*, No. 10; *b*, No. 11; *c*, No. 12; *d*, Gillette shape D; and *e*, No. 15.

Convenient periosteal elevators for use in oral surgery are illustrated in *Fig.* 3.14.

The mucoperiosteal flap is raised from the bone by inserting the sharp end of a periosteal elevator under the anterior edge of the flap just above the gingival margin and stripping the flap from the bone by the use of gentle pressure. This will leave clean bone exposed if the incision has been sufficiently deep (i.e., right down to bone). If not, the flap will resist elevation and the bone will be covered with fibrous strands which must be divided with the scalpel before further attempts are made to raise the flap. An incision of inadequate depth predisposes to separation of the mucous and periosteal layers of the mucoperiosteum during elevation of the flap from the bone. This mishap makes accurate apposition of the soft tissues impossible and postoperative healing is delayed. When difficulty is experienced in finding the subperiosteal plane of dissection the rounded end of either a Mitchell trimmer or a Cumine's scaler (*Fig.* 3.15) will be found to be a more convenient instrument for the purpose of dissection than the larger periosteal elevator.

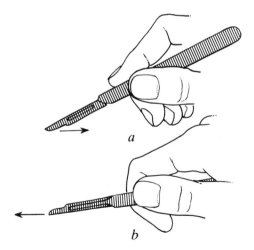

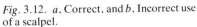

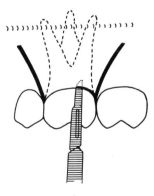

Fig. 3.12. *a*, Correct, and *b*, Incorrect use of a scalpel.

Fig. 3.13. Vertical incision of the cervical margin of a standing tooth.

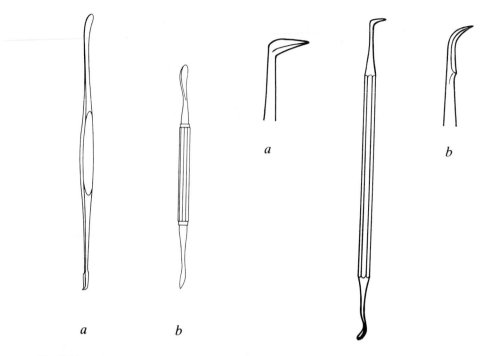

Fig. 3.14. *a*, Howarth's nasal raspatory; *b*, Dial periosteal elevator.

Fig. 3.15. The Mitchell trimmer (*a*) and the Cumine scaler (*b*) differ only in the shape of one end. They are most useful instruments for curettage.

Flaps which are large in the horizontal or anteroposterior dimension (*Fig.* 3.16) heal just as quickly as smaller flaps and have many advantages. Adequate visual and mechanical access is provided without excessive stretching or pulling upon the flap. Thus trauma to the soft tissues is minimized and healing encouraged. The creation of large flaps predisposes to rapid healing by first intention in many cases, by assuring a good blood supply, by ensuring that the flap lies in position when replaced at the end of the operation instead of falling into the bony defects created during the surgical procedure, and because the size of the flap permits the suture lines to lie upon a firm bony base instead of lying over blood clot. The dental surgeon must always remember that incised wounds heal across the incision rather than along it and so an incision 2 inches long heals at the same rate as an incision ¼ inch long, always provided that the edges of both wounds are accurately apposed.

There are, however, disadvantages to over-extending flaps in a vertical dimension, although occasions arise when such disadvantages have to be accepted either in order to obtain adequate access (*see Fig.* 4.15) or during the closure of an oroantral opening by means of an undercut buccal periosteal-lined flap (*see Fig.* 8.7). Over-extension of a flap in the vertical dimension severs the attachment of the buccinator muscle to bone and is accompanied by an increase in postoperative swelling which is more marked extra-orally. Organization of the

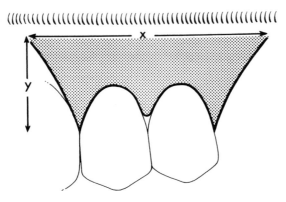

Fig. 3.16. Horizontal (x) and vertical (y) dimensions of a mucoperiosteal flap.

resultant haematoma may reduce the depth of the buccal sulcus and thus create a prosthetic difficulty. Such a complication readily occurs in edentulous areas and every effort should be made to minimize it. Vertical over-extension of a mandibular mucoperiosteal flap may result in damage to the nerves and vessels passing through the mental foramen. Surgical access can often be improved without over-extending a flap in the vertical dimension by increasing the anteroposterior length of the incision. This practice should always be followed when a lingual muco-periosteal flap is raised from the mandible. It is often more difficult to raise flaps cleanly in edentulous areas, especially if the gum is either atrophic or easily distorted by pressure.

Care should be taken to ensure that all the layers of the gum are divided when the initial incision is made. The rounded end of the Mitchell trimmer or Cumine's scaler is particularly useful for defining the subperiosteal plane of cleavage in these circumstances. Fibrosis resulting from chronic inflammation may make elevation of a flap difficult and care should be taken to make the initial incision and to define the plane of dissection in an area free from scarring. Perforation of a flap, often called 'button-holing' (*Fig.* 3.17), prejudices the blood supply of the tissue

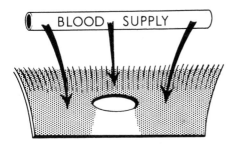

Fig. 3.17. A 'button-holed' flap. The blood supply of the non-shaded area is prejudiced by the artefact.

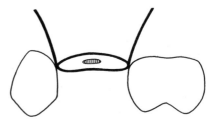

Fig. 3.18. The excision of a sinus during the outlining of a flap.

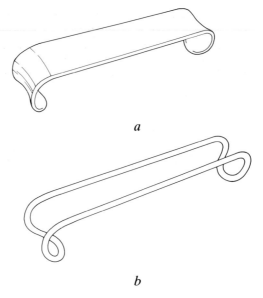

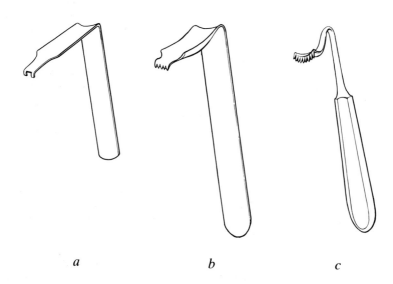

Fig. 3.19. Cheek retractors. *a*, Kilner's pattern; *b*, Sword pattern.

Fig. 3.20. Flap retractors. *a*, Austin's pattern; *b*, Cradock Henry pattern; *c*, Bowdler Henry pattern.

distal to the hole and care should be taken to avoid this complication during the elevation of the soft tissues from the bone. The presence of a sinus must be taken into account when flaps are designed. It is often possible to incorporate a sinus in the incision and thus avoid having the flap 'button-holed' by the sinus (*Fig*. 3.18).

Once the flap has been freed from the bone a metal retractor should be inserted under it and gentle traction applied so that the site of operation is adequately exposed. It is important to ensure that the end of the retractor is both inserted and held in firm contact with the surface of the bone under the periosteum if damage to the flap is to be avoided. The handle or shank of the ideal retractor should gently displace the cheek and lip, thus facilitating the surgeon's view and be comfortable to hold. Those illustrated in *Figs*. 3.19 and 3.20 have been found to be both convenient and useful in oral surgery. That illustrated in *Fig*. 3.20*a* is malleable enough to allow minor adjustments to suit individual patients and yet substantial enough to afford adequate protection to the soft tissues during instrumentation.

The removal of bone

When the mucoperiosteal flap is raised, the bone which invests the tooth, roots, or other lesion to be removed will be exposed. In most cases some of this bone must be removed and not infrequently bone is excised in a haphazard fashion rather than in the planned and systematic manner which should be employed. Bone removal may be indicated prior to the delivery of the tooth, root, or lesion in order to improve exposure of the tooth, root, or lesion, to provide either a point of application for an elevator or sufficient access to permit the use of forceps or a dissecting instrument, or to provide a space into which the tooth, root, or other lesion may be displaced. After delivery of the tooth, root, or lesion, further bone removal may be required in order to remove loose fragments, sharp edges, and bony projections, to reduce the size of the bony socket or cavity, or to ensure that no postoperative prosthetic problem results from the surgical procedure. The amount of bone excised should be limited to that amount required to attain these objectives and should be carefully sited and systematically performed.

Several techniques of bone removal can be employed by the dental surgeon and each method has indications, contra-indications, advantages, and disadvantages. The wise dental surgeon learns to use each technique efficiently, to assess the merits and demerits of each method in his hands, and to employ a particular technique in those cases in which its use is indicated. If is often good practice to employ more than one method of bone removal during one operation. Thus the use of a chisel is a quick clean method of removing young elastic bone provided that the instrument is sharp and used skilfully. However, its use is contra-indicated when the bone to be removed is sclerotic or a tooth or root is deeply embedded in a thin atrophic mandible. Bone removal with burs is more time consuming and messy and care must be taken to ensure that the bur is kept cool by an efficient jet of either sterile water or normal saline. Nevertheless, it is a precise, efficient and useful technique.

Bone, like wood, has a 'grain' which is most marked in young adults and decreases as age advances. The carpenter uses a chisel upon wood only after determining the direction in which the grain runs in the particular piece that he is cutting. In the same way the surgeon should pay due regard to the direction in which the grain runs when he is using a chisel upon bone. In the mandibular third

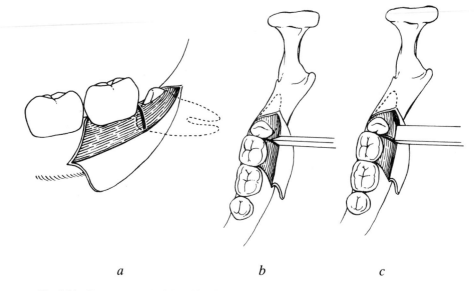

a   *b*   *c*

Fig. 3.21. Bone removal with a chisel is performed utilizing the grain of the bone in lower third molar region (*see* text for explanation).

molar region the grain runs in an anteroposterior direction in both the lingual and buccal plates. Therefore, a vertical stop-cut must be placed at the mesial end of the portion of bone to be removed if accidental splitting of the buccal alveolar plate enclosing the lower second molar is to be avoided (*Fig*. 3.21*a*).

A chisel has a bevelled and a flat surface and these two surfaces affect the direction in which the instrument cuts through bone (*Fig*. 3.22). In most instances the chisel is used with the bevel towards the bone to be sacrificed, thus ensuring that a clean-cut non-bruised bone edge is left after bone removal (*Fig*. 3.21*b*). An exception to this rule is illustrated in *Fig*. 3.21*c*, which depicts the 'use of the bevel' to overcome the difficulty of access in the lower third molar region. The chisel must be held at right-angles to the bone surface if splintering of the bone which is to be retained is to be avoided. Unfortunately, the soft tissues of the lips and cheeks combine to render such an application of the chisel impossible in all but a minority of patients. By using the chisel with its bevel downwards, i.e., towards the bone to be retained, the line of cut is angled correctly and the bone may be cut cleanly (*Fig*. 3.21*c*). Other ways in which the grain of the bone is utilized to assist surgery are illustrated in *Figs*. 4.15 and 5.39.

On occasions even comparatively young patients have dense sclerotic bone in which the 'grain' is not well marked. In these cases chisels rapidly become blunted and the bone tends to flake like 'marble chips'. This occurrence is most frequently found in patients over 45 years of age and in these cases a dental bur should be used to remove bone. Very thin bone can be cut with a sharp chisel, the only kind which should ever be used, and hand pressure alone. More commonly, however, a surgical mallet must be employed (*Fig*. 3.23) and should be used to give the chisel sharp light taps and not heavy blows. The chisel should be carefully controlled and guarded with the left hand whenever it is in use.

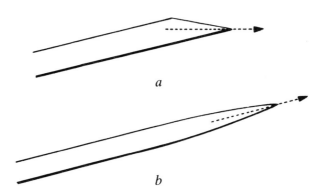

a

b

Fig. 3.22. Ends and line of cut of, *a*, a chisel, and *b*, an osteotome.

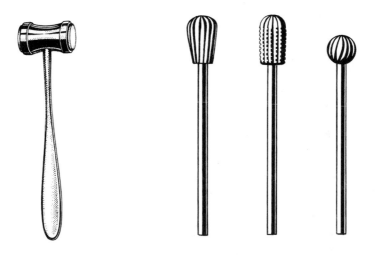

Fig. 3.23. Surgical mallet (Fry's pattern).

Fig. 3.24. 'Vulcanite' burs (Ash's acrylic trimmers. Patterns 8, 6, 20R).

Whilst the chisel, when correctly used, affords a competent operator a clean quick method of bone removal, most general dental surgeons are more experienced and skilled in the use of burs. Although many operators use fissure burs in a right-angle or contra-angle handpiece, the author prefers to use a round bur in a straight handpiece, for such a bur is easier to control and clogs less readily, whilst the straight handpiece is easier to strip, clean, maintain, and sterilize after use. Air motors and handpieces such as that illustrated in *Fig.* A.1, p. 404 provide torque and have the advantage that they can be sterilized by autoclaving. The excellent Ash surgical burs (Toller's pattern) cut even the most dense mandibular bone quickly and efficiently. The removal of such bone with a mallet and chisel under local anaesthesia can be an uncomfortable, tiring, and unpleasant experience for the patient. This problem can be avoided by the use of such a bur. Great care must be taken to ensure that the bur never overheats when cutting bone. It should be run slowly under an efficient jet of sterile water or normal saline to prevent any danger of the bone being damaged by heat. The use of the Cutter pressure bag illustrated in *Fig.* A.1, p. 404 ensures that a constant stream of sterile saline bathes the bur as it cuts. Bone may be removed either piecemeal with a large bur (size 12 round burs or the 'vulcanite' burs illustrated in *Fig.* 3.24 are useful for this purpose) or by the 'postage-stamp' method (*Fig.* 3.25). In this technique a small round bur (e.g., size No. 3) is used to make a series of holes outlining the portion of bone to be sacrificed and then joined up by either bur or chisel cuts. This is a neat and precise method of bone removal but may be time-consuming. No. 6 round burs may also be employed to create a gutter in the bone alongside the crown of the tooth or in the plane of the periodontal membrane (*Fig.* 3.26). This is an extremely useful technique in the removal of lower molars and roots for it leaves a ridge of buccal cortical bone to serve as a fulcrum for an elevator during the delivery of the tooth. A flat-bladed retractor should be employed to hold the mucoperiosteal flap away from the site on which the bur is to be used (*Fig.* 3.20). Flaps of adequate size facilitate this procedure which prevents the occurrence of the common 'accident' of the bur burying itself in the soft tissues. When it is decided to divide a mandibular molar using a bur (*Fig.* 3.25*b*) sufficient buccal

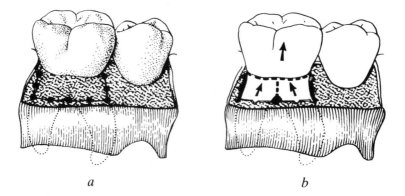

a   *b*

Fig. 3.25. The removal of buccal bone by the 'postage-stamp' method and 'lines of section' used when tooth division is required.

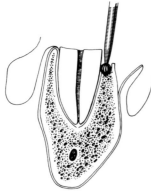

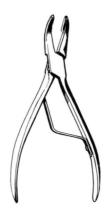

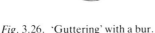

Fig. 3.26. 'Guttering' with a bur.   *Fig*. 3.27. Rongeur forceps.

bone must be removed to expose the bifurcation of the roots. The buccal wall of mandibular molar sockets thickens rapidly towards the root apices. Thus, if the roots were divided transversely at the level of the bifurcation the application of elevators to them would be impeded by the thickness of the cut edge of the buccal plate. For this reason once the bifurcation has been exposed the crown should first be cut off from the root mass. The same round bur can then be used to divide the roots from the bifurcation upwards towards the cut surface of the root mass. Root division in this direction makes it possible for the operator to know with certainty that the line of cut has separated the root mass. If desired the division can be completed by inserting a straight elevator into the cut and twisting it to split the lingual cementum. The roots can then be delivered along their individual lines of withdrawal.

The use of a jet of sterile water or normal saline to cool the bur makes it essential to employ a suction apparatus throughout the procedure. The assistant should hold the tip of the sucker at the most dependent part of the wound in such a way that it neither obstructs the view of the surgeon nor comes too close to the revolving bur. It should be kept still and on bone in order to minimize noise and the chance of obstruction by tags of soft tissue. The sucker should not be employed as a retractor or to deliver solid debris from the wound.

Two kinds of cutting forceps or rongeurs are illustrated in *Figs*. 3.27 and 11.15. These instruments are extremely useful for trimming off sharp bony projections or removing thin plates of compact bone during saucerization of a bone cavity (*see below*). They should have sharp blades and be used with a clean cutting action and not a twisting motion which causes bone to fracture instead of being cut.

The delivery of the tooth, root, or other intra-bony lesion

When the necessary bone removal has been completed the delivery of the tooth, root, or lesion should be effected. Teeth and roots may be extracted by the use of dental forceps if a firm grip of the tooth or root can be obtained. It is better to use forceps rather than elevators when removing either a retained tooth or root from a thin atrophic and otherwise edentulous mandible. The risk of a fracture of the jaw occurring can be minimized by removing bone with burs rather than chisels and using gentle rotation of a tooth, such as that illustrated in *Fig.* 3.28, around its vertical long axis to effect delivery. In those cases in which forceps extraction proves impracticable, elevators may be used to force the tooth or root out of its

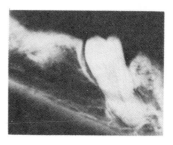

Fig. 3.28. The root of this unerupted mandibular second premolar is grooved by the inferior dental nerve and close to the mental foramen.

socket and along the line of least resistance, i.e., the 'line of withdrawal'. Soft-tissue lesions such as granulomata or cysts should be 'shelled out' from the walls of the bony cavity in which they are situated by the use of a bone curette, a Cumine's scaler, or a Mitchell trimmer (*see Fig.* 3.15). The author finds the latter instruments most useful for this purpose and often uses an angled Warwick James elevator (*see Fig.* 3.31) to deliver very small lesions. Elevators are used to force the tooth or root out of its socket and along the line of least resistance. It is essential to have a fulcrum and to ensure that it is a bony one and not an adjacent tooth, unless that tooth is to be extracted at the same visit.

The line of withdrawal of a tooth or root is the path along which it will move out of its socket when minimal force is applied to it and is largely determined by the long axis of the root or roots.

Elevators may be applied either mesially, buccally, or distally to the tooth to be extracted and the line of withdrawal of the tooth or root determines the site at which force is applied to the root to effect its delivery, i.e., the point of application.

In many multi-rooted teeth the lines of withdrawal of the various roots conflict. When this occurs the tooth may yield to either forceps extraction or the application of an elevator to the buccal surface of the root mass of the tooth. These methods are aimed at forcing the roots along a mean line of withdrawal and can only succeed if the alveolar bone is yielding and the lines of withdrawal of the individual roots do not conflict too severely. It is sometimes necessary to create a point of application for the elevator on the buccal side of the root mass (*Fig.* 3.29).

If a tooth resists elevation the elevator should be put down and the cause of the difficulty sought and remedied. In most instances it will be necessary to divide the root mass and remove the separated roots along their individual lines of withdrawal. Teeth may be conveniently divided by means of burs or osteotomes.

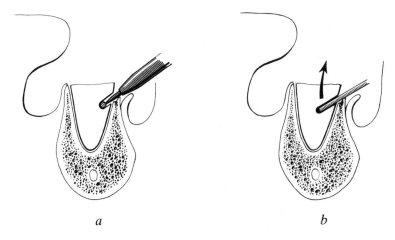

Fig. 3.29. Creation of a buccal point of application for an elevator. *a*, Round bur correctly applied at an angle of 45° to the long axis of the root. *b*, Blade of elevator inserted.

The osteotome differs from the chisel by having a bi-bevelled cutting end (*see Fig.* 3.22*b*). This feature enables the surgeon to apply force along a linear contact and to cut straight forwards and makes the osteotome the ideal instrument for splitting teeth. If the operator knows both the 'lines of cleavage' of a tooth and the correct site to which the cutting edge of an osteotome should be applied to the crown, it is possible to split many teeth in the desired direction by means of a sharp 'pulled' tap of the mallet (*Fig.* 3.30). It cannot be emphasized too strongly that the exhibition of force is not required and is in fact a disadvantage, for excessive and wrongly applied force may either drive a tooth through the lingual plate or cause a fracture of the alveolar bone or jaw.

A tooth which has been previously loosened in its socket cannot be split with an osteotome, for the sharpness of the mallet blow is cushioned by movement of the tooth. The technique has the advantage of being both quick and clean when being performed by those skilled in its use but has the disadvantage that it does not create any space for manipulation and is entirely dependent on the lines of

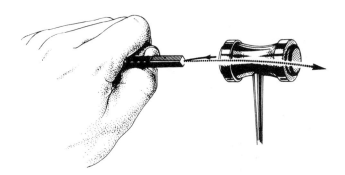

Fig. 3.30. Sharp 'pulled' tap with the mallet.

cleavage of the particular tooth being divided. Most practising dental surgeons are more proficient in the use of a bur than an osteotome and prefer to use the former instrument for tooth division. Although bur division is more time-consuming and creates much more debris, it does permit the operator to place and angle his cut in the exact position he desires and leaves a wide cut through the tooth substance rather than a linear crack. The room thus provided facilitates delivery of the individual fragments of the sectioned tooth (*Fig.* 5.38*c*). Bur division of a tooth is illustrated in *Figs.* 3.25*b*, 5.38*c* and 5.42, whilst osteotome division is shown in *Fig.* 5.38*b*.

In many instances it is convenient to begin tooth division with a bur and complete it with an osteotome split, thus combining the advantages of both methods. Many operators waste time when using the bur to section teeth by failing to be systematic and purposeful during the procedure. One of the most time-consuming tooth divisions is the horizontal sectioning of a mandibular third molar along the amelocemental junction. This procedure can be both effectively and speedily performed if the operator applies a small round surgical bur to the middle of the cervical margin of the tooth and cuts straight through the dental tissues into the pulp cavity and a little beyond. The resultant hole is then enlarged by the use of a larger round bur, which is then employed to extend the cut both medially and distally until only the intact lingual enamel unites the crown and the root mass. Division of the tooth can then be completed either by inserting a straight elevator into the groove and rotating it around its long axis or by the use of an osteotome. Care should be taken to create individual points of application for the crown and

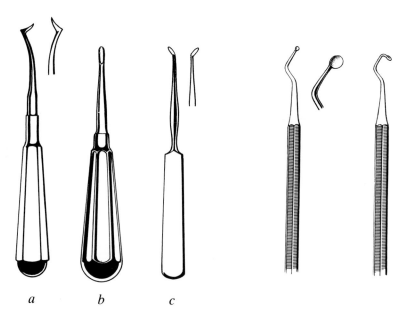

a *b* *c*

Fig. 3.31. Elevators. *a*, Cryer's pattern; *b*, Lindo Levien pattern; *c*, Warwick James' pattern.

Fig. 3.32. Spoon-ended dental excavators. (N.B. Single-ended instruments are preferable to double-ended ones in the practice of oral surgery.)

each of the roots prior to sectioning the tooth. The line and level of the cuts dividing the tooth should be such that no root is left completely embedded in bone.

After teeth or roots have been extracted, any retained periapical granuloma should be removed. As previously stated, the round end of either a Mitchell trimmer or a Cumine's scaler is useful for this purpose when dealing with larger lesions, whilst small lesions can often best be 'winkled out' with the blunt end of an angled Warwick James elevator (*Fig.* 3.31*c*) or a spoon-ended dental excavator (*Fig.* 3.32).

Débridement

Once the removal of any residual soft-tissue lesion has been completed the operator should irrigate the bony cavity with a sterile normal saline solution, and remove any loose bony fragments or other foreign bodies, before deciding whether any trimming of the bony socket is required. Whilst most oral surgeons agree that all sharp bone edges should be smoothed, bone spurs excised, and only a residual blood clot of minimal size left in the wound, there is a divergence of opinion concerning the value of, and indications for, saucerization of the bony cavity. *Fig.* 3.33*a* illustrates the size of the blood clot which follows the removal of a tooth with forceps, whilst *Fig.* 3.33*b* and *c* shows how the size of the blood clot can be reduced if the tooth is dissected out, and the buccal mucoperiosteal flap either sutured or tucked into the wound and held against the bone with either a pom-pom (*Fig.* 3.34) or a pack. *Fig.* 3.33*d* illustrates the size of the blood clot

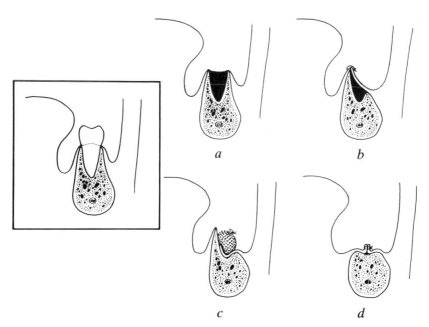

Fig. 3.33. Size of residual blood clot after differing techniques of tooth removal (*see* text for explanation).

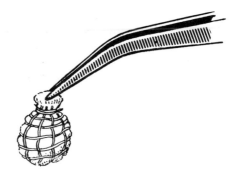

Fig. 3.34. A pom-pom.

which remains following the removal of a tooth by means of the split-bone technique (*see Fig.* 5.39, p. 137), in which both buccal and lingual plates of bone are sacrificed and the wound closed. This latter procedure is an extreme example of saucerization by means of the removal of bone to reduce the size of blood clot, and is only really practicable in areas, such as the lower third molar regions, in which the need for a reduction in the size of the blood clot outweighs the need of preservation of the alveolar ridge form for prosthetic purposes.

Whilst so radical a removal of bone is seldom indicated in the practice of minor oral surgery, the judicious removal of small amounts of bone from strategic sites will often serve to reduce the size of blood clot and facilitate the primary closure of wounds. Primary closure has the advantage of speeding healing and requiring less after-care on the part of both patient and dentist, whilst packing is employed when either sclerosis and avascularity of bone or potential infection of the blood clot makes healing by granulation (secondary intention) the aim. Rongeur forceps (*see Fig.* 3.27) are very useful instruments for the removal of bone in these circumstances. The blades of these instruments should be closed with a firm cutting motion and not a twisting action, which tends to fracture the bone.

Wound closure and packing

When the removal of debris and all the sharp bone edges has been completed, the mucoperiosteal flap must either be accurately sutured in its original position or be tucked into the bony cavity and held against the bone with either a ribbon-gauze pack or pom-pom. For dental purposes ½ inch wide ribbon gauze is the size usually preferred and, after being impregnated with either Whitehead's varnish or bismuth iodoform paste, is packed into the wound.

Pigmentum Iodoformi Compositum BPC

(Pig. Iodof. Co., Whitehead's varnish)

Benzoin, sumatra in coarse powder	44 gr (3 g)
Prepared storax	33 gr (2 g)
Balsam of Tolu	22 gr (1·5 g)
Iodoform	44 gr (3 g)
Solvent ether	to 1 fl oz (28·4 ml)

1 fl oz (28·4 ml) to be dispensed unless otherwise directed

Any excess of medicament should be removed prior to the insertion of the pack by passing the ribbon gauze through a lightly held gauze swab. The cavity should be packed systematically from one end to the other and when almost full any excess of ribbon gauze should be cut off, and the cut end carefully tucked into the wound. The packing is then completed by tucking the remaining bight of the ribbon gauze into the cavity. A pom-pom (*Fig.* 3.34) is a piece of cotton-wool enclosed within an outer layer of gauze, the free edges of which are secured by means of a ligature of either dental floss or suture material. A number of sterile pom-poms of various sizes should be available for use when oral surgery is undertaken. The insertion of a pom-pom rather than a ribbon gauze pack into an intra-oral wound is often more convenient for the operator and more comfortable for the patient. Small intra-oral gauze packs not infrequently become loose and cause either discomfort or annoyance to patients during the healing period. Impregnation of either a pom-pom or a pack with either Whitehead's varnish or bismuth iodoform paste prevents the wound dressing from becoming foul when left in the mouth for 2 or 3 weeks. By this means the need for frequent and repeated changing of dressings in intra-oral wounds may be avoided.

During the operation sutures may be used to control or retract flaps. At the end of an operation they may be used to either assist healing by first intention, or to minimize wound contamination by loosely apposing the soft tissues, or to control haemorrhage, and they should only be inserted if required to achieve one of these three objectives.

Many suture materials and suturing techniques are advocated for use in the practice of oral surgery, but for most purposes sterile black silk, gauge 000, is the material of choice, and the insertion of either simple interrupted sutures (*Fig.* 3.35) or interrupted horizontal mattress sutures (*Fig.* 3.36) suffices. Mattress sutures are more trouble to insert, but do not cut out of friable tissues so readily and may also be used to evert flap margins when required. A Lane's No. 3 (22 mm) cutting needle is widely used in dentistry (*Fig.* 3.37*a*). The silk can be held in the needle, without a knot, if it is threaded through the eye twice. Reverse cutting needles have their cutting edge on the outer curve (*Fig.* 3.37*b*). They actually make a small

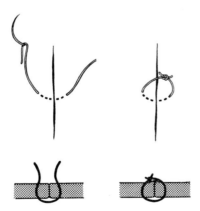

Fig. 3.35. Simple interrupted suture.

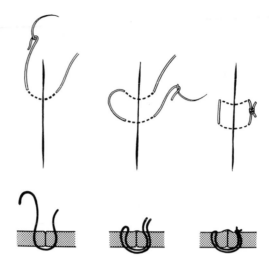

Fig. 3.36. Interrupted horizontal mattress suture.

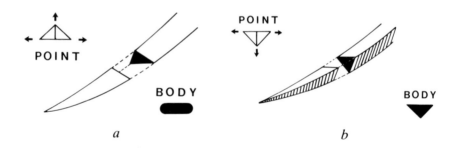

Fig. 3.37. Needles used for suturing. a, Conventional cutting needle. b, Reverse cutting needle.

cut in the tissues to allow smooth passage of the needle and the suture and so penetrate tough tissues, such as palatal mucoperiosteum, more readily than conventional cutting needles. As the cut is made in the direction away from the wound edge the suture does not tend to tear out so readily as when conventional needles are used.

The technique of suturing is as follows. The area to be sutured is first freed of blood, by means of either a sucker or a swab, so that the cut edges are clearly visible. Then the needle is passed through sound tissue at a point which is at least one-eighth of an inch (3 mm) from any free margin and sited nearer the free end of the flap rather than its base. It is the usual practice to pass the needle through the mobile flap first close to the beaks of the toothed dissecting forceps (Fig. 3.38), with which the flap is held firmly. An exception to this rule is that when placing a suture in the mandibular lingual mucoperiosteum, the needle is passed in a linguobuccal direction away from the tongue. Firm but gentle pressure should be employed to rotate the needle through each portion of mucoperiosteum in turn in a definite arc, so that the needle emerges in a situation where it can be grasped with ease. The needle must never be held by either its eye or its point. Needle-holders should be applied just below the eye (*Fig.* 3.39).

Care should be taken not to drive the needle-point into bone if either bending or fracture of the needle is to be avoided. When passing a needle through attached gingiva it is sometimes difficult to pick up both layers of the mucoperiosteum without driving the point of the needle into the underlying bone. In these circumstances the margin of the soft tissues should be separated from the bone by gentle dissection with a periosteal elevator, a Cumine's scaler, or a Mitchell trimmer before insertion of the suture. Tension should be applied to the suture before it is tied in order to ensure that the soft tissues are correctly apposed. If the mucoperiosteal flap does not assume the desired position when tension is applied, the suture should be withdrawn and reinserted at a more appropriate site. Sutures should never be tied tightly, for some oedematous swelling of the soft tissues invariably complicates the postoperative period. Knots must be placed to one side of the incision if healing is not to be delayed. *Fig.* 3.40 illustrates an 'instrument

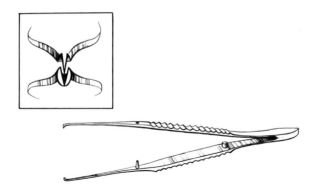

Fig. 3.38. Toothed dissecting tweezers. Inset shows a magnified view of the 'mouse-toothed' beaks.

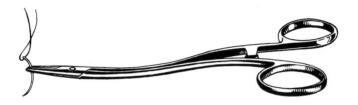

Fig. 3.39. Needle correctly held in Kilner needle-holders. N.B. It should never be grasped by either its eye or its point.

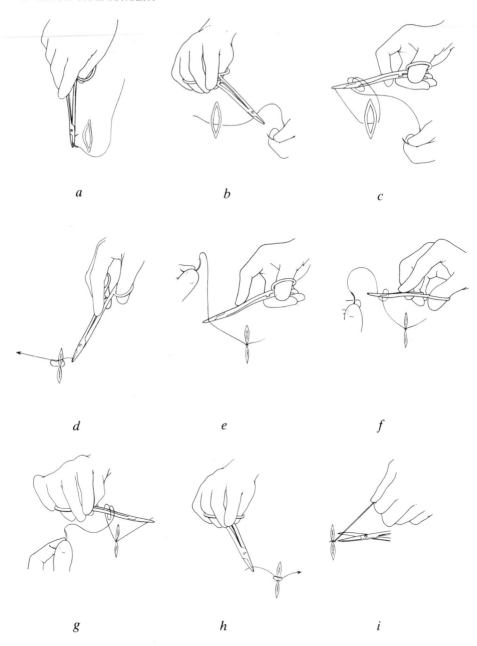

a

b

c

d

e

f

g

h

i

Fig. 3.40. 'Instrument tie'. *a, b,* The tip of the needle-holder is pointed at the needle and passed over the silk twice. *c, d,* The tip of the short end of the silk is grasped and drawn through the loops. *e, f,* The needle-holders are pointed towards the needle once again and passed *under* the silk once or twice. *g,* The tip of the short end is then grasped and pulled through the loops, thus completing the knot. *h,* The loose ends are used to draw the knot to one side of the incision and, *i,* then cut with scissors.

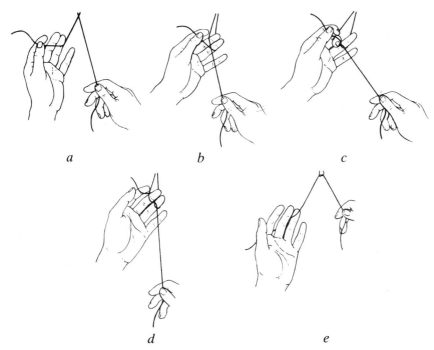

Fig. 3.41. 'One-handed tie'. *a*, The short end of the silk passes across the palmar surfaces of the fingers of the left hand and is grasped between the index finger and thumb. *b*, The bight of the long end of the silk is passed between the left index and second fingers and, *c*, *d*, is pulled under the short end of the silk by flexing the second finger. *e*, Then traction on both ends of the silk tightens the tie. This sequence must be repeated three times to give a secure knot.

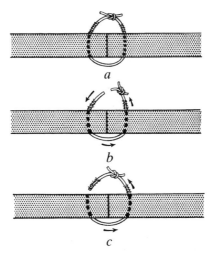

Fig. 3.42. An intra-oral suture is loose and impregnated with food detritus after being in situ for 1 week. If it is cut just below the knot as in *b*, the wound is contaminated as infected silk is pulled through the tissues. *c*, This complication is avoided if the silk is cut just as it enters the tissues.

tie' of a surgeon's knot, whilst *Fig.* 3.41 illustrates a 'one-handed tie'. During use scissors, like other hinged instruments, should be held with the operator's index finger over the hinge in order to provide maximum stability. When they are used in the mouth the danger of damaging the lip can be minimized by opening and closing the blades vertically rather than horizontally.

In the mouth sutures are usually left in situ for between 3 and 7 days. When removing the suture the dentist should grasp the knot in a pair of toothed tweezers, and cut the suture just below the knot at the point where the suture enters the tissues. The cut suture is then withdrawn from the tissues by traction on the knot, thus avoiding wound contamination (*Fig.* 3.42).

After-care

The dental surgeon's duty to his patient does not end with the placing of a pack or the insertion of the last suture. He has a responsibility to ensure that the patient's postoperative period is as pain-free and uneventful as possible. A suitable analgesic should be prescribed for use as required. Some popular preparations used for this purpose are as follows.

1. Paynocil, a proprietary product, containing aspirin gr 10 (600 mg) and amino acetic acid gr 5 (300 mg) in each tablet. The adult dose is 1 or 2 tablets 4-hourly to control pain.

2. Codeine compound tablets BP (Tab. Codein Co.). Each tablet contains: codeine phosphate 8 mg; acetyl salicylic acid 250 mg; phenacetin 250 mg. The dose is 1 or 2 tablets every 4 hours.

3. Codeine compound soluble tablets BP (Tab. Codein Co. Sol.) contain the same ingredients as the above with the addition of calcium carbonate, anhydrous citric acid, and saccharin sodium. The dose is 1 or 2 tablets 4-hourly.

The efficacy of aspirin is known to be dose related and when given in single doses of 1000 mg or more the drug has been described as the analgesic of choice. However, aspirin may have topical erosive effects on the gastro-intestinal tract and so may cause iron-deficiency anaemia, haematemesis, nausea, or vomiting. Sensitivity reactions which can occur include rashes, swellings, asthma, and even an anaphylactoid reaction in rare instances. Even small doses of salicylates may prolong the prothrombin time in patients on anticoagulant therapy. The prescription of aspirin, or mixtures containing aspirin, is contra-indicated in anyone giving a history of sensitivity to the drug, asthmatics, patients afflicted with either peptic ulceration, a haemorrhagic disease, or those on anticoagulant therapy. In all these instances aspirin-free analgesics must be used, such as:

4. Codeine phosphate tablets BP, each tablet containing 31 mg codeine phosphate. The dose is 10–60 mg (gr $1/_6$–1). Constipation may complicate the repeated use of these tablets, and patients should be counselled against the ingestion of large amounts of this drug. It has been suggested that this drug is more effective when used in combination with others as in Codeine compound tablets BP.

5. Paracetamol tablets BP, each tablet containing 500 mg of paracetamol. The dose is 1 or 2 tablets 4-hourly, which in rare instances may cause dizziness, sleepiness, and gastro-intestinal disturbances. The pain relief afforded by paracetamol is not dose related and in view of the danger of hepatotoxicity in overdosage patients should be warned not to exceed the stated dose.

These tablets have been found to be of value only in the control of mild pain and other aspirin-free proprietary preparations are usually employed when a patient is expected to have more severe pain.

The first of these (Antidol) contains phenacetin 200 mg, caffeine 50 mg, and salicylamide-(2-ethoxy ethyl)-ether 250 mg in each tablet and has been found to be effective in an adult dosage of 2 tablets every 4 hours. Another preparation is mefenamic acid (Ponstan), which has been found to be effective in an adult dosage of two kapseals (500 mg) orally followed by one kapseal (250 mg) every 6 hours. This drug should be used with caution in patients with renal impairment or peptic ulceration, and its use should be discontinued if diarrhoea or skin rashes occur, or there is depression of the white-cell count. It should not be prescribed for either epileptic or pregnant patients.

Diflunisal (Dolobid) is a non-steroidal anti-inflammatory analgesic with a relatively long duration of action. It has peripheral analgesic, anti-inflammatory and weak antipyretic effects, and inhibits synthesis of prostaglandins and platelet aggregation less than aspirin. The recommended adult dose is 1000 mg followed by 500 mg twice a day and in this dosage the drug appears to be more effective than aspirin and its effects last from 8 to 12 hours. It causes less gastric irritation than aspirin but should be used with caution, if at all, in pregnant women.

Other than in hospital practice there is seldom a need for a dental surgeon to use addictive drugs which are subject to legal control.

The patient should be instructed to avoid vigorous mouthwashing, violent exercise, stimulants, or very hot food and drink for the rest of the day in an attempt to minimize the risk of postoperative haemorrhage. Before the patient is discharged he should be shown how to place either a gauze pressure pack or a clean folded handkerchief upon the intra-oral wound and to bite upon it firmly in order to arrest any haemorrhage which might occur.

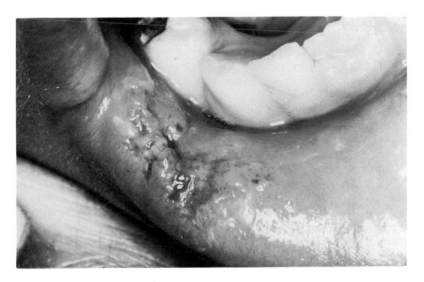

Fig. 3.43. An example of ulceration of the lower lip in a child who bit it after receiving an inferior dental injection. (*By courtesy of Mr M. A. Young.*)

The intra-oral wound should be cleansed by rinsing the mouth with warm saline immediately before going to bed on the day of operation. Healing may be aided by the use of hot saline mouth baths frequently during the next 2 or 3 days. The solution is prepared by dissolving half a teaspoonful of salt in a tumbler of hot, but not scalding water. Copious amounts should be taken into the mouth as frequently as is practicable and held over the site of operation for as long as is possible. The use of mouth-baths is particularly helpful when undertaken immediately after meals and before going to bed. Following the use of local anaesthesia the lips, tongue, or cheeks may remain numb for 2 or 3 hours during which they may be damaged by biting (*Fig.* 3.43), drinking scalding fluids, or whilst smoking a cigarette. The patient should be warned of these dangers and instructed to return for consultation should anything untoward complicate the healing period. Whenever it is practicable to do so, verbal postoperative instructions should be supplemented by giving the patient either a printed or written copy of the instructions.

It is courteous to notify the patient's general medical practitioner of any surgery performed upon his patient and it is a good practice to instruct the patient to return to the dentist without delay should anything untoward complicate the healing period.

MINOR ORAL SURGICAL PROCEDURES INVOLVING ONLY SOFT TISSUES

Most of the principles enumerated above are of equal importance when an oral surgical operation involving soft tissues alone is being performed. The exact size and extent of the excision should be determined prior to embarking upon surgery and the operation planned step by step before it is undertaken. When an operation is being performed upon the lips, tongue and/or cheeks, haemostasis is of particular importance and the insertion of stay sutures (i.e., sutures enclosing a mass of tissue and rendering it ischaemic) or the continuous application of firm pressure to the part with the fingers and thumbs by an assistant will do much to aid the surgeon. Local infiltration with a solution containing a vasoconstrictor such as adrenaline (1 in 80 000) can also be of value in this respect, but unless it is done with discretion it may cause ballooning of the tissues and render the recognition of landmarks more difficult. Mopping the wound with dry gauze swabs or the skilled use of an efficient suction apparatus by an assistant are effective means of ensuring a dry operative site (*Fig.* 3.44). Care must be taken not to contaminate other swabs when removing those required for use from a storage jar or sterile drum (*Fig.* 3.45).

Although the No. 15 scalpel blade is useful when incising the soft tissues, the Gillette shape D blade (*see Fig.* 3.11*d*) cuts the mucosa more readily with minimal pressure and enables the surgeon to determine the depth of his incision more accurately. This facilitates soft-tissue surgery by aiding the operator to both find and stay in the correct tissue planes at all times. Dissection is made easier if the soft tissues are made and kept tense throughout the operation, as for instance when a soft-tissue lesion is transfixed with a suture and raised from its bed by traction (*Figs.* 3.46 and 13.4). Blunt dissection with scissors is often of value.

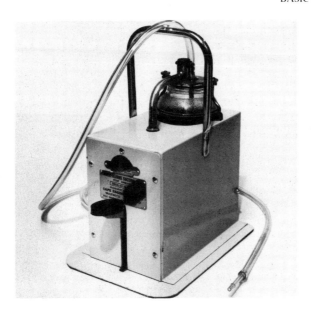

Fig. 3.44. Smith Clarke foot-operated suction apparatus.

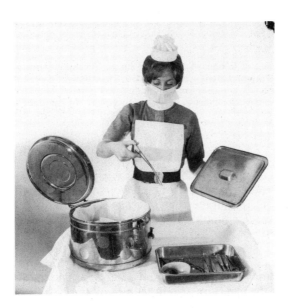

Fig. 3.45. Sterile swabs being transferred from drum to sterile tray. N.B. The way in which the lid of the tray is held.

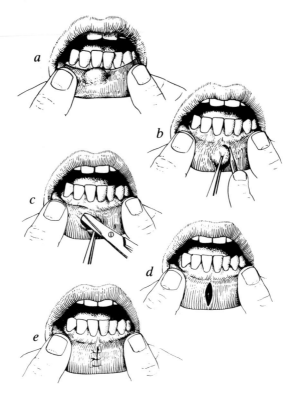

Fig. 3.46. Excision of a mucous cyst of the lip. *a*, The lip is compressed and held out between the fingers and thumbs of an assistant. *b*, The cyst is grasped in dissecting tweezers, the overlying mucosa is incised and the lesion and the attached mucous glands are *c*, separated from their attachments by blunt dissection. *d*, Resulting defect. *e*, Sutures inserted.

A pair of scissors of the type illustrated in *Fig*. 3.47 are plunged into the tissues with the blades closed, opened within the wound, and then withdrawn whilst still open. By this means the surgeon can dissect widely without the risk of damage to either nerves or vessels. Should bleeding make dissection difficult it can usually be readily dealt with, either by picking up small bleeding points with curved 'mosquito' artery clips or by continuous pressure on a hot saline pack (49° C) held against the bleeding tissues for a timed 3 min. It is seldom necessary to tie off a small bleeding point when a haemostat has been applied to it for 5 min or so, and only very rarely is the insertion of a stay suture required to secure a bleeder. When the dissection of the soft-tissue lesion is complete, the surgical specimen should be lifted from the wound and placed in a previously labelled specimen jar containing formol saline, and sent to a pathologist for examination (*see Fig*. 3.48*b* and p. 336).

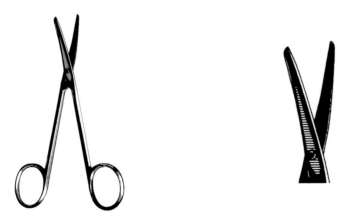

Fig. 3.47. Curved dissecting scissors.

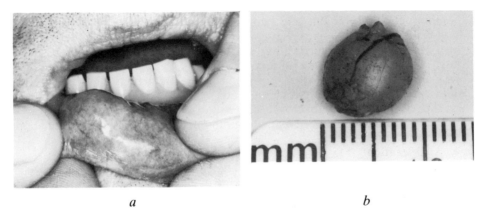

a   b

Fig. 3.48. Mucous extravasation cyst of lip. *a,* Preoperative appearance. *b,* Excised specimen. N.B. Glandular tissue.

The preoperative treatment plan should include a decision as to whether the wound is to be either closed or left to heal by granulation. Careful undercutting of the mucosa at the margins of a wound will enable the surgeon to utilize the inherent elasticity of the mucous membrane to cover defects of considerable size and to approximate the edges of the wound without tension. Whenever this is not possible, the undercut mucosa should be advanced as far as its inherent elasticity permits and then sutured to the underlying exposed muscle, thus reducing the area of mesodermal tissue left to granulate. Some dental surgeons like to cover such an exposed area by sewing a pack soaked in Whitehead's varnish over the wound, but this measure is seldom required if the patient uses hot saline mouth-baths frequently during the postoperative period in the manner described on p. 86.

SUMMARY

Most of the problems in oral surgery can be solved, the difficulties overcome, and the possible complications either completely avoided or effectively dealt with if the dental surgeon employs a systematic approach when undertaking oral surgery. Such a scheme may be summarized as follows.

1. Diagnosis History and clinical examination enable a provisional or presumptive diagnosis to be made which, when combined with special methods of examination, provides a definitive diagnosis.

2. Treatment Planning In those cases in which an operation is indicated, determination of the amount of surgery required, followed by an appreciation of possible difficulties which may be encountered and any complications which may ensue, will enable the correct type of surgical procedure to be planned.

3. Decisions to be taken prior to Surgery

a. Outpatient or inpatient procedure? Determined by:

i. General medical condition of patient.

ii. Probable duration of operation.

iii. Type of anaesthesia indicated.

b. Any special arrangements required?

i. Instructions to patient (e.g., not to drive motor-vehicle, whether to take meals, probable length of incapacity, whether he should be accompanied, etc.).

ii. ? Desirability of premedication.

iii. ? Any indication for antibiotic cover.

iv. ? Any need for other forms of medical treatment (e.g., anticonvulsants, insulin, anticoagulant or steroid therapy, etc.).

v. Are containers available for specimens?

vi. Have arrangements been made for both the transport and the examination of specimens?

4. At Operation

a. Ensure all instruments which may be needed are available and sterilized. (Requirements may be compiled by thinking of each stage of the procedure and listing the instruments needed to perform it.)

b. Lay out instruments in a regular order on a sterile trolley top or in a sterile tray.

c. When single-ended instruments are used, only the handles should be touched.

d. After use instruments should be returned to their former place on the trolley top or in the tray. Soiled swabs should be placed in a separate receptacle.

e. Have *labelled* specimen containers ready for use.

f. Other requirements: good light, skilled assistance, radiographs of operation site, effective anaesthesia, and an operation plan designed to cope with difficulties and avoid complications.

5. Postoperative

a. Prescribe analgesics as required.

b. Give clear instructions regarding:

i. Oral hygiene including the use of hot saline mouth baths.

ii. Haemorrhage, after-pain, and postoperative swelling.

iii. Indications for emergency treatment and arrangements available for it.

c. Make a follow-up appointment.

SUGGESTED READING

Duvall A. E. (1960) Minor oral surgery. *Br. Dent. J.* **109**, 303–9.

Holroyd S. V., Watts D. T. and Welch J. T. (1960) The use of epinephrine in local anaesthetics for dental patients with cardiovascular disease: a review of the literature. *J. Oral Surg.* **18**, 492–503.

McLundie A. C., Kennedy G. D. C., Stephen K. W. et al. (1968) Sterilisation in general dental practice. *Br. Dent. J.* **124**, 214–18.

O'Neil R., Verril P. J., Aeillig W. H. et al. (1970) Intravenous diazepam in minor oral surgery. *Br. Dent. J.* **128**, 15–18.

Seymour R. A. and Walton J. G. (1982) Analgesic efficacy in dental pain. *Br. Dent. J.* **153**, 291–8.

Shovelton D. S. (1982) The prevention of cross infection in dentistry. *Br. Dent. J.* **153**, 260–4.

Walker R. O. and Geddes Dorothy A. M. (1965) The sterilisation of syringes. *Br. Dent. J.* **118**, 151–7.

Chapter 4

Illustrative oral surgical procedures

The value of preoperative assessment and treatment planning in oral surgery cannot be overemphasized. The early recognition of difficulties which may be encountered during the operative procedure together with careful consideration of possible complications which may occur enables the dental surgeon to formulate a treatment plan, by the use of which the difficulties may be overcome and the complications either avoided altogether or promptly and effectively treated. The application of these principles is best illustrated by examples.

THE MANAGEMENT OF 'DIFFICULT' EXTRACTIONS

Difficulties may be encountered during the removal of a tooth for a variety of reasons and the dental surgeon should never ignore any warning of the possibility that such difficulties may be encountered during any proposed tooth extraction. If the patient states that difficulty has been experienced when teeth have been removed on previous occasions, this may indicate the presence of some factor such as dense sclerotic unyielding bone or hypercementosis of the roots (*see Figs*. 1.16 and 1.17).

Sometimes the likelihood of difficulty can be diagnosed on clinical grounds. Thus a mandibular second molar affected by cervical caries, and with an occlusal surface worn flat by attrition, which is firmly set in dense alveolar bone with a convex buccal surface in the square jaw of a bull-necked heavyweight boxer, is liable to be more difficult to extract than a non-carious second mandibular molar, the bony support of which has been destroyed by periodontal disease. Although this would appear to be a statement of the obvious, such clinical warnings are frequently ignored, and injudicious and ineffectual attempts are made to extract such a tooth with forceps, often under nitrous-oxide anaesthesia.

Good pre-extraction radiographs may also provide evidence of the presence of such causes of difficulty as hypercementosis or an unfavourable root pattern, and whenever it is possible to do so a radiographic examination of the tooth and its supporting and surrounding structures should be undertaken prior to extraction being attempted (*Figs*. 4.1–4.4).

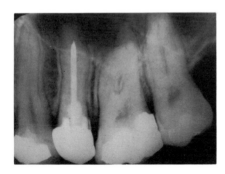

Fig. 4.1. The root-filled second premolar is heavily filled and hypercementosed. The apex of the root is closely related to the maxillary antrum, the bony floor of which has been eroded due to periapical inflammation.

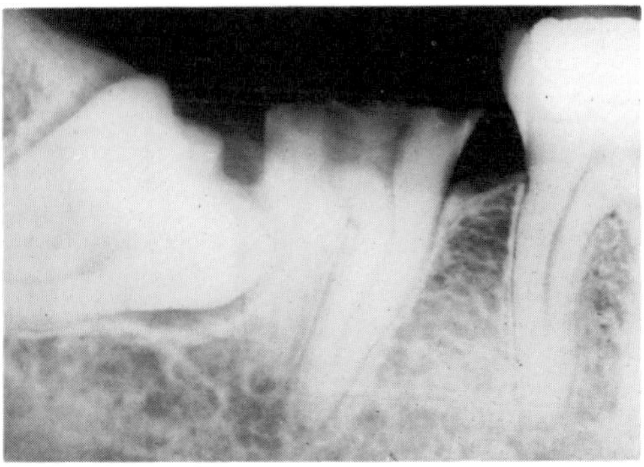

Fig. 4.2. The lower right second molar resisted extraction with forceps and its crown was fractured. This radiograph reveals that an unerupted mandibular third molar was impacted into the tooth.

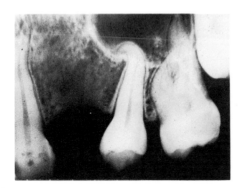

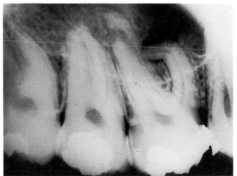

Fig. 4.3. A maxillary second premolar with a hooked root in close relationship to the maxillary antrum.

Fig. 4.4. A pulpless heavily filled maxillary first permanent molar with widely splayed roots. The mesiobuccal root is unfavourably curved.

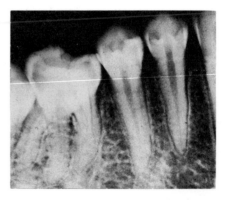

Fig. 4.5. This right lower first permanent molar resisted extraction with forceps. A periapical radiograph revealed the presence of three roots and the tooth was removed by the transalveolar method of extraction.

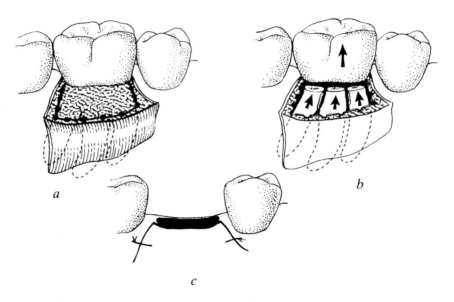

Fig. 4.6. The removal of the tooth shown in *Fig.* 4.5.

In everyday practice the dentist may only realize that the extraction of a tooth is going to be difficult when he encounters abnormal resistance during an attempt to remove the tooth with forceps. In these circumstances it is good practice to abandon the attempt at forceps extraction and to try to determine the cause of difficulty by means of a careful clinical and radiographic assessment. The tooth can then be removed by a planned surgical procedure under conditions which guarantee success (*Figs.* 4.5, 4.6).

THE REMOVAL OF UNERUPTED OR SEMI-ERUPTED MAXILLARY THIRD MOLARS

Although maxillary third molars cause symptoms less frequently than mandibular third molars, the extraction of these teeth may be indicated if either caries or pericoronal infection supervene. In the majority of cases the long axis of such a tooth is inclined distobuccally (*Fig.* 4.7), but many variations in position may be seen (*Figs.* 4.8, 4.9, 4.10).

In the maxillary molar region the buccal sulcus is related to the inner surface of the coronoid process of the mandible, which moves forwards as the mouth is opened, and so the main difficulty which confronts the dental surgeon when extracting such a tooth is the limited access, both visual and mechanical. The roots of a maxillary third molar are usually fused and conical in form but occasionally hooked roots or wide divergence between the buccal and palatal roots may cause difficulty (*Figs.* 4.11, 4.12).

Extraction of a maxillary third molar may be complicated by fracture of the tooth, a root, the maxillary tuberosity, the creation of an oro-antral communication, or the displacement of the tooth into either the antrum or the pterygopalatine fossa.

Unfortunately, intra-oral periapical radiographs are often of limited value in the determination of root shape of maxillary third molars due to the superimposition of bony structures. In these circumstances an extra-oral lateral oblique radiograph is sometimes more helpful (*Fig.* 4.13). Surgical access is improved if the mouth is only opened partially, thus limiting the forward movement of the coronoid process. If a co-operative and conscious patient deviates his jaw towards the side being worked upon, the resulting increase in the room available for

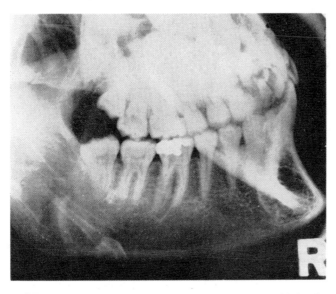

Fig. 4.7. Disto-angular impactions of right upper and lower third molars.

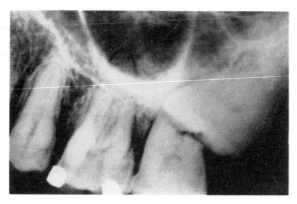

Fig. 4.8. Mesio-angular impaction of maxillary third molar associated with resorption of the roots of the second molar.

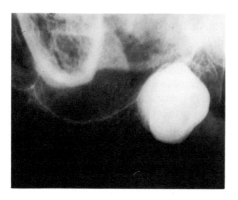

Fig. 4.9. An unerupted maxillary third molar lying transversely in the tuberosity with its occlusal surface on the palatal side and its apex on the buccal side.

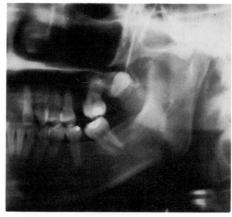

Fig. 4.10. An unerupted inverted maxillary third molar.

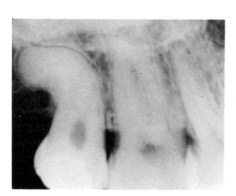

Fig. 4.11. An upper third molar with a fused hooked root.

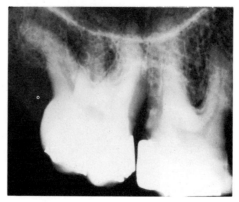

Fig. 4.12. A maxillary third molar with five widely splayed roots.

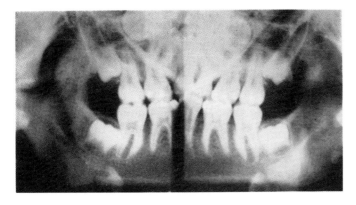

Fig. 4.13. Bilateral mesio-angular impaction of upper and lower third molars.

instrumentation is of great assistance. If a large buccal mucoperiosteal flap is raised access is improved and any oro-antral communication which may occur can be readily repaired. To this end a vertical incision should be made at the level of the mesial surface of the second molar and an incision around the gingival crevice of the second molar extended distally to the buccal side of the hamular process (*Fig.* 4.14*a*). A periosteal elevator is inserted in the vertical incision and the mucoperiosteal flap outlined by this incision is then elevated from the underlying bone in the usual manner, thus affording adequate surgical exposure. If the more widely used incision (*Fig.* 4.14*b*) is employed the bone mesial to the third molar root remains covered by gingiva, whilst the soft-tissue flap is difficult to control and is inadequate for the repair of an oro-antral communication.

In order to minimize the risk of displacing the tooth into the antrum no upwards pressure should be applied to it during bone removal and delivery of the tooth. Buccal and mesial bone may be removed with either a bur or a chisel used with hand pressure applied in either an anteroposterior or palatal and downwards direction (*Fig.* 4.15*c*). The use of a large flap facilitates bone removal and, in those cases in which difficulty is experienced, exposure can be further improved by extending the vertical incision as shown in *Figs.* 4.14*c* and 4.15*a*. The palatal soft tissues should be freed from the distal surface of the neck of the second molar and elevated from the palatal surface of the crown of an unerupted or semi-erupted third molar.

It is important to expose the entire crown of a maxillary third molar prior to attempting to deliver it. The crowns of these teeth are frequently of an abnormal shape which often takes the form of an increase in buccopalatal width due to the presence of an extra cusp situated palatally (*Fig.* 4.16). Unless such a cusp is freed of bone before an attempt is made to elevate the tooth from its socket, fracture of the alveolar bone and tuberosity may occur. When forceps are employed to deliver such a tooth, care must be taken to ensure that the inner blade is applied to the palatal surface of the crown and not to the occlusal surface of such a cusp, if displacement of the tooth into the antrum is to be avoided. In most instances maxillary third molars can be delivered by the application of force distally and downwards by means of an elevator applied to the mesial surface of the tooth at

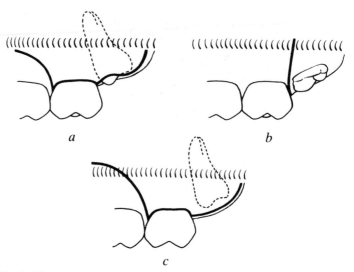

Fig. 4.14. Incisions employed during the removal of maxillary third molars (*see* text for explanation).

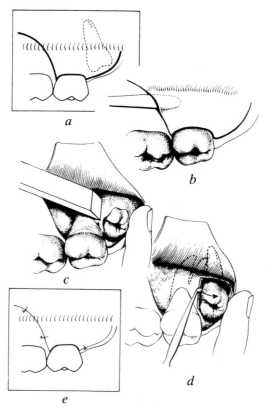

Fig. 4.15. The removal of an unerupted maxillary third molar (*see* text for explanation).

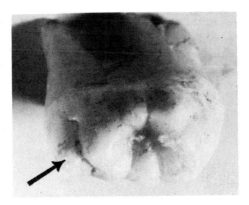

Fig. 4.16. A large extra palatal cusp is commonly present on maxillary third molars and must be exposed before delivery of the tooth is attempted.

the level of its amelocemental junction (*Fig.* 4.15*d*). Some bone removal is usually required to create a point of application, and during bone removal with a chisel and elevation of the tooth from its socket, either a finger or a periosteal elevator should be placed behind the tooth to prevent excessive distal movement towards the pterygo-palatine fossa (*Fig.* 4.15*c, d*).

After delivery of the tooth and the removal of any follicular remnants which may be present the socket margins are smoothed and the soft tissues apposed, care being taken to replace accurately the soft tissues around the neck of the second molar. In most instances a single suture placed in the vertical incision is all that is required, but on occasions this should be supplemented by a suture inserted between the buccal and palatal soft tissues distal to the second molar (*Fig.* 4.15*e*). On the rare occasions when a large oro-antral communication is created, it should be repaired by the use of an undercut buccal flap as described on p. 211.

THE EXTRACTION OF INSTANDING SECOND PREMOLARS

The loss of space in the dental arch which can follow early loss of the deciduous predecessor may result in the second premolar assuming a position lingual to the other standing teeth when it erupts. It is then described as being instanding, and the extraction of such a tooth may be indicated either for caries, orthodontic reasons, or to eliminate an interdental food-trap.

The choice of the method which should be employed to remove an instanding second premolar is governed by the amount of eruption and lingual tilt of the tooth, the root shape and line of withdrawal of the tooth, the presence of tooth impaction (*see* p. 124), and the amount of space between the first premolar and the first permanent molar (*Figs.* 4.17–4.19).

Completely erupted premolars lying lingually to the standing teeth can often be removed with Read pattern forceps applied from the opposite side of the mouth (*Fig.* 4.20). If fine-bladed forceps are used and sufficient space exists between the

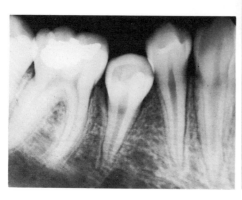

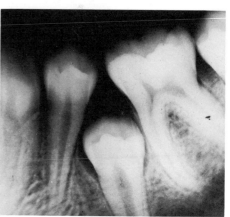

Fig. 4.17. Slightly instanding mandibular second premolar.

Fig. 4.18. Lower second premolar impacted between the first premolar and first molar, which are almost in contact.

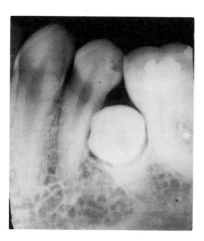

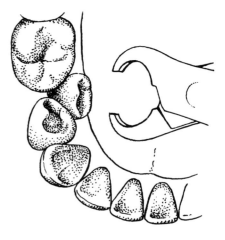

Fig. 4.19. Mandibular second premolar in marked lingual obliquity.

Fig. 4.20. The extraction of an instanding second premolar with Read pattern forceps.

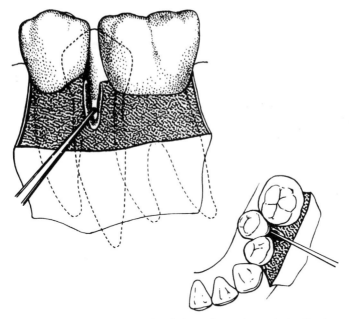

Fig. 4.21. So-called 'broken instrument' technique of removing an instanding lower second premolar.

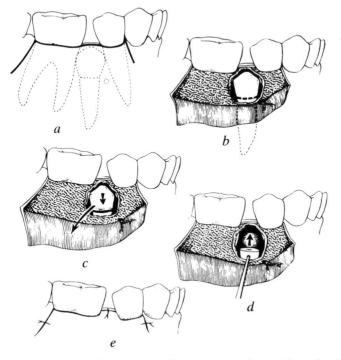

Fig. 4.22. The removal of an impacted lower premolar (*see* text for explanation).

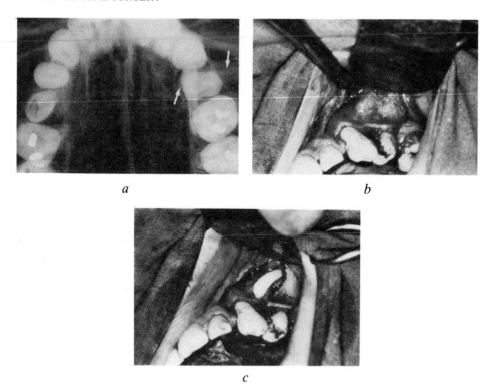

Fig. 4.23. *a*, Occlusal radiograph showing the left first maxillary premolar lying across the arch (arrowed). *b*, The buccal plate is elevated by the root of the tooth. *c*, Root exposed by removal of the overlying bone.

first premolar and first molar the forceps may be applied in the conventional manner, but in other cases it is necessary to grip the mesial and distal surfaces of the tooth. Delivery is effected by a combination of lingual movements and rotation around the long axis of the tooth.

When an instanding premolar is more deeply embedded, a lingual muco-periosteal flap is raised and lingual bone removed to expose the maximum convexity of the crown. A buccal mucoperiosteal flap is then raised and any bone covering the crown removed. If the line of withdrawal of the tooth permits, the tooth is elevated from its socket by the use of either a distal or a buccal application of force. The so-called 'broken instrument' technique is a useful way of applying force to such a tooth from the buccal side. A rosehead bur is used to create a buccal point of application on the premolar root. A fine-bladed elevator, or a suitably modified dental instrument such as one of those employed in conservative dentistry, is applied to this buccal point of application. A few sharp light taps on this instrument suffice to effect delivery of the tooth (*Fig.* 4.21).

If the instanding premolar is tooth-impacted between the first premolar and the first molar, it will be necessary to divide the tooth in order to effect its delivery. The buccal surface of the crown and the cervical portion of the root are widely exposed by removal of bone, care being taken to avoid damage to the mental nerve and the adjacent teeth. A bur is then used to divide the crown of the premolar from its root (*Fig.* 4.22). The separated crown is then moved towards the cut surface of the root and delivered either buccally or lingually. The root is elevated from its socket, the bone edges are smoothed, and the soft tissues repositioned and sutured into place.

The hooked apex of a maxillary premolar lying in marked lingual obliquity is sometimes palpable above the reflection of the mucous membrane in the buccal sulcus. It may be necessary to resect the hooked apex via an 'apicectomy type' window (*see* p. 323) in the bone before the remainder of the tooth can be delivered (*Fig.* 4.23).

THE REMOVAL OF BURIED ROOTS

The mere presence of a buried root should never be regarded as a positive indication that it should be removed. Whilst every endeavour should be made to avoid fracturing roots during tooth extraction, there are times when this mishap occurs despite every care having been taken. In these circumstances the excision of a large amount of alveolar bone to facilitate the removal of a small fragment of the root of a vital tooth is often unjustifiable. Every root which is associated with infection, a cyst or a granuloma should be removed, whilst the extraction of any root which is liable to be exposed as resorption of the alveolar bone progresses is a sensible precaution. As it has been shown that root fragments of vital teeth usually retain their vitality and are not infected, many of those which are less than 5 mm in their greatest diameter and have not been mobilized to such a degree as to prejudice their blood supply can safely be 'put on probation' in otherwise healthy patients. In the rare case in which it is required, removal can be undertaken if and when symptoms supervene.

The dental surgeon should never attempt to remove a root until he has localized it as precisely as is possible. If it is known which root of which tooth is retained, adjacent teeth and/or sockets can often be utilized to determine its position. For this reason the dentist should always make a note in his records of the precise details of any root which he leaves in situ. He should also inform the patient that a root has been left. When retained roots cause symptoms they are usually found to be lying in a superficial position and are often in communication with the oral cavity by means of a sinus. Careful clinical examination may enable the dental surgeon to locate a root. After drying the mucoperiosteum a thorough search should be made for the presence of a sinus either patent or healed. If the sinus is patent and the tip of a probe is passed down it, the characteristic hard surface of a root can often be felt. There can be no more precise or certain way to locate a root. Palpation of edentulous ridges may yield valuable information, especially if related to radiographic findings, but too much reliance should not be placed upon this form of examination for it may prove to be misleading.

In cases of difficulty at least two radiographs should be taken in two planes at right-angles to each other whenever this is practicable (*Fig.* 4.24). Careful examination of the films enables the dental surgeon to assess accurately the relationship between the retained root and adjacent structures, such as erupted teeth or the mental foramen. Localizing plates are often employed in an attempt

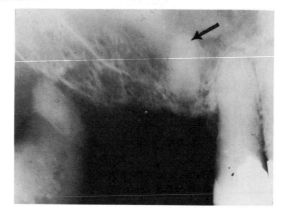

a

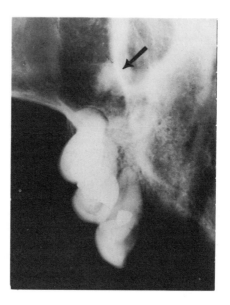

b

Fig. 4.24. A dentist attempted to remove this maxillary root via a buccal flap and opened up the antrum without finding the root. *a*, In the periapical radiograph the apex of the root lies above that of the first premolar suggesting that it was the palatal root of a molar. This impression was confirmed by an occlusal radiograph (*b*) and at operation.

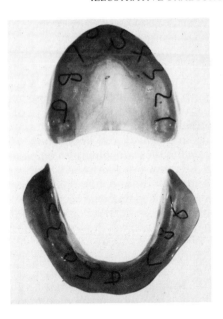

Fig. 4.25. Localizing plates.

to determine the position of buried roots in edentulous jaws. An impression of the jaw is taken and a wax or acrylic resin base-plate containing wire figures constructed (*Fig.* 4.25). Radiographs are then taken with the plate in situ and the position of the roots determined by reference to the radio-opaque shadows made in the film by the wire figures. The technique is time-consuming and its accuracy is entirely dependent upon the positioning of the central beam of X-rays. Ill-founded confidence in the precision of localization by this technique may lead the operator into the error of creating inadequate surgical exposure. A hole is made in the base-plate over the estimated position of the root. The plate is then inserted prior to surgery and the gum pricked via the hole to mark the estimated site of the root. Once the soft tissues have been reflected it is very difficult to use the localizing plate again. Most experienced oral surgeons have abandoned the use of localizing plates and employ a method similar to that described below.

After the position of the buried root has been estimated by means of clinical and radiographic examination, large mucoperiosteal flaps are raised, thus ensuring good exposure of the underlying bone. The exposed alveolar bone is dried and a careful search is made for the presence of either a root or a bony defect related to the root. Roots usually have a greenish-yellow tinge in relationship to the bone surrounding them and are easily seen in the vast majority of cases undertaken by non-specialist dental surgeons. On the rare occasions when the root is not obvious, acriflavine solution should be applied to the alveolar bone. The bone, being porous, takes up the orange stain whilst the non-stained root becomes more obvious against the darker background. The test is not specific, for sclerotic areas of bone also fail to take up the dye. Every dental surgeon is familiar with the characteristic feel of dental tissues when a sharp probe is passed over their surface, and such an examination of a suspected root may resolve the difficulty.

Only rarely do these measures fail and in these circumstances two radiographs should be taken in planes at right-angles to each other using radio-opaque markers. Straight and bent pins or thin wire may be stuck into the anaesthetized gum and used for this purpose. It is safer to use suture needles threaded with silk as markers provided that the silk is knotted in the eye of the needle and that the free end of the silk is brought out of the mouth. Soft wire can be moulded to the mucosa and held firmly in place by the application of an intra-oral adhesive bandage. More refined techniques which may be employed include the insertion into the soft tissues of the radio-opaque thread removed from 'raytec' surgical swabs or marking the gum with radio-opaque paint composed of silver-tin alloy mixed with copal varnish. This paint can be removed by the application of chloroform when the purpose for which it was applied has been fulfilled. If the radiographs are examined whilst still wet these techniques take only a few minutes to perform.

In most cases no difficulty is experienced in locating roots provided that careful preoperative clinical and radiographic examination is followed by adequate surgical exposure, and the technique employed may be illustrated by the removal of some completely buried mandibular premolar roots from an otherwise edentulous jaw. The dental surgeon's main problem when operating on such a case is locating the roots, whilst the possible complications which may occur are damage to the mental nerve and the creation of prosthetic difficulties due to loss of sulcus depth or ridge height or both. In the absence of a sinus the relationship between the roots and the mental foramen is noted in the radiograph. When the premolar region is palpated in most thin and atrophic mandibles the thickened and superficial mental nerve can be rolled under the examining finger-tip. If it can be felt, the position of the mental nerve should be noted and marked upon the overlying soft tissues.

After anaesthesia has been secured a long incision, down to bone, is made along the crest of the ridge from the molar to the lateral incisor region. The incision should be curved slightly lingually in the premolar region in order to minimize the danger of damage to the mental nerve (*Fig.* 4.26*a*). A vertical incision, down to bone, is made at the anterior end of the anteroposterior incision. Elevation of the mucoperiosteal flap thus outlined from the bone should be started well behind and well in front of the site of the nerve (*Fig.* 4.26*a*). Blunt subperiosteal dissection enables the nerve to be identified and preserved intact. A metal retractor should be used to protect the nerve whenever a bur is used to remove bone related to it (*Fig.* 4.26*b*, *c*). When removing bone in this manner to expose premolar roots the risk of damage to the nerve is minimized if the maximal removal is at the expense of the mesial bone when dealing with first premolar roots, and distal bone when second premolar roots are being removed. Whenever possible bone should be removed from the buccal aspect in such a way as to preserve ridge form. The root is then delivered by means of an elevator applied buccally to it and the wound closed with black silk sutures after removal of any debris or pathological tissue and smoothing of bone edges (*Fig.* 4.26*d*, *e*).

The removal of deeply embedded teeth and roots from thin atrophic mandibles should only be undertaken by very experienced operators working under optimum conditions, for these procedures may tax the skill of the oral surgeon to the full.

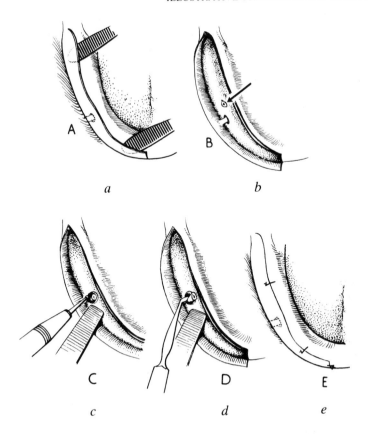

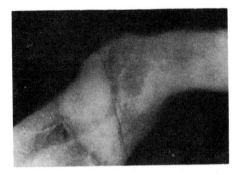

Fig. 4.26. The removal of a buried premolar root from an otherwise edentulous mandible (*see* text for explanation).

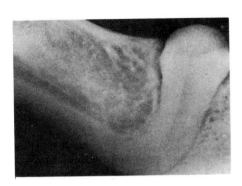

Fig. 4.27. Unerupted second premolar with unfavourable root pattern in an edentulous mandible.

Fig. 4.28. This mandibular second premolar root is grooved by the inferior dental nerve and lies close to the mental foramen.

The difficulties are not only local problems such as localization of the tooth or root and ankylosis, but also the fact that as many of these patients are elderly they do not stand prolonged surgical procedures well, and they have friable tissues which heal only slowly. Grooving of the roots of such teeth by the neurovascular bundle is not unusual (*Fig.* 4.28). In addition to the danger of damage to the inferior dental and mental nerves occurring, there is also the risk of the jaw fracturing either during or after surgery. For these reasons the dental surgeon is advised to refer any patient presenting with teeth or roots such as those shown in *Figs.* 3.28, 4.27, and 4.28 to a specialist for treatment (*see* Chapter 16).

SUGGESTED READING

Dachi S. F. and Howell F. C. (1961) Survey of 3874 routine full mouth radiographs. *Oral Surg.* **14**, 916–24, 1165–9.

Helsham R. W. (1960) Some observations on the subject of roots of teeth retained in the jaws as a result of incomplete exodontia. *Aust. Dent. J.* **5**, 70–7.

Howe G. L. (1960) The use of pre-extraction radiographs in the management of difficult extractions. *Dent. Prac.* **10**, 196–201.

Moore J. R. and Gillbe G. V. (1968) Removal of roots. *Br. Dent. J.* **125**, 272–4, 310–11.

Moore J. R. and Gillbe G. V. (1969) Unerupted mandibular premolars. *Br. Dent. J.* **126**, 33–5.

Chapter 5

The management of impacted mandibular third molars

Many members of most civilized races exhibit a disproportion between jaw size and tooth size in that they possess jaws which are too small to accommodate their teeth. The third molar is the last tooth to erupt and so it may readily become either impacted or displaced if there is insufficient room for it within the dental arch. The frequency of this occurrence is illustrated by one study which revealed that 65·6% of males with an average age of 19½ years had 1–4 embedded third molars equally divided between the four quadrants of the dental arches. Thus the removal of impacted mandibular third molars is one of the most important and most frequently performed oral surgical procedures. In most instances these patients are first seen by the general dental practitioner who is called upon to decide whether removal of the tooth is indicated.

INDICATIONS AND CONTRA-INDICATIONS TO REMOVAL

Many factors govern the decision to advise the extraction of an impacted mandibular third molar, some of which are related to the general condition of the patient and have been discussed in Chapter 2. *Table* 5.1 records the indications for

Table 5.1. Reasons for the Extraction of Wisdom Teeth

Reason for extraction	Number of teeth	Percentage of total number of teeth
Recurrent pericoronitis	790	58·5
Symptomless*	204	15·06
Caries		
With pain	118	8·71
Without pain	80	5·91
Periodontal disease		
(including acute ulcerative gingivitis)	41	3·02
Obscure facial pain	34	2·51
Attempted extraction elsewhere	34	2·51
Exposed under denture	22	1·62
Orthodontic reasons	15	1·11
Apical abscesses	9	0·67
Cysts	8	0·6
Total	1355	100

* Includes 118 teeth extracted because they were present when a general anaesthetic was administered for the removal of the opposite mandibular third molar which had given symptoms.

which teeth were removed in a personal series of 1355 consecutive unselected extractions.

Recurrent pericoronitis

Even cursory examination of *Table* 5.1 will suffice to reveal that recurrent pericoronitis is the commonest indication for the removal of impacted mandibular third molars. Paradoxically it is also the commonest contra-indication to surgery, for the extraction must be deferred until the acute inflammation is controlled if a predominantly soft-tissue infection is not to be converted into a bony infection. This important subject is discussed in detail elsewhere in this book (*see* p. 238).

Although bilateral *concurrent* pericoronitis is so rare a clinical entity as to be an indication for the dental surgeon to review his diagnosis, pericoronitis commonly affects bilateral impacted lower third molars at different times. This finding is so common as to make it sound practice to advise the removal of an uninfected contralateral tooth when an impacted mandibular third molar, which has been the site of pericoronitis, is to be removed.

Caries

The impaction of a partially erupted third molar often causes a food-trap which the patient finds impossible to keep clean. The resulting retention of food debris and plaque is first accompanied by an unpleasant taste and odour, but sooner or later caries occurs in either the occlusal surface of the third molar or the adjacent distal surface of the second molar or in both teeth (*Figs*. 5.1, 5.9, 5.19). It may prove impossible to conserve the second molar until the impacted third molar has been removed. In these circumstances the caries should be excavated and a temporary dressing inserted prior to the removal of the third molar. This not only facilitates the extraction of the impacted third molar but enables the dental

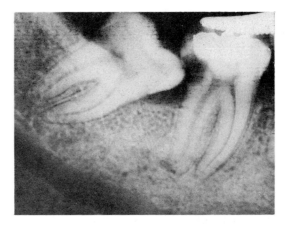

Fig. 5.1. Mesio-angular impaction of lower third molar which has early caries in the crown. The second molar is grossly carious and periapical rarefaction is present.

surgeon to ensure that all caries has been eliminated and the desired cavity form obtained prior to the insertion of the permanent filling.

When the third molar is carious it is sometimes possible to temporize by removing the caries and inserting either a dressing or a permanent restoration. However, caries recurs unless the food-trap is eliminated and if left untreated it may proceed to pulpal exposure and abscess formation. An apically abscessed impacted mandibular third molar should be removed under endotracheal anaesthesia and antibiotic cover if circumstances permit, but in many cases the general condition of the patient, the degree of trismus, and the presence of submaxillary cellulitis make the systemic administration of antibiotics and the institution of surgical drainage the primary treatment (*see* p. 235). The extraction of the diseased tooth is then deferred until the inflammation is controlled.

Periodontal disease

Impaction of the lower third molars is associated with a high incidence of periodontal pocketing distal to the second molar. This incidence increases following surgical removal of the impacted tooth regardless of the technique employed. Pocketing of the gum around a partially erupted and impacted mandibular third molar may be the site upon which relapses are centred following the treatment of periodontal disease. The removal of the tooth is often the only effective way of eliminating the pocketing in such circumstances. This is especially important during the 'cleaning up' phase of treatment for acute ulcerative gingivitis if the insidious progress of the disease is to be halted. Unless all such catchment areas are effectively dealt with the disease persists in its subacute and chronic phases until the teeth are finally lost (*see Fig*. 9.14). Extraction of the tooth in the presence of any acute gingival inflammation will produce at the least an infected tooth socket and at the most acute osteomyelitis of the mandible. It is thus obvious that the acute phase of any periodontal infection must be effectively treated before any dental extractions are undertaken.

It is good practice to remove all impacted or potentially impacted third molars as early in their development as possible utilizing the technique of lateral trepanation (*see* pp. 140–3) thus preserving the periodontal tissues distal to the second molar in a healthy state.

Obscure facial pain

Completely embedded or partially erupted mandibular third molars are not uncommonly detected and are often incriminated during a search for the cause of an obscure facial pain. In the absence of detectable pathology it is wise to adopt a conservative approach, although in practice the dental surgeon can often only guarantee that such a tooth is not the cause of pain by eliminating it. The patient should be given a guarded prognosis, with regard to relief of the pain, before an extraction is peformed in these circumstances.

Previous attempted extraction

If a previous unsuccessful attempt has been made to extract an impacted mandibular third molar a thorough preoperative investigation into the causes of failure is indicated. The particular causes of the difficulty should be diagnosed and a plan of campaign designed to deal with them formulated and implemented (*see* p. 52).

Prosthetic considerations

These may influence the management of the impacted mandibular third molar. Before undertaking a dental clearance it is a wise precaution to radiograph all 'edentulous' areas, especially the canine, premolar, and third molar regions, unless the operator has good reason to be certain that no buried teeth or retained roots are present in these sites. Sometimes it is sound judgement to leave a deeply embedded tooth in situ unless symptoms supervene. Many prosthetists claim that it is essential to leave buried maxillary third molars to erupt, when young patients have a dental clearance performed, if the maxillary tuberosity is to be retained. Whilst, in some circumstances, it is sound practice to leave buried teeth and roots in the jaws 'on probation', it is bad practice to retain them because a defect in diagnosis has failed to reveal their presence.

As resorption of the mandible progresses some retained teeth become more superficial and may either interfere with the fit of a full lower denture or cause pain due to either caries or a gum infection (*see Figs*. 5.2 and 9.24). These teeth should be removed as soon as the gingival inflammation has been effectively treated.

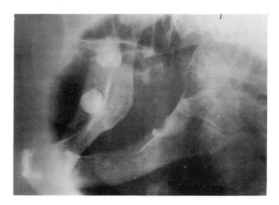

Fig. 5.2. Lateral oblique radiograph of mandible showing carious embedded mandibular third molar. N.B. The radiographic superimposition of an intervertebral space simulates the appearance of a fracture of the angle of the mandible.

Orthodontic reasons

Orthodontists are divided in their opinions concerning the value of prophylactic removal of mandibular third molar tooth germs in children in whom there is a marked disproportion between the tooth size and the jaw size. As long ago as 1934 Bowdler Henry described an operation for the enucleation of third molar germs at an early age when they were still superficial, together with the use of an elaborate system of measurements taken from radiographs to decide whether the operation was indicated.

The enucleation of tooth germs which is quick, simple and atraumatic, if peformed before the calcified cusps have united, has never enjoyed widespread favour, for many dentists have reservations about committing a patient to the loss of third molars during the early mixed dentition stage when there is still an appreciable amount of growth to occur, and there is a risk that other teeth in the quadrant may be lost either due to caries or for other reasons.

More recently the development of computer-based and other predictions of growth has rekindled interest in the removal of mandibular third molars at an early age. However, controversy still rages over the efficiency and accuracy of growth prediction. A consensus conference on the subject held in 1980 concluded that whilst there are cogent orthodontic reasons for early removal of third molars the group thought that the suggested practice of enucleation of third molar buds, based on predictive studies at age 7–9 years, is not currently acceptable. However, it was agreed that postoperative pain, swelling, infection and other possible consequences of surgery are minimized in patients in whom the third molar roots are approximately two-thirds developed at the time of surgery.

In 1969 Bowdler Henry described a method of removing the lower third molars at a later stage of development when the formation of the crown is completed. At this stage there is a much better chance of assessing correctly the potential for impaction and both the orthodontic and caries status of the patient are more clearly defined. This operation is known as lateral trepanation and it has been utilized to remove unerupted lower third molars in which as much as one-third of the roots have been formed, but the hard and soft tissues overlying the tooth were still intact. The operation is undertaken earlier than the conventional surgical approach and before the third molar can have an deleterious effects on either the periodontal condition of the second molar or on crowding in the lower arch. It thus affords the dentist the opportunity to make the decision whether or not to remove an unerupted third molar as late as 16 years of age combined with the advantages of performing such surgery on the dentally young patient. The technique is described on p. 140.

Some orthodontists believe that imbrication of the lower incisors may be produced by the ineffectual attempts of impacted mandibular third molars to erupt. Whether these teeth do produce imbrication or not, clinical experience reveals that whilst the removal of the impacted molars may prevent the imbrication becoming more severe, it is not followed by realinement of the incisors in most cases.

The presence of a pathological lesion

If an impacted third molar is related to a *pathological lesion* this relationship may be either an indication or a contra-indication to extraction. If the tooth is related to a *cyst* or is in a *fracture line*, it is usually better removed. If, however, an impacted tooth situated in the line of fracture is preventing the displacement of the bony fragments, it may be wiser to leave it in situ at least until some callus has formed.

If the tooth is related to a *malignant lesion* which is to receive therapeutic irradiation, its removal is usually indicated, whilst if the tooth is situated in a bone which has been irradiated it is usually best left alone, unless symptoms supervene, because of the risk of osteoradionecrosis complicating the extraction. When such an extraction becomes necessary it should be performed with minimal trauma to the investing tissues under general anaesthesia and antibiotic cover (*see* p. 37).

The removal of an impacted lower third molar is sometimes required before a physician can be given an assurance that no *oral focus of sepsis* exists (*see* p. 329). If the impaction causes a food-trap, halitosis may result which can be remedied only by the elimination of both the tooth and the associated food-trap.

Social and economic factors

These may influence the management of an impacted mandibular third molar. Patients with busy, full lives may wish either to defer the extraction or have a symptomless tooth removed at a particular time in order to minimize the inconvenience. Others, due to travel to areas devoid of hospital or other facilities, may request extraction as a prophylactic measure.

It is usual to avoid undertaking oral surgery at the extremes of age and the vast majority of impacted mandibular third molars are removed from patients aged between 15 and 35 years.

PREOPERATIVE ASSESSMENT OF THE IMPACTED MANDIBULAR THIRD MOLAR

After deciding that the removal of an impacted mandibular third molar is indicated the dental surgeon must next determine whether he ought to extract the tooth himself or refer the patient to a colleague specializing in oral surgery. This decision should be based upon a thorough assessment of the difficulties which would be encountered and the possible complications which might occur during the removal of the tooth. Unless the dentist can prepare an operation plan which is designed to deal with such difficulties and avoid possible complications, and is certain that he possesses both the necessary skill and the facilities to complete the operation successfully, he should refer the patient to a colleague for treatment. The degree of difficulty experienced during the removal of an impacted lower third molar may be influenced by both general and local factors. The patient's age, temperament, or general medical condition may cause problems and these are noted during history-taking and clinical examination and have been discussed in Chapter 2.

If the patient has a small mouth, or a mandibular retrusion, the opening is limited and access to the operation site is poor. These conditions make the extraction more difficult to perform, especially when the movement at the temporo-mandibular joint is mainly of the 'hinge' variety. If the patient has a large mouth, or a mandibular protrusion, the access to the third molar region is good and this facilitates the extraction, especially if the head of the condyle glides freely over the articular eminence when the mouth is opened. During clinical examination access may be assessed by palpating the external oblique ridge with the finger-tip and noting its relationship to the third molar. When the ridge is situated behind the tooth access is good, whilst if the ridge is either alongside or in front of the third molar access is poor and the extraction more difficult.

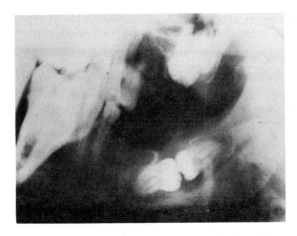

Fig. 5.3. Lateral oblique radiograph of mandible showing horizontal impaction of second and third permanent molars.

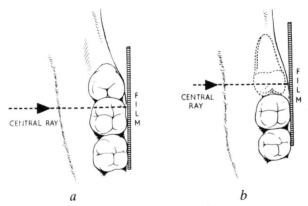

a   *b*

Fig. 5.4. Position of film packet and angulation of central ray seen from above. *a*, Average case. *b*, In the presence of a horizontal impaction.

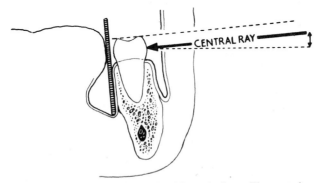

Fig. 5.5. Angulation of central ray when viewed from the front. The central ray is parallel with the transverse occlusal plane which is usually at an angle of 3 to 4 degrees above the horizontal plane (lower dotted line).

Most of the local factors causing difficulty may be diagnosed by the careful interpretation of a preoperative radiograph. It is not possible to plan the removal of an impacted mandibular third molar unless an accurate radiograph showing the whole tooth and its investing structures is available. Extra-oral lateral oblique views of the mandible may indicate the amount of bone which exists below a buried tooth in a thin mandible, but the inevitable distortion, introduced by the need to rotate the opposite side of the mandible out of the path of the central ray during exposure of the film, renders these films of limited value in the diagnosis of local factors causing difficulty (*Fig.* 5.3). Despite this limitation they should be used if it proves impossible due to retching or some other cause, to include the entire area to be examined on an intra-oral radiograph. An orthopantomogram is useful in such circumstances. A standard accurate intra-oral periapical radiograph is the most suitable film for use during preoperative assessment and such a film may be taken by any general dental practitioner who takes the trouble to master the following technique.

The patient is seated in such a position that the occlusal plane of his mandibular teeth is horizontal and parallel to the floor when his mouth is open. In most patients the upper anterior corner of the film packet is gripped with either a Worth film holder or a pair of straight 'mosquito' haemostats and then inserted on the lingual side of the mandibular teeth, with its anterior edge in line with the mesial surface of the first permanent mandibular molar (*Fig.* 5.4*a*). In those cases in which clinical examination has revealed the mandibular third molar to be horizontally impacted, the film packet should be inserted more posteriorly so that the root apices can be examined (*Fig.* 5.4*b*). The X-ray tube is then positioned so that the central ray will be parallel to the occlusal surface of the second molar (*Fig.* 5.5), and pass through the distal cusps of the second molar at right-angles to the film packet (*Fig.* 5.4). If the central ray is correctly angled, a radiograph is obtained in which the lingual and buccal cusps of the second molar are superimposed upon one another in the same vertical and horizontal plane.

Fig. 5.6 shows a standard accurate intra-oral periapical film in which the angulation of the rays has been correct and a typical 'enamel cap' appearance of

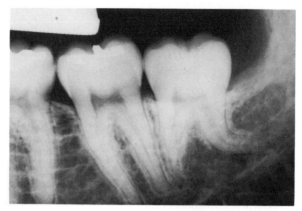

Fig. 5.6. Standard periapical radiograph. Note the unfavourable root pattern of the lower third molar.

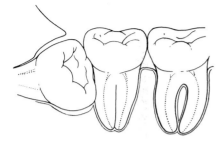

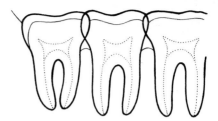

Fig. 5.7. The enamel cap of the second molar is absent when the central ray is not parallel to the transverse occlusal plane (*see Fig.* 5.5).

Fig. 5.8. If the central ray does not pass at right-angles to the film packet in the horizontal plane, overlapping of the contact points is seen (*see Fig.* 5.4).

the second molar is seen. *Figs.* 5.7 and 5.8 are drawings of poor films in which an incorrect angulation has been employed. The radiographic appearances of the second lower molar are used to determine whether an intra-oral film is suitable for use during the critical analysis of the local factors causing difficulty during the removal of an impacted mandibular third molar. If an undistorted view of the second mandibular molar is present and is surmounted by an 'enamel cap' the film may be used with confidence (*see Figs.* 5.1, 5.6, 5.11, 5.20, 5.31). Care must be taken to ensure that any lingual tilt or rotation of the second molar which may be present is noted during clinical examination, for such a finding may influence both the positioning of the tube and the interpretation of the radiograph (*see Fig.* 5.33).

Interpretation of the standardized intra-oral radiograph
When the technique described is employed, the resulting periapical radiograph may be used in the diagnosis of most of the local factors causing difficulty during removal of an impacted mandibular third molar.

Access
Ease of access to the site of operation may be determined by noting the inclination of the radio-opaque line cast by the external oblique ridge. If this line is vertical access is poor (*see Figs.* 5.10, 5.12, 5.18), whilst if it is horizontal access is excellent (*see Figs.* 5.1, 5.14, 5.20, 5.31).

Position and depth
The position and depth of the impacted tooth within the mandible are determined by means of a method first described by George Winter, in which three imaginary lines are drawn on the standard radiograph. In order to facilitate discussion these imaginary lines are given distinctive colours and are described as the 'white', 'amber', and 'red' lines respectively.

In most instances the long axis of the impacted tooth is seen in the radiograph to be either horizontal, vertical, or mesially or distally inclined, and so these

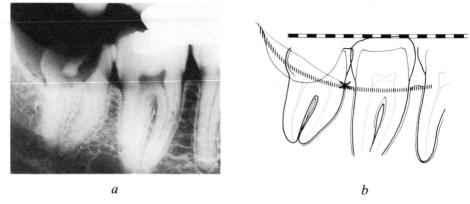

Fig. 5.9. *a*, Radiograph of carious vertically impacted mandibular third molar. *b*, Tracing of the radiograph (*see Fig.* 5.10*b*).

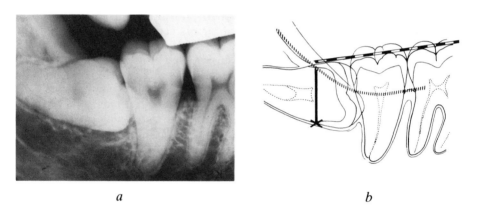

Fig. 5.10. A horizontally impacted mandibular third molar. *a*, Radiograph. *b*, Tracing on which the 'white' line (chequered), the 'amber' line (cross-hatched), and the 'red' line (heavy black) have been drawn. Note that the posterior end of the 'amber' line is drawn on the shadow cast by the bone in the retromolar fossa and not that cast by the external oblique ridge which lies above and in front of it.

impactions are described as being vertical, horizontal, mesio-angular or disto-angular impactions respectively (*Figs.* 5.9–5.12). One of the most serious errors made by dental surgeons undertaking the removal of impacted lower third molars is to misdiagnose a disto-angular impaction as a vertical impaction. The path of withdrawal of a disto-angularly impacted tooth inclines distally and it is essential to ensure that space exists, or is created, into which the tooth may be displaced before elevation is commenced.

Many vertical impactions can be delivered by the use of a straight elevator applied to the mesial surface of the tooth, but if this technique is employed to deliver a disto-angular impaction the tooth engages on the bone lying distal to it. A further application of force applied in these circumstances may fracture the

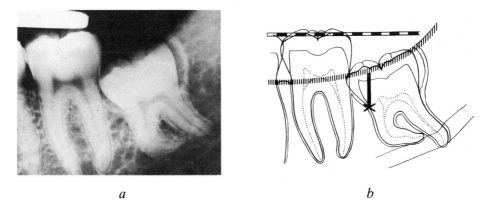

Fig. 5.11. *a*, Radiograph and, *b*, tracing of a mesio-angularly impacted mandibular third molar.

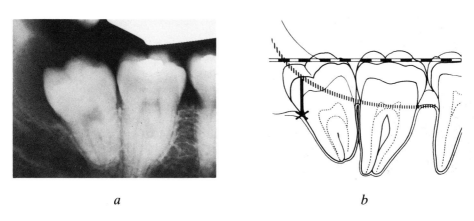

Fig. 5.12. *a*, Radiograph and, *b*, tracing of a disto-angularly impacted mandibular third molar.

mandible (*Fig*. 5.13). This error may be avoided by careful interpretation of the standard radiograph. When a vertical impaction is present the anteroposterior width of the interdental septum between the second and third molars is similar to that of the septum between the first and second molars (*see Figs*. 5.9, 5.23). If, however, a disto-angular impaction is present, the interdental septum between the second and third molars is much narrower than that between the first and second molars (*see Figs*. 5.12, 5.17, 5.32).

When the first or 'white' line of Winter is drawn along the occlusal surfaces of the erupted mandibular molars and extended posteriorly over the third molar region, the axial inclination of the impacted tooth is immediately apparent. The occlusal surface of a vertically impacted tooth is seen to be parallel to the 'white'

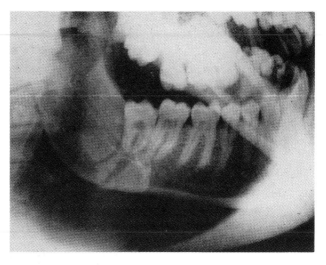

Fig. 5.13.   Fracture of the mandible complicating the extraction of an impacted third molar.

line (*see Figs.* 5.9, 5.23), whilst when a disto-angular impaction is present the occlusal surface of the tooth and the 'white' line are seen to converge as if to meet in front of the third molar (*see Figs.* 5.12, 5.17).

The relationship of the occlusal surface of the impacted tooth to those of the erupted molars may also be estimated by the use of the 'white' line and this provides an indication of the depth at which the tooth is lying in the mandible.

The second imaginary line, called for convenience the 'amber' line, is drawn from the surface of the bone lying distally to the third molar to the crest of the interdental septum between the first and second mandibular molars (*see Fig.* 5.10). When drawing this line it is essential to differentiate between the shadow cast by the external oblique ridge and that cast by the bone lying distal to the tooth, if errors are to be avoided. The 'amber' line indicates the margin of the alveolar bone enclosing the tooth and so when the soft tissues are reflected, only that portion of the tooth shown on the film to be lying above and in front of the 'amber' line will be visible, for the remainder of the tooth will be enclosed within the alveolar bone.

The third or 'red' line is used to measure the depth at which the impacted tooth lies within the mandible. It is a perpendicular dropped from the 'amber' line to an imaginary 'point of application' for an elevator. With the solitary exception of disto-angular impactions (*see below*), the amelocemental junction on the mesial surface of the impacted tooth is used for this purpose. The more deeply embedded the tooth, the longer the 'red' line and the more difficult the extraction is to perform. Clinical experience reveals that every time that the length of the 'red' line increases by 1 mm, the extraction becomes about three times more difficult to complete, even if factors other than depth alone are ignored.

As a general rule, any tooth with a 'red' line 5 mm or more in length is better removed under an endotracheal anaesthetic. If the 'red' line is 9 mm or more in length the inferior surface of the crown of the impacted third molar may be either

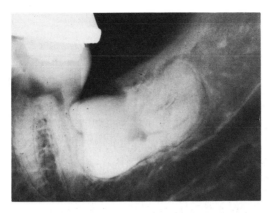

Fig. 5.14. Deeply embedded horizontally impacted mandibular third molar.

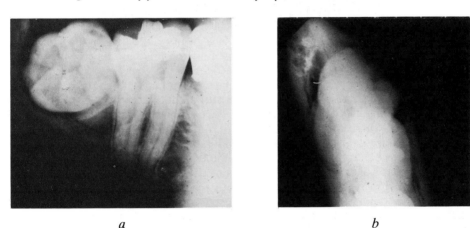

a   *b*

Fig. 5.15. *a*, Periapical and, *b*, occlusal radiographs of tooth lying in marked lingual obliquity.

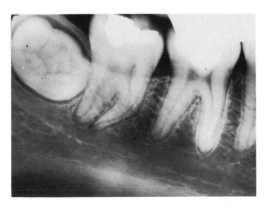

Fig. 5.16. 'Bull's-eye' appearance seen in periapical film when tooth is lying in complete lingual obliquity.

level with or even below the apex of the second molar. In such a case the dental surgeon must estimate the amount of bone which will be left distal to the second molar after the third molar has been extracted. If care is taken at operation to preserve the bone and soft tissue lying distal to the second molar in good condition, a considerable amount of bone regeneration occurs after operation. Nevertheless, if it appears likely that the distal surface of the root of the second molar will be denuded of bone, it is better to remove the second molar at the time the third molar is extracted rather than to be compelled to do so a few weeks or months later, either by persistent pain or abnormal mobility of the tooth (*Figs.* 5.14, 5.21, 9.21).

When estimating the depth of *disto-angular* impactions the perpendicular 'red' line must be dropped to the amelocemental junction on the distal surface of the buried tooth. Examination of *Figs.* 5.12 and 5.32 will reveal that the use of the amelocemental junction on the mesial surface of a disto-angularly impacted tooth for this purpose would give a grossly misleading estimation of depth. As a general rule a disto-angularly impacted tooth is always a little more difficult to remove than a mesio-angular impaction of similar depth and root pattern.

If in the standard film the third molar is seen in profile and an 'enamel cap' surmounts its crown, then the long axis of that tooth is parallel to the antero-posterior axis of the erupted teeth in the dental arch (*see Figs.* 5.1, 5.11). If, however, the occlusal surface of the tooth faces the tongue, the tooth is said to lie in *lingual obliquity*, whilst if the occlusal surface faces the cheek the tooth is described as being in *buccal obliquity*. Lingual obliquity increases the difficulty of extraction whilst buccal obliquity reduces it. Unfortunately, the vast majority of impacted mandibular third molars which exhibit obliquity lie in lingual obliquity. It is often possible to distinguish between the two types of obliquity by using the standard periapical radiograph, thus avoiding the need to take an occlusal radiograph (*Fig.* 5.15a). The portion of the tooth nearest to the film packet is always more sharply defined and more radio-opaque and so if, after allowing for the difference in density between enamel and cementum, the crown of the buried tooth is seen to be sharply defined and radio-opaque, that tooth is lying in lingual obliquity (*Fig.* 5.16), whilst if the apices are the more sharply defined portion of the tooth, that tooth is lying in buccal obliquity.

Root pattern of an impacted mandibular third molar

This may affect both the 'line of withdrawal' of the tooth and the decision concerning which 'point of application' would be appropriate when an elevator is selected to deliver the tooth. The radiograph should be carefully examined in a good light so that the number and shape of the roots may be determined and the presence of hypercementosis detected (*Figs.* 5.17–5.19, 5.23). The use of a hand lens may greatly assist the detection of small ancillary roots, especially when they are inclined in either a buccal or lingual direction. When the apical portion of a root takes a sharp bend in the direction of the X-ray beam, the root often appears to have a blunt rounded end in radiographs, and such an appearance should always be regarded as an indication for further meticulous examination of the film. The presence of roots with conflicting lines of withdrawal may indicate the need for tooth division (*see Fig.* 5.18).

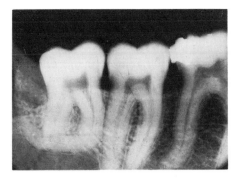 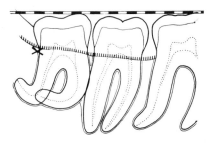

Fig. 5.17. This disto-angularly impacted mandibular third molar has hooked roots.

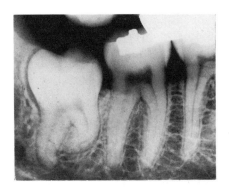 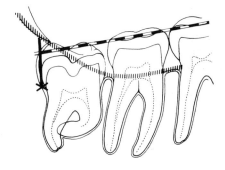

Fig. 5.18. The roots of this tooth have conflicting lines of withdrawal.

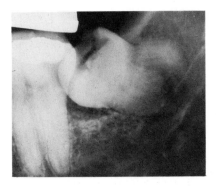 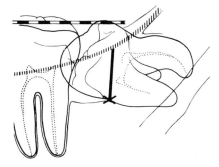

Fig. 5.19. 'Tooth impaction' of three-rooted mesio-angularly impacted mandibular third molar.

Shape of crown

Although the shape of the crown of an impacted lower third molar is seldom a major cause of difficulty during its removal, teeth with large square crowns and prominent cusps (*see Figs.* 5.14, 5.31) are more difficult to remove than teeth with small conical crowns and flat cusps (*Fig.* 5.20). Crown and cusp shape are of especial importance when the 'line of withdrawal' of the third molar is completely obstructed by the presence of a part of the second molar, a condition known as *'tooth impaction'*. When 'tooth impaction' is present the cusps of the third molars are superimposed upon the distal surface of the second molar in the standard intra-oral radiograph (*see Figs.* 5.10, 5.14, 5.19, 5.20). In these circumstances the application of force to the mesial surface of the impacted tooth will either cause damage to the supporting structures of the second molar or even displace the tooth from its socket. This mishap is most likely to occur when the second lower molar has a single conically shaped root and especially so if the first molar has been lost (*see Fig.* 5.10). This complication can be avoided by sectioning the impacted tooth with either a bur or an osteotome. Whichever method of tooth division is employed it inevitably prolongs the operating time.

On rare occasions resorption of the root of the second molar may be related to the impaction of a mandibular third molar (*Figs.* 5.21, 5.22). This rare complication can be distinguished from the more frequently occurring 'tooth impaction' by the presence of a break in the continuity of the shadow cast by the distal surface of the second molar root in the standard radiograph (compare *Fig.* 5.20 with *Fig.* 5.21).

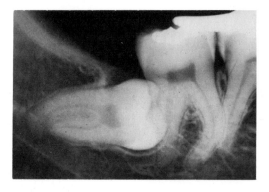

Fig. 5.20. In this case the distal inclination of the mandibular second molar increases the degree of 'tooth impaction' of the third molar.

Texture of the investing bone

This varies between individuals, and with age and site in the same individual. Bone tends to become more sclerosed and less elastic as age advances. The texture of the bone can be accurately determined by radiography only if rigid standardization of exposure and developing technique is practised. In most instances this is not practicable and so it is fortunate that some indication of the texture of the bone can be gained by noting the size of the cancellous spaces and the density of the bone structure enclosing them in the standard film. Thus, if the spaces are large

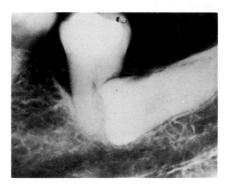

Fig. 5.21. Resorption of the distal root of a lower second molar related to a horizontally impacted third molar.

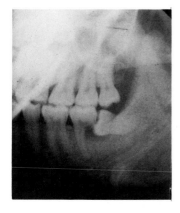

a

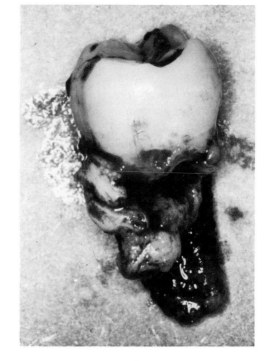

Fig. 5.22. Complete resorption of the distal root of a second molar. *a*, Radiograph. *b*, Surgical specimen.

b

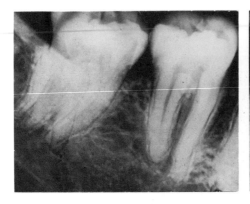

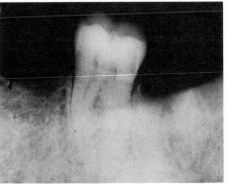

Fig. 5.23. Fully erupted four-rooted lower third molar in a young patient. The blurred shadow of the pulp chamber is due to rotation of the tooth around its long axis. The second molar has three roots.

Fig. 5.24. Retained hypercementosed roots of lower third molar surrounded by dense sclerotic bone.

and the bone structure fine, the bone is usually elastic (*Figs*. 5.10, 5.12, 5.23), whilst if the spaces are small and the bone shadow dense, the bone is sclerotic (*Figs*. 5.1, 5.24).

Position and root pattern of the second molar

Both of these may create difficulty in the extraction of an impacted mandibular third molar. Thus a distal tilt of the long axis of the second molar may either create or increase 'tooth impaction' of the buried tooth (*see Fig*. 5.20).

If the second molar has a simple conical root it may be dislodged very easily during removal of the third molar by the use of an elevator applied to its mesial surface, even in the absence of tooth impaction. As has been mentioned already, this complication is more likely to occur if the first molar is missing from the arch.

Inferior dental canal

This is often seen to be crossing the roots of the mandibular third molar in the standard film. In most instances this appearance is due to radiographic super-imposition, but on occasions either grooving or even perforation of the root of the third molar is present. It is possible to distinguish between these two states in the standard film by noting whether certain signs are present or not (*Fig*. 5.25). A band of decreased radio-opacity crossing the roots and coinciding with the outline of the inferior dental canal indicates that the tooth root is grooved by the inferior dental canal and its contents. This sign is probably due to the decreased amount of tooth substance between the source of X-rays and the film at the level of the groove.

The condensed bone forming the roof and floor of the canal is represented on the radiograph by parallel lines of radio-opacity (*Fig*. 5.25). Interruption of the continuity of one or both of these lines of radio-opacity as they cross the tooth root

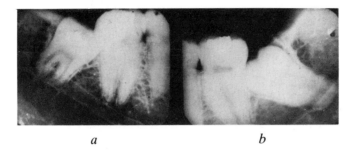

a   *b*

Fig. 5.25. *a*, Radiographic superimposition. *b*, Radiograph of tooth in 'true relationship'.

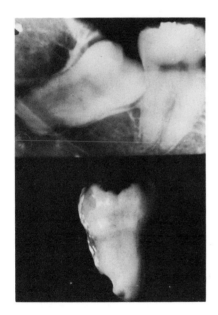

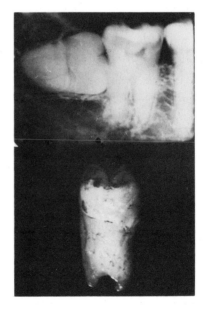

Fig. 5.26. Radiograph and specimen of tooth with 'grooved root'.

Fig. 5.27. Radiograph and specimen: 'Apical notch'.

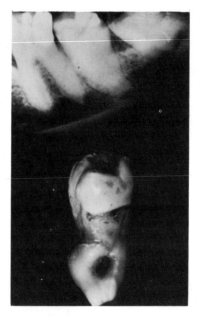

Fig. 5.28. Radiograph and specimen: 'Perforated root'.

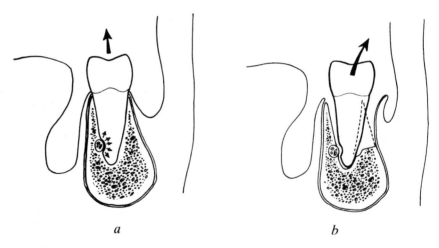

a   *b*

Fig. 5.29. The incidence of nerve damage complicating the removal of 'grooved' teeth can be reduced by removing the buccal plate and delivering the tooth through the resultant defect.

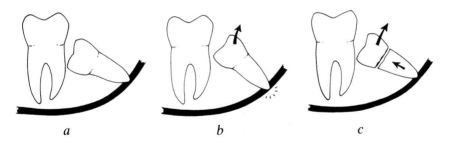

Fig. 5.30. *a*, Mesio-angular impaction of a notched ⌐8. *b*, Mesial application of force crushes canal contents. *c*, Tooth division minimizes the risk of damage to the canal contents.

is seen when deep grooving is present (*Fig.* 5.26). Grooves caused by the inferior dental canal and its contents are usually situated on the lingual surface of the roots (*Fig.* 5.26). If the radiolucent band crosses the apex of the tooth root and only the upper white line is broken, an 'apical notch' is present (*Fig.* 5.27). Very rarely the contents of the inferior dental canal actually perforate the tooth root and in these cases a characteristic narrowing of the radiolucent band with loss of the white lines is noted in the standard radiograph (*Fig.* 5.28).

If the tooth is seen to be in close relationship to the inferior dental canal and its contents, the patient should be warned preoperatively of the possibility that impairment of labial sensation may complicate the extraction. This factor should be taken into consideration when the decision to remove a symptomless third molar is made. Every endeavour should be made to avoid damaging the inferior dental nerve during the removal of an impacted mandibular third molar which is intimately related to it. Inevitably such attempts to minimize damage to the nerve prolong the operation. As has already been stated, grooving due to the inferior dental canal is usually situated on the lingual surface of the roots. In these cases the risk of nerve damage may be minimized by removal of a generous amount of the bone lying on the buccal side of the tooth, which is then delivered through the resultant defect (*Fig.* 5.29). An apical notch is most frequently associated with mesio-angular or disto-angular impactions. Bur division of the tooth should be employed to minimize the risk of nerve damage (*Fig.* 5.30).

When the contents of the inferior dental canal actually perforate the root their continuity may sometimes be preserved by widely exposing the site of perforation by removal of buccal bone. The enclosing root is then divided at the level of the neurovascular bundle by making a deep groove with a bur and completing the division by inserting an elevator into the groove and twisting it. The root fragments are then delivered separately. When it proves impossible to preserve the continuity of the neurovascular bundle in this way, a sharp scalpel should be used to sever the inferior dental canal contents. If the cut ends are placed close to each other in the bottom of the socket, normal sensation is often restored to the lower lip within 6 months of operation.

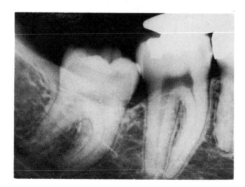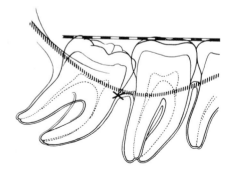

Fig. 5.31. Specimen preoperative assessment: Access, good; Angulation, mesio-angular; Obliquity, nil; Depth, 1 mm 'red' line; Root pattern, favourable; Crown shape, square, deep fissures; Tooth impaction, minimal; Second molar, slight distal tilt; Rotation, present; Inferior dental canal, superimposition only; Bone texture, elastic. Conclusion: Tooth could be removed under regional anaesthesia without difficulty. N.B. Rotation is indicated by a loss of definition of the outline of the pulp chamber and canal.

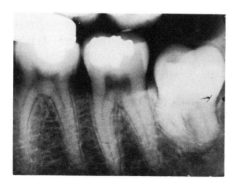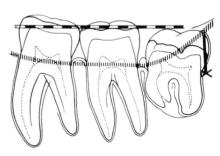

Fig. 5.32. Specimen preoperative assessment: Access, restricted; Angulation, disto-angular; Obliquity, mild degree of lingual obliquity; Depth, 4 mm 'red' line; Root pattern, two mesial roots curved favourably but distal root unfavourably curved; Crown shape, square; Tooth impaction, absent; Second molar, normal; Rotation, present; Inferior dental canal, not related; Bone texture, elastic. Conclusions: In view of a combination of factors (restricted access, unfavourable angulation and obliquity, depth, root pattern, and rotation) it would be preferable to extract this tooth under endotracheal anaesthesia. Other extractions which might be indicated could be performed under the same anaesthetic.

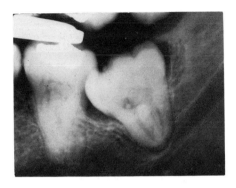
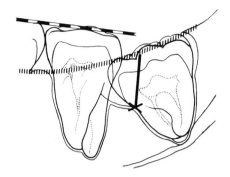

Fig. 5.33. Specimen preoperative assessment: Access, fair; Angulation, mesio-angular; Obliquity, nil; Depth, 4 mm; Root pattern, conical; Crown shape, bulbous; Tooth impaction, present; Second molar, rotated, two fused roots; Rotation, nil; Inferior dental canal, shallow 'apical notch'; Bone texture, elastic. Conclusions: Tooth should be sectioned in order to relieve tooth impaction and minimize risk of nerve damage. Patient should be warned of this possible complication before surgery is undertaken and advised to lose the impinging upper third molar, which will be unopposed when the lower tooth is lost. This surgery could be performed under regional anaesthesia in a co-operative patient.

Upon completion of his preoperative assessment the dental surgeon must first decide whether it would be in the best interests of his patient to refer him to a specialist oral surgeon (*see* Chapter 16). In those cases in which the dental surgeon decides to perform the extraction himself, he must make an operation plan designed to deal with any difficulties that are foreseen, and either to avoid or to cope with the complications diagnosed during preoperative assessment (*Figs.* 5.31–5.33).

THE REMOVAL OF MANDIBULAR THIRD MOLARS

As every one of the plethora of techniques which are available for the removal of mandibular third molars can be divided into the stages described in Chapter 3 (*see* p. 64), it is convenient to discuss these procedures in general terms before describing specific techniques.

Mucoperiosteal flap

This should be outlined in the manner shown in *Fig.* 5.34. The anterior incision curves forwards from the distobuccal corner of the crown of the second molar and ends alongside the mesiobuccal cusp of that tooth. The incision should be made through the mucoperiosteum and down to the bone with firm pressure on a scalpel blade and, if possible, should not extend into the reflection of the mucous membrane. The incision is then extended distally level with the buccal side of the tooth to the external oblique ridge. If the anterior part of the flap is elevated from the bone, one blade of a pair of scissors may be inserted on to the surface of the bone and the incision completed by closing the blades. The posterior part of the

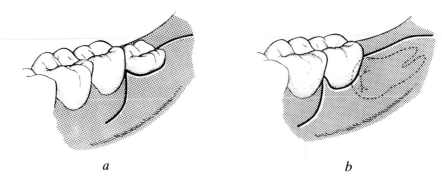

Fig. 5.34. Ward's incisions for the removal of lower third molars. *a*, Standard incision. *b*, Modified incision for use when improved access is required at the anterior end of the bony wound.

incision must slope outwards as well as backwards, for the ascending ramus lies to the lateral side of the body of the mandible. The mucoperiosteal flap created in this manner provides excellent visual and mechanical access and can be closed by means of a suture inserted between the buccal and lingual soft tissues alone. This avoids the need to insert a suture in the buccal sulcus, a procedure which at times may give rise to considerable difficulty. When a portion of the crown is visible during preoperative inspection (*Fig.* 5.34*a*) and it is decided to close the operation wound by approximating the buccal and lingual flaps, any epithelium present in the gingival crevice must be excised by making a reverse bevel incision of appropriate length before the soft tissues are elevated (*see* p. 358 and *Fig.* 5.35). A No. 12 scalpel blade is ideal for this purpose (*see Fig.* 3.11). The risk of a periodontal pocket developing distal to the second molar during the postoperative

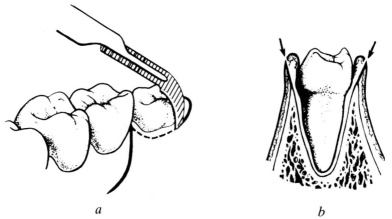

Fig. 5.35. Epithelium lining the gingival crevice surrounding a semi-erupted mandibular third molar should be removed by a reverse bevel incision if primary closure of the wound is planned. *a*, Viewed from the side. *b*, Viewed from the front (incision lines arrowed).

period can further be minimized by siting a transverse suture as far forward in the buccal and lingual flaps as is possible (*Figs.* 5.39*h* and 5.42*g*). Primary closure of the wound should not be attempted unless a band of buccal-attached muco-periosteum at least 5 mm in width is present in the third molar region prior to operation. In the absence of such soft tissue it is only possible to obtain primary closure by abolishing the buccal sulcus and so producing a periodontal problem. In such cases a better result is obtained by leaving the wound to heal by second intention (*see* p. 78).

Occasionally, it may be necessary to reflect a larger buccal mucoperiosteal flap than the one described in order to obtain adequate access. In these circumstances, the anterior incision should be commenced at the distobuccal corner of the crown of the lower first molar and extended forwards alongside that tooth. A vertical incision should then be made through the buccal gingival crevice of the second molar before the remainder of the incision is completed as previously described (*Fig.* 5.34*b*). Especial care must be taken to ensure that such a mucoperiosteal flap is carefully replaced at the end of the operation. On occasions the use of suture placed interdentally is indicated. If the anterior part of the incision is commenced half-way along the gingival crevice of the second molar, healing is not so satisfactory as when the incision is made in front of the tooth.

After the buccal flap has been elevated from the bone the lingual soft tissues should be reflected. This may often be accomplished by carefully inserting the tip of the periosteal elevator under the periosteum distal to the tooth, and passing it in a distolingual direction to reach the lingual border of the mandible at the point where it flares buccally. When this has been achieved, the same instrument may be used to elevate the tissues overlying the tooth by means of blunt dissection. Provided that the tip of the instrument is kept under the periosteum and close to bone, the lingual nerve and soft tissues will not be damaged by this manoeuvre. It is absolutely essential that the distolingual spur of bone should be seen (*Fig.* 5.36), and this can be ensured by reflecting the lingual soft tissues so that at least 5 mm of the bone lying behind the tooth is exposed. Lengthening the lingual flap anteriorly after making a vertical incision through the lingual gingival crevice of a standing second molar relieves tension and thus minimizes trauma to the soft tissues during retraction. The Bowdler Henry retractor provides an excellent means of retracting the buccal soft tissues from the field of operation (*Figs.* 3.20*c* and 5.40).

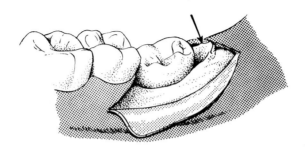

Fig. 5.36. Soft tissues reflected to reveal the distolingual spur of bone (arrowed).

Bone removal

Bone removal to expose the crown of the impacted tooth will not be required in those cases in which the whole crown lies above and in front of the 'amber' line in the standard radiograph. When required it may be performed with either a chisel or a bur or both (*see* p. 69 and *Figs.* 3.25, 5.39, 5.41, 5.42). A bur may also be used to create a gutter around the tooth neck (*see* p. 72 and *Figs.* 3.26, 5.41), and a point of application for an elevator. If a mesial point of application is adequate the elevator should stand up at an angle of 45° to the body of the mandible without support (*Fig.* 5.37). No attempt to elevate the tooth should be made until the operator has ensured that a space exists into which the tooth may be displaced. Such a space may be created either by cutting off a portion of the crown of the tooth or by removing bone. Whilst distolingual bone is being removed with a bur, the lingual soft tissues should be protected with a retractor (*see Fig.* 5.41c). A chisel can also be used to remove the distolingual spur of bone (*see Fig.* 5.39d).

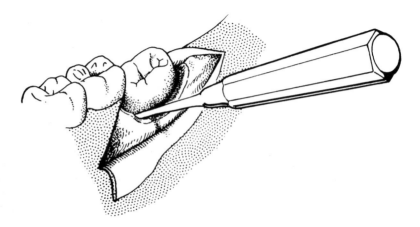

Fig. 5.37. An elevator applied to an adequate mesial point of application should remain in situ without support.

Delivery of the tooth

This must be preceded by tooth division in those cases in which tooth impaction exists or the roots have unfavourable or conflicting lines of withdrawal (*see* p. 74). If sufficient force is applied by means of an elevator to the mesial surface of the tooth-impacted lower third molar illustrated in *Fig.* 5.38a, the tooth will rotate in an arc, the centre of which is situated at the apex of the distal root. As the mesial cusps are impacted below the distal convexity of the second molar the attachments of this tooth will be damaged. Vertical division of the third molar with either an osteotome or a bur (*Fig.* 5.38b) permits the distal root and the portion of crown attached to it to be picked out of the socket. As the remainder of the tooth will rotate along an arc, the centre of which is the tip of the mesial root, it can then be delivered with an elevator. Splitting teeth with an osteotome is a quick and

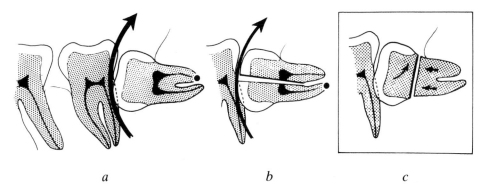

Fig. 5.38. Diagrams to show how tooth division may be used to relieve tooth impaction (*see text* for explanation).

efficient technique of tooth division, but requires the exercise of considerable skill and judgement based on extensive experience to be effective.

The occasional oral surgeon is advised to use bur division (*Fig.* 5.38*c*) to relieve this kind of tooth impaction, especially when the third molar has a square crown and prominent cusps or the second molar has either a conical root or a distal tilt. If the third molar is divided at the amelocemental margin by means of a bur, the separated crown may be moved backwards into the space so created before delivery from the wound. The roots may then be elevated into the space formerly occupied by the crown. It is sometimes necessary to divide the root mass with a bur and deliver each root separately. It is sound practice to protect the lingual investing tissues by leaving the lingual enamel intact when dividing the tooth with a bur. The blade of a straight elevator is then inserted between the cut dentinal surfaces and twisted to fracture the lingual enamel. The angulation of such a cut should be at right-angles to the long axis of the tooth in both the mesiodistal and linguobuccal planes. It should be made at a level which ensures that a point of application is left on the separated root mass or roots. After delivery of the various portions of the tooth the individual fragments should be related to each other in order to confirm that the whole tooth has been removed.

Wound toilet

A careful wound toilet should then be performed and particular attention paid to the area under the base of the buccal flap where bone debris frequently collects.

If healing by primary intention is desired, the wound should be closed with sutures, care being taken to insert the most anterior transverse suture as close to the distal surface of the second molar as possible. If healing by granulation is the aim, the buccal flap should be turned into the wound and held against the bone with either a ribbon-gauze pack or a pom-pom impregnated with Whitehead's varnish (*see* p. 78).

There is no agreement concerning either the value or the efficacy of the host of dressings and medicaments which have been claimed to minimize postoperative discomfort and speed healing and recovery after surgery. However, there can be no doubt that gentle handling of both the hard and soft tissues during the operation is of great importance in this respect. The patient should be instructed to use hot saline mouth-baths frequently and suitable analgesic drugs should be prescribed for his use (*see* p. 84). A single intramuscular injection of 1·3 ml of triplopen given 20 min before surgery has been shown to reduce the incidence of 'dry socket' following the removal of impacted mandibular third molars. However, the use of long-acting penicillins for this purpose is often criticized on the ground that should the patient develop a sensitivity reaction it is liable to be a prolonged one. In one trial betamethasone in an oral dosage of 14·5 mg decreasing over 4 days reduced postoperative pain by 80%, swelling by 65% and trismus by 40% when compared with a placebo and so appears to be a worthwhile form of therapy. Before the patient is discharged he should be instructed to avoid violent exercise, stimulants, or very hot food or drink for the rest of the day, in an attempt to minimize the risk of postoperative haemorrhage, and shown how to place either a gauze pressure pack or a clean folded handkerchief upon the intra-oral wound and to bite upon it in order to arrest any haemorrhage which might occur. The patient should be encouraged to consult the dentist without delay if anything untoward should complicate the postoperative period, and told how any necessary professional aid may be obtained after normal surgery hours in an emergency. An appointment should be arranged in order that the patient's postoperative progress may be reviewed.

SOME ILLUSTRATIVE PROCEDURES

1. The split-bone technique of Sir William Kelsey Fry

This is a quick, clean technique which has the advantage of reducing the size of the residual blood clot by means of saucerization of the socket. It is only suitable for use in young patients with elastic bone in which the grain is prominent. Although it can be performed under regional anaesthesia, endotracheal anaesthesia is preferable in most cases. A slight increase in the incidence of transient lingual anaesthesia during the postoperative period complicates the use of this technique. The procedure is illustrated in *Fig.* 5.39, in which, for the purposes of illustration, the soft-tissue retractor has been omitted. The use of a Bowdler Henry retractor to keep the buccal soft tissues out of the operative field is shown in *Fig.* 5.40.

After a standard incision has been outlined (*Fig.* 5.39*a*) the soft tissues are reflected to expose the bone enclosing the impacted tooth. A chisel is used to make a vertical 'stop cut' at the anterior end of the wound (*Fig.* 5.39*b*). Then with the chisel bevel downwards a horizontal cut is made backwards from a point just above the lower end of the 'stop cut' (*Fig.* 5.39*c*), thus enabling the buccal plate to be removed. A point of application for an elevator is made with the chisel by excising the triangular piece of bone bounded anteriorly by the lower end of the 'stop cut' and above by the anterior end of the horizontal cut (*Fig.* 5.39*d*). The distolingual bone is then fractured inwards by placing the cutting edge of a chisel along the dotted line shown in *Fig.* 5.39*c*, with the chisel held at an angle of 45° to the bone surface and pointing in the direction of the second lower premolar on the other side. Provided that the cutting edge of the chisel is kept parallel to the external oblique line a few light taps with a mallet suffice to separate the lingual plate from the rest of the alveolar bone and to hinge it inwards on the soft tissues

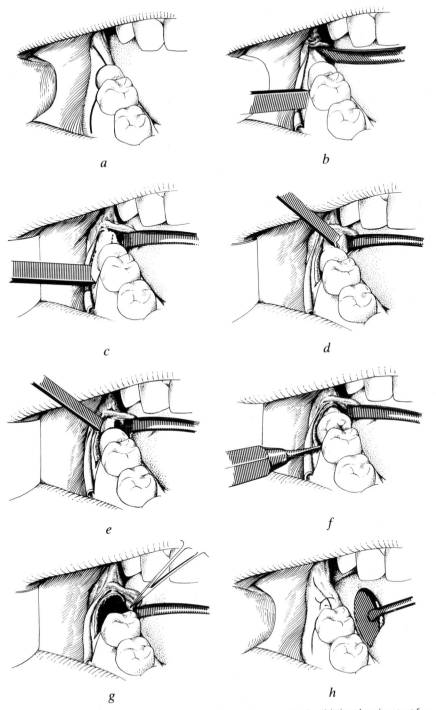

Fig. 5.39. Split-bone technique of removing impacted mandibular third molars (*see* text for explanation).

attached to it (*Fig.* 5.39*d*). Especial care should be taken to ensure that the cutting edge of the chisel is not held parallel to the internal oblique line, for this error in technique may result in extension of the lingual split to the coronoid process. The 'peninsula' of bone which then remains distal to the tooth and betwen the buccal and lingual cuts is excised (*Fig.* 5.39*e*).

A sharp-pointed, fine-bladed straight elevator is then applied to the mesial surface of the tooth and the minimum of force used to displace the tooth upwards and backwards out of its socket (*Fig.* 5.39*f*). As the tooth moves backwards the fractured lingual plate is displaced from its path of withdrawal, thus facilitating delivery of the tooth. After the tooth has been removed from its socket, the lingual plate is grasped in fine haemostats and the soft tissues are freed from it by blunt dissection (*Fig.* 5.39*g*). The fractured lingual plate is then lifted from the wound, thus completing the saucerization of the bony cavity.

After smoothing the cut bone edges with a bone file the wound is irrigated with sterile normal saline and closed with sutures. In most cases the solitary suture illustrated in *Fig.* 5.39*h* suffices and the curved anterior part of the incision comes together, and so the insertion of a suture in this site is seldom required.

2. The removal of an impacted mandibular third molar using a bur

These teeth may be removed with a bur in a variety of ways. The Moore/Gillbe collar technique sacrifices a similar amount of bone to that removed when the split-bone chisel technique is employed. A more conventional technique using a bur is performed in the following manner. A mucoperiosteal flap of standard design is elevated exposing the underlying bone (*Fig.* 5.41*a*). A rose-head bur is used to create a 'gutter' along the buccal side (*Fig.* 5.41*b*) and distal surface of the tooth. The lingual soft tissues should be protected with a periosteal elevator during the removal of the distolingual spur of bone (*Fig.* 5.41*c*). A mesial point of application is created with the bur, and a straight elevator is used to deliver the tooth (*Fig.* 5.41*d*).

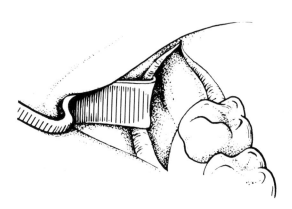

Fig. 5.40. Bowdler Henry retractor in use during the removal of an impacted mandibular third molar.

After delivery of the tooth has been effected the sharp bone edges are smoothed with a vulcanite bur (*Figs*. 3.26 and 5.41*e*), and the cavity is irrigated. Either the wound may be closed with sutures or the buccal flap may be tucked into the cavity and held against the bone with a pom-pom soaked in Whitehead's varnish (*Fig*. 5.41*f*).

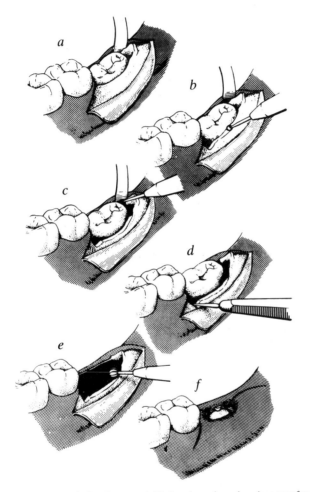

Fig. 5.41. The removal of an impacted third molar using a bur (*see* text for explanation).

3. The removal of a tooth-impacted mandibular third molar using tooth division

Improved access to this horizontally impacted mandibular third molar is obtained by making the anterior part of the incision alongside the first molar (*Fig*. 5.42*a*). The removal of the bone lying buccally to the tooth is started with a chisel (*Fig*. 5.42*b*) and then a bur is used to complete the exposure of the crown, to remove distal bone, and to provide two points of application—one under the crown and the other on the buccal side of the roots (*Fig*. 5.42*c*).

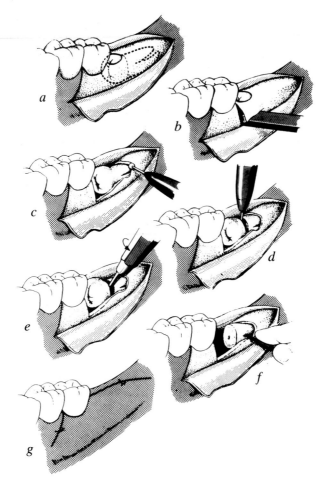

Fig. 5.42. The removal of a tooth-impacted lower third molar by means of tooth division (*see* text for explanation).

The crown is separated from the root mass by using a bur to divide all of the tissue other than the lingual enamel, which is severed by inserting an elevator into the resultant slot and twisting it around its long axis (*Fig*. 5.42*d, e*). The separated crown is then delivered by means of an elevator applied to its mesial surface, leaving the cut surface of the root mass projecting from the alveolus. After the roots have been delivered by the use of either a straight or an angled elevator (*Fig*. 5.42*f*), a careful wound toilet is performed and the wound closed with sutures (*Fig*. 5.42*g*).

4. The lateral trepanation technique of Bowdler Henry

This procedure can be employed to remove any partially-formed unerupted third molar that has not breached the hard and soft tissues overlying it and has been employed to remove such teeth from patients from 9 to 18 years of age. It can be performed under either general or regional anesthesia with sedation. The use of endotracheal anaesthesia permits both sides to be treated on one occasion if desired. After-pain is minimal although virtually every patient has some post-operative buccal swelling for 2 or 3 days after surgery which is occasionally accompanied by some bruising or soreness. Bone healing is excellent and there is no loss of alveolar bone around the second molar.

Postoperative radiographs reveal that the alveolar crest distal to the second molar is preserved intact and that bone regeneration in the third molar region is excellent (*Fig.* 5.43).

Soft-tissue healing is uneventful and provided that the incision is correctly sited the preoperative periodontal condition of the standing second molar is unchanged (*Fig.* 5.44).

The operation is performed as follows: After palpating the external oblique ridge an extended S-shaped incision is made from the retromolar fossa, across the external oblique ridge curving down through the attached mucoperiosteum to run along the reflection of the mucous membrane to the anterior border of the first permanent molar (*Fig.* 5.45*a*). Experience has revealed the importance of leaving a cuff of attached mucoperiosteum 5 mm in width distobuccally to the second molar.

The soft tissues lying behind and below the incision are then readily elevated from the surface of the bone and held away with a Bowdler Henry retractor (*Fig.* 5.45*b*). A round Toller bone bur in a straight handpiece is then used to trephine the position of the crypt of the third molar which appears to lie further forwards than one would think. When the anteroposterior length of the crypt has been determined in this manner, the same bur is used to make a vertical cut through the external plate at its anterior margin. A second cut through the outer plate is made at the posterior end of the crypt at an angle of 45° from the row of trephine holes (*Fig.* 5.45*c*).

A chisel applied in a vertical direction is used to outfracture the buccal plate, which is then delivered with a curved haemostat thus exposing the crown of the third molar lying in its crypt (*Fig.* 5.45*d*). A Warwick James elevator is applied to

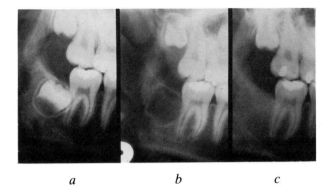

a   *b*   *c*

Fig. 5.43. Radiographs of the third molar area (*a*) 1 month before, (*b*) 3 weeks and (*c*) 15 months after the removal of a third molar by lateral trepanation.

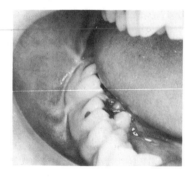

Fig. 5.44. Soft tissues 15 months after lateral trepanation. N.B. The position of the scar.

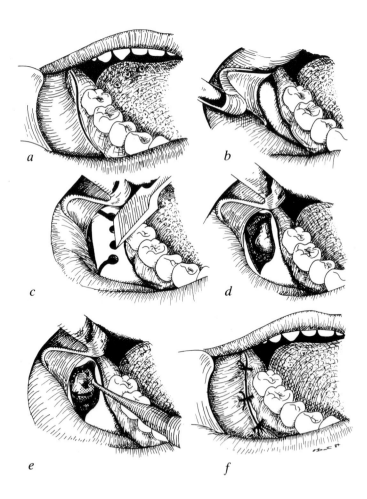

Fig. 5.45. The removal of a partially formed unerupted third molar by lateral trepanation (*see* text for explanation).

the occlusal surface of the tooth and used to deliver it (*Fig. 5.45e*). If difficulty is experienced it is usually overcome by removal of bone at the distal and lower corner of the bony window. Any follicular remnants are removed by carefully curetting the upper part of the bony cavity. Curettage of the lower part of the cavity is contra-indicated due to the presence of the contents of the inferior dental canal. The bone margins are then smoothed, the wound irrigated and closed with two or three black silk sutures (*Fig. 5.45f*). It is important to carefully record the number of sutures inserted and to identify and remove all of them 7–10 days later.

No technique is ideally suited to every case and the dentist is advised to master all of the practical skills that have been described. He will then be in a position to adapt his technique to deal with the particular problems presented by different cases, and provided that he adheres to sound surgical principles excellent results should be obtained.

SUGGESTED READING

Burgess P. T., Houston W. J. B. and Howe G. L. (1971) Orthodontic and surgical observations on the removal of mandibular third molars by lateral trepanation. *Dent. Pract.* **22**, 69–72.

Durbeck W. E. (1957) *The Impacted Lower Third Molar*, 2nd ed. London, Kimpton.

Finne K. and Klamfeldt A. (1981) Removal of lower third molar germs by lateral trepanation and conventional technique. A comparative study. *Int. J. Oral Surg.* **10**, 251–4.

Groves B. J. and Moore J. R. (1970) The periodontal implications of flap design in lower third molar extractions. *Dent. Pract.* **20**, 297–304.

Guralnick W. C. and Laskin D. M. (1980) NIH consensus development conference for removal of third molars. *J. Oral Surg.* **38**, 235–6.

Hardman F. G. (1952) Bilateral horizontal impaction of mandibular molars. *Dent. Pract.* **2**, 307–8.

Henry C. B. (1969) Excision of the developing mandibular third molar by lateral trepanation. *Br. Dent. J.* **127**, 111–18.

Howe G. L. (1958) Tooth removed from lingual pouch. *Br. Dent. J.* **104**, 283–4.

Howe G. L. and Poyton H. G. (1960) Prevention of damage to the inferior dental nerve during the extraction of mandibular third molars. *Br. Dent. J.* **109**, 355–63.

Killey H. C. and Kay L. W. (1965) *The Impacted Wisdom Tooth*. Edinburgh, Livingstone.

Moore J. R. and Gillbe G. V. (1968) The extraction of lower third molars in mesioangular impaction. *Br. Dent. J.* **125**, 454–6.

Poyton H. G. (1958) Radiographic technique for third molars. *Br. Dent. J.* **104**, 241–4.

Rood J. P. (1983) Degrees of injury to the inferior alveolar nerve sustained during the removal of impacted mandibular third molars by the lingual split technique. *Br. J. Oral Surg.* **21**, 103–16.

Rud J. (1983) Third molar surgery: relationship of root to mandibular canal and injuries to the dental nerve. *Tandlaegebladet.* **87**, 619–31.

Ward T. G. (1955) The radiographic assessment of the impacted lower wisdom tooth. *Dent. Delin.* **6**, 3–7.

Winter G. B. (1926) *Impact Mandibular Third Molar*. St Louis, American Medical Book Co.

Chapter 6

Surgical aids to orthodontics

The extraction of healthy, normal, fully erupted teeth is frequently an essential part of an overall orthodontic treatment plan. Furthermore, during a course of regulation treatment surgery may also be employed to deal with unerupted, semi-erupted, or misplaced teeth, supernumerary teeth, dilacerated and submerged teeth, and persistent abnormal frenum labii.

These procedures seldom present any problems if a systematic approach is employed. Prior to surgery being undertaken, a complete diagnosis, assessment, and treatment plan must be made: not just a surgical plan, not just an orthodontic plan, but a complete dental treatment plan which embraces all the conservative, periodontal, prosthetic, orthodontic, and surgical treatment required. A carious exposure of the pulp may make radical revision of an orthodontic treatment plan essential and it is preferable to know about it before the die is cast by surgical intervention. 'Vitality testing' of adjacent teeth, especially upper lateral incisors, prior to surgery should be undertaken as a routine procedure. It is better to discover that an unerupted canine is related to a pulpless lateral incisor of dens invaginatus type before surgery than after operation. Proper treatment planning enables any necessary preliminary orthodontic treatment to be performed before surgery, whilst any extractions which are required as part of the treatment plan can often be performed under the same anaesthetic.

These comments should not be interpreted as a plea for procrastination, for although surgery performed in conjunction with orthodontic treatment may be undertaken at any time, experience shows that it is most successful when performed during the eruption phase of any involved displaced tooth. The importance of early recognition and correct diagnosis of any abnormality involving the eruption of teeth cannot be overemphasized.

THE LOCALIZATION OF UNERUPTED TEETH

Orthodontic surgery requires precision both in planning and in execution. It is not enough for the dental surgeon to know that an unerupted tooth is present, for before surgery can even be considered the exact position of the tooth and its precise relationship to other unerupted or erupted teeth must be determined.

Although clinical examination, especially palpation, is often of some value, accurate localization is largely dependent upon the careful interpretation of good radiographs. It is of particular importance to determine whether a buried tooth is

144

lying labiobuccally or palatally to the standing teeth, so that the surgeon knows whether to use a labiobuccal or a palatal approach. If the buried tooth actually lies within the arch of standing teeth the use of both a buccal and a palatal approach may be indicated.

Careful radiographic assessment is essential and at least two views taken at right-angles to each other are required. The dental surgeon must know both the value and the shortcomings of each of the radiographic views available for his use if an accurate estimate of the position of the buried tooth is to be made. All radiographs should be examined meticulously on a good viewing box and the use of a hand lens aids interpretation considerably.

Periapical films

These reveal the condition of teeth adjacent to the buried tooth together with the size, shape, and root pattern of the unerupted tooth (*Figs*. 6.1, 6.2, 6.11). The presence of cysts, odontomes, or supernumerary teeth can also be detected in a periapical film, which may also give some indication of the relationship between the buried tooth and the adjacent erupted teeth in the *vertical* plane. Whilst the relative definition and radiopacity of the crown may assist in the determination of the tooth position (*see* p. 122), a more reliable estimate can be made by the use of the so-called parallax method. In this technique a periapical radiograph of the area is taken and the X-ray tube is then moved in either a mesial or a distal direction before a second periapical film is taken. The two radiographs are then compared and if the buried tooth is seen to move in the same direction as the X-ray tube it is lying palatally to the standing teeth, whilst if it moves in the opposite direction it is lying on the labial side of them (*Figs*. 6.3, 6.10).

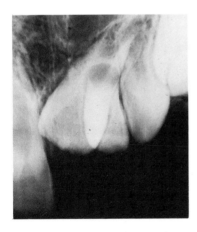

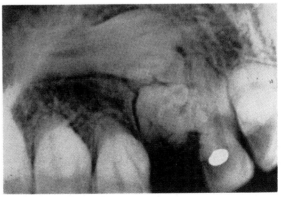

Fig. 6.1. Periapical film showing un-erupted left permanent central and lateral incisors and the presence of a supplemental tooth.

Fig. 6.2. Periapical radiograph of a 20-year-old patient showing a compound odontome and a buried canine lying high in the alveolar bone.

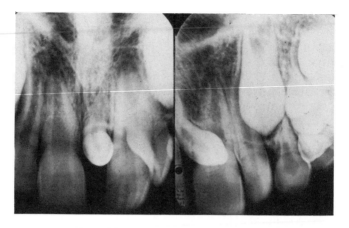

Fig. 6.3. Localization of a buried tooth by parallax. At operation this mesiodens was found to be lying between the central incisors with the crown on the palatal side and the apex on the labial side of these teeth.

Occlusal films

A number of occlusal views are available for use and the value and shortcomings of each should be clearly appreciated. When an *anterior* occlusal radiograph is taken the X-ray tube is sited at nasion and the central ray is angled as shown in *Fig.* 6.4. This produces a film showing much detail, which is useful for diagnostic purposes but of no value in determining the relative position of teeth due to the inevitable distortion which occurs.

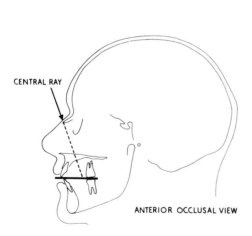

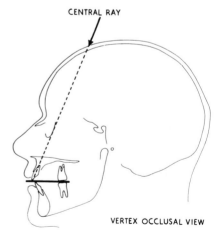

Fig. 6.4. Angulation of the central ray when an anterior occlusal radiograph is taken.

Fig. 6.5. Angulation of the central ray when a vertex occlusal radiograph is taken.

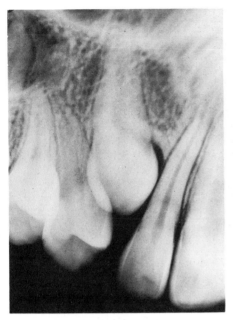

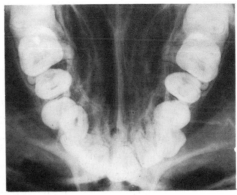

b

Fig. 6.6. *a*, Periapical and, *b*, Vertex occlusal radiographs of a tooth-impacted canine.

a

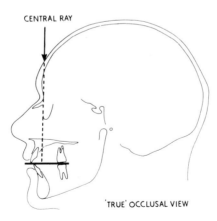

Fig. 6.7. Angulation of the central ray when a so-called 'true' occlusal radiograph is taken.

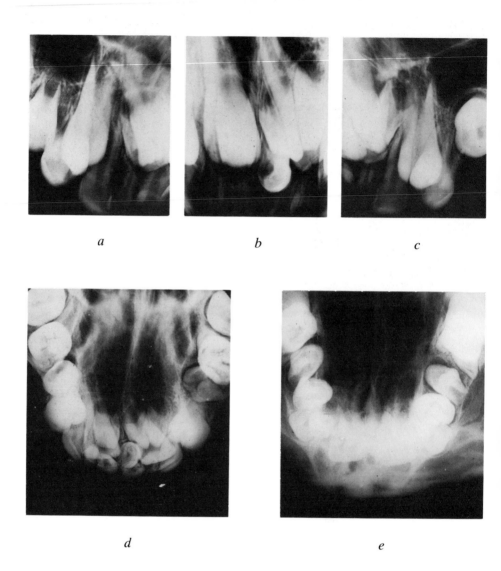

Fig. 6.8. The radiographic localization of buried teeth. *a, b, c,* Periapical views showing 4̲2̲B̲A̲|A̲B̲2̲4̲ erupted, and 5̲3̲1̲|̲1̲3̲5̲ and some supernumeraries unerupted. *d,* Four super-numeraries are clearly seen on the anterior occlusal radiograph on which the canines appear to be lying above the standing teeth. *e,* Vertex occlusal film showing that the unerupted 3̲1̲|̲1̲3̲ are lying labially to the dental arch, whilst the supernumeraries are lying on the palatal side of the unerupted permanent teeth. These findings were confirmed at operation.

When taking the *vertex* occlusal view the X-ray tube is arranged so that the central ray passes along the long axis of the central incisors (*Fig.* 6.5). If the central incisors are shown in cross-section, the film is an accurate one and may be used with confidence to determine the true position of a buried tooth. As the rays have to pass through the skull and facial bones to reach the film, this type of radiograph lacks both contrast and detail and is useful only for determining the relative position of the teeth. A longer exposure to X-rays is required and an intra-oral cassette containing an intensifying screen should be used to reduce the dose of radiation as much as possible. The patient's gonads must be protected with a lead apron.

The proximity of the buried tooth to the roots of standing teeth can be determined from this type of radiograph and the presence of tooth impaction is readily detected. If the crown of the buried tooth impinges upon the roots of the standing teeth, the unerupted tooth must be sectioned and removed in pieces if damage to the standing teeth and their attachments is to be avoided (*Fig.* 6.6).

The so-called 'true' occlusal film is taken with the X-ray tube positioned so that the central ray is at right-angles to the film packet when viewed from the sides and front of the patient (*Fig.* 6.7). It is a valueless film, for it gives a distorted view in which the shadow cast by the supra-orbital ridges is often superimposed upon the area it is desired to examine.

In the practice of oral surgery periapical radiographs and a vertex occlusal film are all that are required in most cases (*Fig.* 6.8), although if lateral and postero-anterior views of the skull have been taken for orthodontic purposes they may provide much useful information. Thus, if the crown of an unerupted canine is seen in the lateral skull radiograph to be lying in front of the anterior surface of the root of the central incisor, a labial approach should be employed (*Fig.* 6.9), whilst if the canine lies behind this surface a palatal approach is indicated.

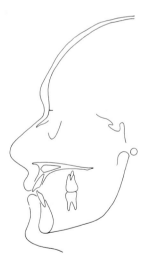

Fig. 6.9. Tracing of lateral skull radiograph in which the tip of the cusp of the canine is shown to be lying in front of the apices of the incisors. The tooth was removed via a labial approach.

COMPLICATED EXTRACTIONS

When patients exhibit marked crowding of the teeth it is often necessary to extract one or more teeth for orthodontic purposes. The problems differ in every case and must be resolved by means of preoperative diagnosis and treatment planning. On occasions the removal of a misplaced buried tooth may shorten treatment considerably if it can be performed without the adjacent teeth being damaged. This is only possible if the buried tooth is carefully localized preoperatively and the utmost caution is exercised during its removal (*see Fig.* 6.22).

The removal of the tooth germs of lower third molars for orthodontic reasons is discussed on p. 112.

THE MANAGEMENT OF THE UNERUPTED CANINE

The dental surgeon should make a practice of notating the teeth present in the mouth whenever he performs a routine dental examination. In this way the eruption pattern and dental age of his child patients will at once be apparent and, if the eruption of any tooth is delayed, the reason for this abnormality can be promptly sought. If there is no sign of a maxillary canine in a patient who is 12 years of age the case should be investigated systematically (*Fig.* 6.10).

A careful history should be taken, the eruption dates of other teeth determined, and a note made whether the deciduous canine is retained or missing and, if the latter, when it was either shed or extracted. Inquiries should reveal at once if the permanent tooth has been removed or if there is a family history of either malpositioning or absence of teeth. Inspection and palpation of the alveolar bone may reveal the presence of bulges due to the buried tooth or the roots of either the deciduous predecessor or the neighbouring teeth. Tilting and displacement of adjacent teeth may provide a clue to the position of the unerupted canine. Thus, if the crown of the lateral incisor is displaced distally and labially, the canine is usually found to be related to the labial surface of the apex of the erupted tooth (*Fig.* 6.10*a*).

In addition to assessing the general condition of the patient's mouth and the state of oral hygiene, especial care should be taken to test all of the adjacent teeth including any retained deciduous canine for mobility and to determine the condition of the periodontal tissues (*Fig.* 6.11). The 'vitality' of the teeth should be checked by means of either thermal or electric pulp testing before and after operation. This is particularly important in the case of lateral incisors which may exhibit dens invaginatus, a condition which predisposes to pulpal death (*Fig.* 6.12). If a sinus is present a silver probe should be passed along it in an attempt to feel any underlying tooth. The maxillary canine area is a rare site for supernumeraries but occasionally a dentigerous cyst is found to be present in relation to the crown of an unerupted canine (*see Figs.* 6.14, 6.48, 7.1).

Radiographic examination should reveal the direction of the long axis of the canine as well as the position of both its crown and root apex relative to the adjacent teeth, in the vertical, mesiodistal, and labiopalatal dimensions. No single film can supply all this information and so several views are required. Two or three periapical views are often needed to show the whole length of the canine, and the maxillary incisor, canine, and premolar regions should be examined.

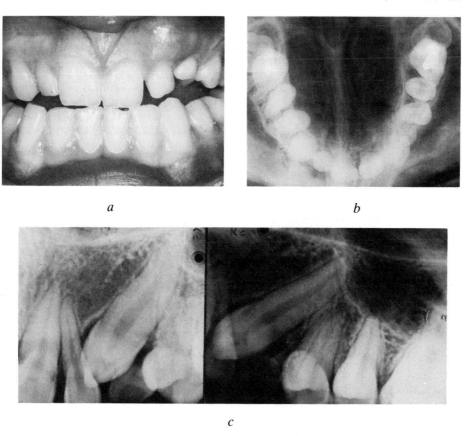

Fig. 6.10. *a*, Retained deciduous canine in a 12-year-old boy. Note the inclination of the left lateral incisor. *b, c,* Vertex and periapical occlusal radiographs confirm the clinical impression that the canine is lying on the labial side of the standing teeth.

These films reveal the condition of neighbouring teeth (*see Figs.* 6.6*a*, 6.11, 6.12) and give some indication of the vertical position of the canine in relationship to adjacent standing teeth. They will also show any cyst or supernumerary tooth which happens to be present.

Unerupted canines often have hooked roots and the periapical film should be carefully examined for signs of this. In some instances the root appears to be straight with a blunted end, and in these cases a hook is usually present, the long axis of which coincides with the path of the X-rays (*Fig.* 6.13). Prior to surgery it is essential to determine whether the tooth is lying buccally to, palatally to, or directly above the standing teeth, and the methods employed to do this have already been discussed on pp. 144–9. Many patients with an unerupted canine have other orthodontic abnormalities and for this reason a complete orthodontic diagnosis and treatment plan should be made prior to surgery. Once a diagnosis has been made usually only three or four courses of action are available to the

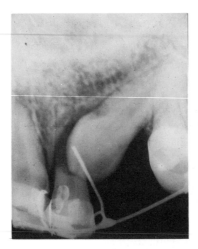

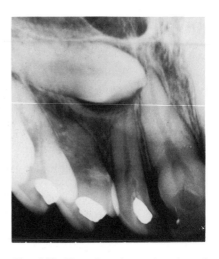

Fig. 6.11. Resorption of the root of a permanent lateral incisor related to a buried canine.

Fig. 6.12. Dens invaginatus in a lateral incisor related to an unerupted canine.

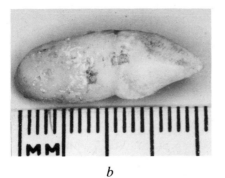

a

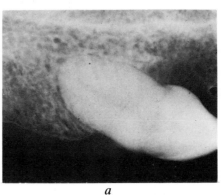

b

c

Fig. 6.13. *a*, The apex of this canine root looks blunt and rounded in this periapical radiograph. *b*, When viewed from the side the tooth gives a similar appearance, but, *c*, when viewed from above the true configuration of the root is seen.

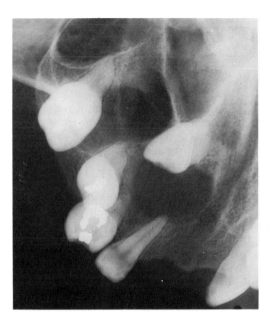

Fig. 6.14.   Dentigerous cyst related to an unerupted maxillary canine and involving the apex of a vital lateral incisor.

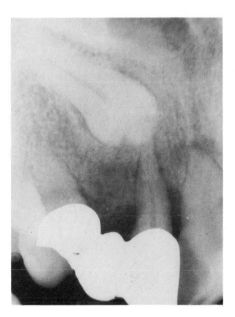

Fig. 6.15.   Resorption of the crown of an unerupted misplaced maxillary canine.

dental surgeon. Treatment should not be planned until both the patient's concern about the condition and desire for it to be treated have been carefully assessed. In a minority of cases the dentist may decide to leave the buried tooth in situ, for in some patients an impacted tooth may act as a buttress for an adjacent erupted tooth which is carrying an excessive occlusal load, and its removal may prejudice the retention of other teeth in a healthy state. In making such a decision it should be remembered that few retained deciduous canines remain in situ after 40 years of age and that the appearance of most of them leaves much to be desired long before that. Any canine left in situ should be radiographed at regular intervals to check that no pathological changes are occurring. A dentigerous cyst may form on an unerupted canine (*Fig.* 6.14) and if impacted such a tooth may cause resorption of the root of an adjacent tooth (*Fig.* 6.11) or be affected by resorption itself (*Fig.* 6.15). Spontaneous eruption of a palatally impacted canine is relatively rare and in most instances surgical treatment is indicated. In the majority of cases the canine should be either surgically exposed in an attempt to aid its eruption or removed, and the choice of treatment must be based on both surgical and orthodontic considerations.

When the ipsilateral first premolar and lateral incisor are suitably positioned the planned and timely removal of an unerupted labially placed maxillary canine may produce an acceptable aesthetic result and minimize the length of time for which orthodontic appliances have to be worn (*Fig.* 6.22). In recent years the successful results of autotransplantation of misplaced maxillary canines have been reported by a number of workers and the technique may provide a preferable alternative to extraction in selected cases (*see* p. 162).

Whilst different orthodontists hold varying views concerning the indications for surgical exposure of the unerupted canine, all would agree that there must be room in the arch for the tooth or that room must be created for it either by orthodontic means or by the extraction of either the lateral incisor or the first premolar. The potential path of eruption of the canine must be towards the surface and be unobstructed by other teeth if the treatment is to succeed. When eruption is complete, the apex must be near to the normal position in all planes if

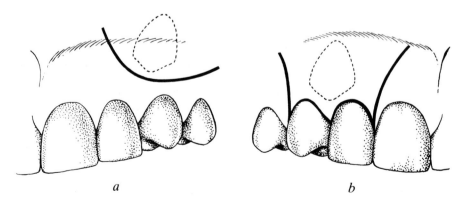

a   *b*

Fig. 6.16. Alternative incisions for use during the removal of a buried canine via a labial approach (*see* text for explanation).

the tooth is not to be unsightly. These criteria are fulfilled only if the path of eruption of the tooth passes through the site at which the canine apex is normally situated.

The dental surgeon should base his decision whether to employ a labial or a palatal approach when removing an unerupted canine upon a careful preoperative radiographic localization of the tooth. Flaps suitable for use during a labial approach are illustrated in *Fig.* 6.16. When such a flap is outlined it is essential to ensure that the margins of the flap are supported by bone at the end of the operation, and that the collar of attached labial gum which is retained is at least 5 mm wide (*Fig.* 6.16*a*). In most instances the incision illustrated in *Fig.* 6.16*b* is to be preferred.

When a palatal approach is employed the palatal gingival margins are incised vertically from at least second premolar to second premolar (*Fig.* 6.17*a*). When the flap outlined by this incision is raised from the bone with a periosteal elevator, it will be found to be tethered in the midline by the nerves and vessels passing through the incisive foramen. In most cases the flap should be freed by severing the neurovascular bundle close to the bone with a sharp scalpel (*Fig.* 6.17*b*). The brisk haemorrhage which results is easily controlled by applying pressure with a gauze pack soaked in hot saline (49 °C) to the bone for a few minutes. Then sufficient bone is removed with either a bur or chisel to expose the entire crown of the tooth, including the tip of the cusp if this is possible without risking damage to the standing teeth (*Fig.* 6.17*c*).

If the unerupted tooth is not tooth-impacted and the root formation permits, it can now be delivered by the use of a Warwick James elevator applied to its mesial surface. When tooth-impaction is present or the root pattern is unfavourable, the crown should be separated from the root by the use of a bur and the fragments delivered separately (*Fig.* 6.17*d*). Whenever elevation of the buried tooth is attempted the index finger of the left hand should be applied to the labial surfaces of the standing teeth, in order to afford them support and to detect any force transmitted to them (*Fig.* 6.17*e*). If the apex of a buried canine fractures during delivery of the tooth it should usually be left in situ.

In a minority of cases the root of a canine in the palate passes between the roots of the standing teeth to form an elevation which is easily palpable high up in the labiobuccal sulcus. In these circumstances after the exposure of the crown of the tooth has been completed in the manner described, a labiobuccal mucoperiosteal flap should be elevated from the bone. The curved root apex is then exposed and excised, thus permitting the buried tooth to be delivered by pressure applied to the cut surface of the root. After all loose fragments of alveolar bone and follicular remnants have been removed from the wound the bone edges are smoothed and the soft tissues replaced. The palatal flap should be moulded to the vault of the palate with a hot saline pack. Sutures are inserted between the teeth and the knots tied on the labiobuccal side to avoid tongue worry (*Fig.* 6.17*f*).

Healing is usually uneventful. Some dental surgeons prefer to construct a clear acrylic resin base-plate with clasps and cribs on it preoperatively, which is inserted at the end of the operation to hold the palatal mucoperiosteal flap firmly against the bone. When such an appliance is used care should be taken to ensure that the tissues underlying it are not rendered ischaemic by pressure from the plate, or necrosis of the flap may follow. The patient is seen 1 week postoperatively and at this visit the sutures are removed and the 'vitality' of the teeth related to the

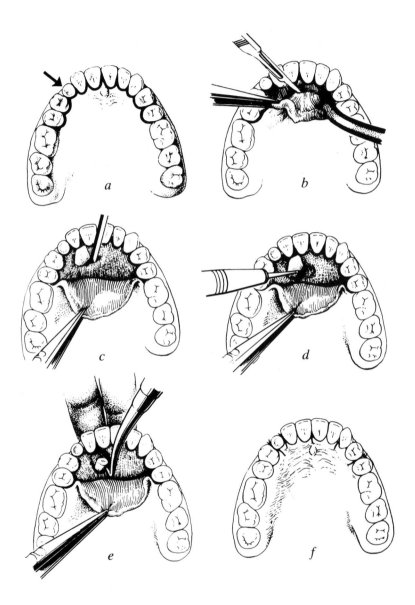

Fig. 6.17. The removal of a buried canine from the palate (*see* text for explanation).

operative site tested by either thermal or electrical methods. Any tooth which fails to respond at this time should be tested again 3 and 6 months later before loss of vitality is assumed.

THE SURGICAL EXPOSURE OF TEETH FOR ORTHODONTIC REASONS

Canines

A technique which has been successfully employed to expose a canine for orthodontic purposes on many occasions is illustrated in *Fig.* 6.18*a–d*.

After the radiographs have been carefully examined a cruciform incision is made with its centre over the estimated position of the crown of the buried tooth (*Fig.* 6.18*b*). The four triangular flaps are raised and after the actual position of the crown has been verified the appropriate extensions are made to the incisions and the resulting flaps excised. Haemorrhage from the palatal vessels can usually be controlled by pressure, and the insertion of a stay suture is seldom required. At the end of the operation the crown of the tooth will be left lying in a saucer-shaped bony cavity and a pack is inserted to prevent the soft tissues growing over the exposed tooth. If the soft tissues are removed in the manner described, the margins of the mucoperiosteal defect remain firmly attached to bone and the insertion of the pack is facilitated, whilst if a flap has been raised and replaced, the pack tends to spread out between the surface of the bone and the periosteum when pressure is applied.

By the use of hand pressure on a sharp chisel, or hand gouge, bone is removed so as to expose the tip of the cusp, the cingulum, and the greatest mesial and distal convexities of the crown (*Fig.* 6.18*c*). Surrounding bone is carefully excised in a similar fashion to saucerize the resultant bony cavity as far as this is practicable without the risk of damaging either adjacent standing teeth or their supporting tissues (*Fig.* 6.19). It is very easy to damage the tooth being exposed if either burs or mallets are employed during bone removal and so it is wise to avoid using these instruments for this purpose if it is practicable to do so.

Some orthodontists believe that removal of the labial mucoperiosteum and bone during the surgical exposure of a tooth may result in the cervical margin of such a tooth being at a higher level than that of its neighbours when eruption is complete (*Figs.* 6.20, 6.21*d*). Other authorities state that this finding is due to the anterior position of the affected tooth in the bone and claim that the condition resolves as the 'passive phase' of eruption, i.e., the rolling back of the soft tissues, proceeds. Nevertheless, care should be taken to keep the removal of labial mucoperiosteum and bone to the minimum amount which is required to expose the tooth satisfactorily. The resultant cavity is then tightly packed with wisps of cotton-wool impregnated with a paste of zinc oxide and oil of cloves, which is built up to form a pack which is left in situ for 10–14 days. Small pieces of the packing material should be inserted into the most inaccessible areas first and a mattress suture may be required to aid the retention of the pack in situ.

Most correctly assessed and adequately exposed canines erupt without the insertion of pins, inlays, or the fitting of celluloid crown forms or stainless-steel bands (*Fig.* 6.21). It is a widely held opinion that the application of traction by such means may be followed by either failure of the tooth to erupt or pulpal death,

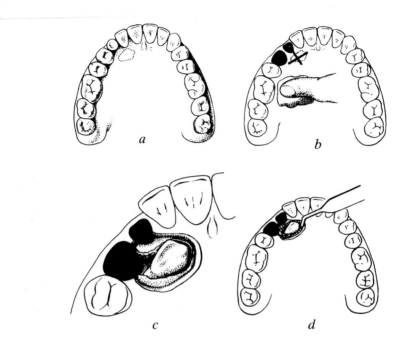

Fig. 6.18. Surgical exposure of a buried canine for orthodontic purposes (*see* text for explanation).

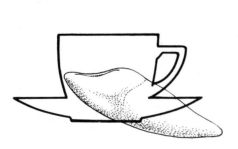

Fig. 6.19. Following exposure, the crown of the tooth should lie in a bony cavity which, as far as is practicable, resembles a saucer rather than a teacup.

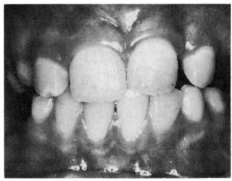

Fig. 6.20. Although this surgically exposed left central incisor has erupted into occlusion, its cervical margin has remained at a higher level than that of the right central incisor for more than 18 months.

or both. However, as these techniques are usually employed in the treatment of badly placed canines or in those cases in which treatment is commenced after the normal time of eruption, such opinions are a matter of debate. If traction is to be employed it is best applied by the use of a bracket cemented to the crown of the canine after the tooth has been acid etched. The eruption of an exposed canine can be aided by cutting away the bone which obstructs the path of movement, e.g., distobuccal bone in the case of a palatally situated canine, to form an 'eruption channel' if this is practicable (*see Fig*. 6.18*c*).

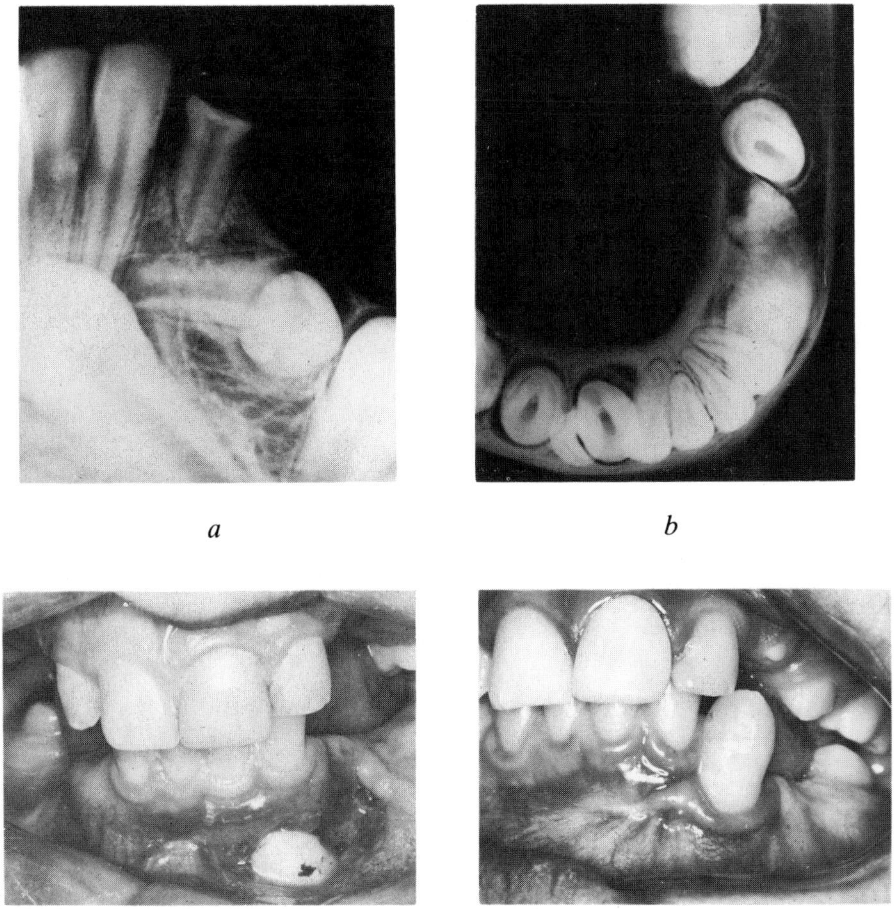

a *b*

c *d*

Fig. 6.21. Master W. Q., aged 12 years. *a*, *b*, Periapical and occlusal radiographs showing ⌈4 dilacerated and ⌈3 buried and lying labial to the standing teeth. *c*, Clinical condition 2 weeks after removal of ⌈4 and surgical exposure of ⌈3. ⌊1 bears a temporary crown. *d*, Clinical condition 15 months later. No appliances were worn.

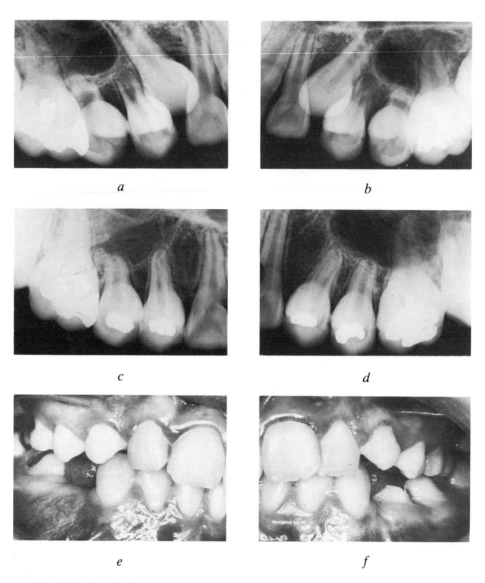

a *b*

c *d*

e *f*

Fig. 6.22. The labially placed unerupted canines were removed from a girl, aged 10 years and 4 months, who was considered to be unsuitable for appliance therapy due to the doubtful efficiency of oral hygiene. *a, b,* Preoperative radiographs. *c, d,* Radiographs and, *e, f,* clinical appearances 1 year after surgery. Note the contact points between the lateral incisors and premolars.

Although adequately exposed canines usually erupt, many orthodontists are tending to request surgical exposure less frequently, perhaps because the end-results do not justify the amount of treatment required in many cases. An alternative treatment involving removal of buried canines at an early age gives excellent results in suitably selected cases (*Fig.* 6.22).

Incisors

The surgical exposure of an unerupted incisor tooth is performed in a similar fashion to that described above, care being taken to expose the entire incisal edge, cingulum, and mesial and distal convexities of the buried tooth.

When incisors are palpable above the reflection of the mucous membrane they may be exposed with ease by incising the mucosa. This, however, may give a shallow labial sulcus with a deficiency of attached mucoperiosteum. If the gum is incised well on the palatal side of the buried tooth and the resultant mucoperiosteal

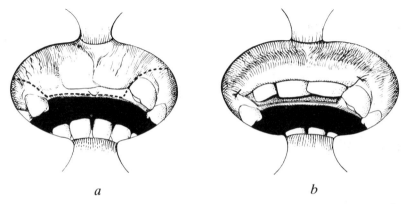

a   *b*

Fig. 6.23. A technique utilizing an apically repositioned labial mucoperiosteal flap is employed to expose unerupted incisors lying above the reflection of the mucous membrane (*see* text for explanation).

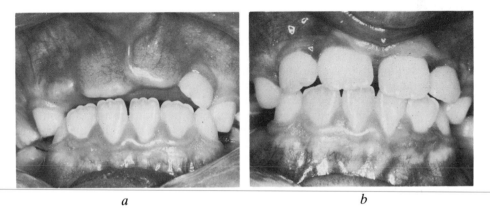

a   *b*

Fig. 6.24. Exposure of three unerupted incisors in the labial sulcus. *a*, Before surgery. *b*, Fourteen weeks after surgery.

flap is widely undermined and rotated forwards and upwards to line a labial sulcus, a better result is obtained (*Figs*. 6.23, 6.24). By using an apically repositioned flap in this manner the amount of attached labial mucoperiosteum is increased and gingival health is preserved.

Cheek teeth

When exposing a cheek tooth the bone and soft tissues should be cleared from the cusps, the occlusal surface, and the crown down to and including the greatest convexity of the tooth. This leaves the cervical portion of the anatomical crown surrounded by a collar of soft tissue and thin bone, which should be packed away from the tooth with an annular pack of zinc oxide and oil of cloves on cotton-wool.

The patient is instructed to keep the site of exposure clean by using hot saline mouth-baths (*see* p. 86) and the pack is removed 2 weeks after operation. Surgical exposure of unerupted teeth followed by any necessary orthodontic treatment is a very successful method of bringing teeth into occlusion. The optimum age for such treatment is from 12 to 14 years and it is seldom successful when used in patients over 17 years of age.

AUTOGENOUS REPLANTATION

Autogenous transplantation of misplaced maxillary canines is now a proven and widely accepted technique and may even be the procedure of choice in some cases. A successful autograft is a superior alternative to a partial denture or a fixed bridge in a young patient and should also be considered a valid option in patients over 17 years of age in whom surgical exposure and prolonged orthodontic treatment to reposition a canine is often only partially successful or completely unsuccessful and/or unacceptable to the patient on aesthetic and social grounds. It is sometimes combined with simple orthodontic treatment designed to achieve either a small increase of space in the maxillar canine region or to re-align an over-erupted opposing mandibular canine, or both, usually by utilizing removable appliances.

The technique is usually successful if care is taken to preserve the periodontal membrane of the transplant and to minimize the time between its removal and re-implantation in a new socket. In a few cases the canine may be surgically repositioned by swinging it into its new position without removing it from the tissues or dividing its nerve and blood supply. More frequently, however, the apex of the canine is in so poor a position that such a procedure is not practicable and the tooth must be delivered and transplanted.

Whilst success cannot, and should not, be guaranteed the transplantation of a misplaced maxillary canine can be attempted at any age provided that there is either adequate room in the arch for the tooth, or it can be created by simple orthodontic treatment, and the tooth can be removed whole with its periodontal membrane intact. It is easier to do this in younger patients who have more elastic bone and a wider periodontal space than in older patients whose bone is more dense, whose periodontal spaces are less well defined and whose teeth are more difficult to remove. Damage sustained by the implant during its removal appears to affect adversely the prognosis of the transplant.

The decision to transplant a canine should be based upon a careful preoperative assessment utilizing radiographs and study models mounted on an adjustable articulator. Periapical and vertex occlusal films should be utilized for this purpose together with a postero-anterior view localized on the canine in the vertical plane and a true lateral view localized on the tooth sagittally. The use of articulated models facilitates measurement of the space in the arch which is available for the transplant, evaluation of the contouring of the alveolus required to enable the crown of the canine to be properly positioned and amount of adjustment of occlusal opponents that is required. This latter objective can be achieved either by judicious grinding or by means of orthodontic treatment. The upper model can be duplicated and utilized to fabricate a splint comprising a contoured horizontal loop of 0·5 mm soft stainless-steel wire. The loop should be constructed at the level of the contact points and should include at least two teeth on either side of the transplant. If there is insufficient space to accommodate the canine in its correct position a removable orthodontic appliance should be fitted to regain the space. Where present the opposite permanent canine can be measured. In cases in which both maxillary canines are unerupted the size of the opposing mandibular canine can be used as a guide. The permanent maxillary canine is approximately one millimetre wider mesiodistally than its mandibular opponent.

Systemic antibiotic cover (p. 256) should be given for at least 5 days. Whilst the procedure can be undertaken using local anaesthesia and premedication it is usually better performed under a general anaesthetic with endotracheal intubation. A large palatal mucoperiosteal flap is raised from the bone after incising the gingival margins from second premolar to second premolar. The neurovascular bundle is divided as it emerges from the incisive foramen thus enabling the flap to be raised to ensure good visual access to the site of operation. The crown of the canine is exposed by careful removal of bone using only a chisel with hand pressure if possible in order to minimize the danger of damaging the tooth. Bi-bevel burs can be obtained which are claimed to cut bone but not enamel. The fragments of bone are stored in the blood collecting between the base of the flap and the bone. Sufficient bone must be removed to enable the tooth to be delivered from its socket in such a way as to avoid damage to its amelocemental junction, periodontal membrane and cementum. This can be a time-consuming and pains-taking process. However, it is probably of great importance to the survival of the tooth and can be achieved in a variety of ways. It may be possible to deliver the tooth by putting traction on its follicle, or by the careful use of right and left Warwick James elevators applied only to the mesial and distal surfaces of the crown just coronally to the amelocemental junction, or the use of a Thonner snare to apply gentle leverage and traction on the canine. This device is illustrated in *Fig.* 6.25 and comprises a stainless-steel tube about 5 cm long and 2 mm external diameter, the end of which is slightly flattened and in which holes are drilled with a rosehead bur. To the other part a cross-bar is soldered in order to enable the tube to be turned. The ends of a soft ligature wire of 0·4 mm stainless steel are inserted in the holes at the flattened end of the tube and passed through the tube to project a few centimetres beyond the other opening. The ends of the ligature are anchored around the cross-bar. At the flattened end a loop is formed that by twisting can be made just large enough to slip over the crown. By further twisting the loop is locked under the crown. Once delivered the tooth is stored along with the bone chips in the blood collecting under the base of the palatal flap. Care must

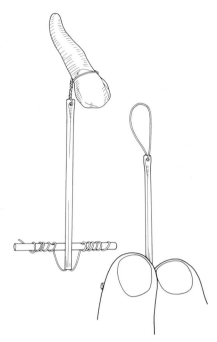

Fig. 6.25. The Thonner snare may be used to harvest canines for transplantation.

be taken to ensure that it does not become dry.

During the creation of the new socket every endeavour should be made to preserve the labiobuccal bone and mucoperiosteum. It may be necessary to create room to place the transplanted tooth in a labiopalatal position which is acceptable from a functional and aesthetic point of view or to provide a canine eminence. These objectives can be achieved by the creation of an osteoplastic flap between the lateral incisor and the first premolar after first removing the deciduous canine, if present.

This flap comprises the labiobuccal mucoperiosteum and the attached compact layer of bone and is created by inserting a chisel vertically with its bevel towards the palate and outfracturing the compact layer of labiobuccal bone on the intact attached mucoperiosteum. The socket is then created using either a chisel or a water-cooled bur taking care not to damage the roots of adjacent teeth. The new socket should not be excessively large but should be made slightly larger than the root of the canine in order to minimize the risk of damage to the periodontal membrane during the insertion and positioning of the tooth. The aim should be to create a socket in which the canine root is a 'friction fit'. After removing any attached follicle from the canine by carefully incising it against the enamel as near to the cementum as possible, the tooth is gently inserted into the new socket. The position of the tooth is adjusted using finger pressure alone, in order to ensure a good appearance and that the canine is free of traumatic occlusal contacts with its mandibular opponent during all excursions of the mandible. Care should be taken to ensure that the tooth is correctly sited in the vertical dimension. It should be placed just, but only just, out of occlusion as no further eruption can be expected after transplantation. Every endeavour should be made to minimize the time between the removal of the tooth from its misplaced socket and its insertion into the newly created socket, for the shorter this time is the better is the prognosis for the transplant. The time taken is normally in the region of 10 min and should never exceed 30 min for the chances of success diminish sharply after this. The transplanted tooth should not be root filled and if less than 1 mm more space is required it is better to grind the proximal surfaces of adjacent teeth rather than the canine in order to minimize handling of the transplant. When the canine is positioned correctly the bone fragments removed earlier are packed around it as necessary and into any residual palatal defect. The palatal mucoperiosteal flap is trimmed to fit the neck of the canine and sutured into place. Pressure on a gauze swab should be used to express blood clot from under the flap.

A decision must then be made whether or not to splint the tooth as in some cases this is not necessary provided that the tooth is firm, free of the bite and the patient exercises care in the postoperative period. If required, the previously constructed wire splint is placed in situ and ligatured to the teeth with fine wire tied interdentally. If further stability is required cold-cure acrylic can be flowed over the splint.

Healing is usually uneventful and gingival reattachment and bone regeneration occur rapidly. The splint should be removed as soon as the tooth is firm, usually in between 2 and 6 weeks. It is important to repeatedly check the occlusion in the immediate postoperative period and at each subsequent visit if excessive mobility of the transplant is to be avoided. The patient is usually seen 1 week, 3 weeks, 6 weeks, and 12 weeks after surgery and then reviewed at 6-monthly intervals for 2 or 3 years (*Fig.* 6.26).

The gingival condition returns rapidly to normal, the gingival crevice around the transplant usually being from 1 to 3 mm in depth within a few weeks provided that there are no traumatic occlusal contacts. Regeneration of bone around the root of the tooth takes longer and does not appear to be related to age. It is usually complete in 6–12 months. Provided that the periodontal membrane has been

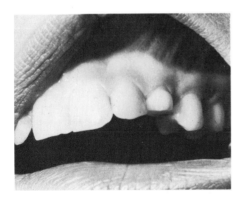
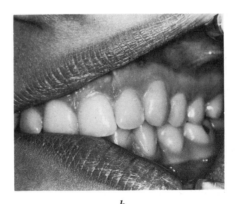

a   *b*

Fig. 6.26. *a*, Retained left maxillary deciduous canine associated with a palatally impacted permanent successor. *b*, Condition 4 years later after autotransplantation of the canine. (*Courtesy of Dr R. M. Cook.*)

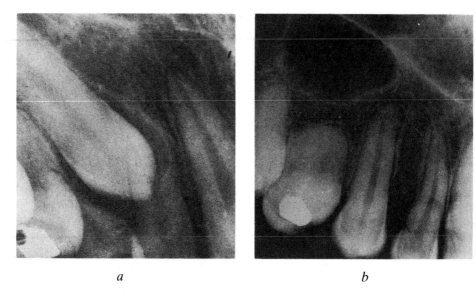

a   *b*

Fig. 6.27. Radiographs showing a misplaced right maxillary canine before (*a*) and after (*b*) autotransplantation. N.B. New intact lamina dura and normal appearance of the periodontal space in *b*. (*Courtesy of Dr R. M. Cook.*)

preserved during removal of the tooth and its subsequent positioning in the new socket both the periodontal space and the lamina dura around it are normal in appearance (*Fig.* 6.27). Even when the root of a transplanted canine is fully developed and the apical foramen is closed the pulp appears to establish a blood supply or some form of cellular nutrition. In some cases calcific replacement of the pulp chamber occurs whilst in others the tooth may react to 'vitality' tests although it is difficult to know whether the pulp or the periodontal membrane responds. Teeth which fail to respond to pulp testing should not be root-filled routinely but followed up clinically and radiographically. Only if pathological changes occur should orthograde endodontic treatment be undertaken. A few transplanted canines show a loss of translucency whilst an occasional tooth darkens in colour.

Resorption may occur in the transplanted tooth and may be either lateral, internal or periapical, and its extent and progression may determine the prognosis of the canine. It usually occurs within 3 years of transplantation. Lateral resorption occurs near the amelocemental junction often on the distal surface of the root and can be detected on radiographs within 6 or 12 months of transplantation. It is thought to be due to injury to the periodontal membrane and/or cementum during the removal and reimplantation of the canine. It usually ceases to progress within 12 months. Internal and periapical resorption are more serious conditions and can be gross and progressive. They are sometimes arrested by root filling the tooth, but may progress until the tooth is lost.

On occasions the position of the unerupted tooth which is to be transplanted renders the preoperative orthodontic treatment required to regain space either difficult or even impossible. Such cases have been treated successfully by means of a two-stage procedure in which the unerupted canine has been removed and stored in a submucosal pouch in the patient's buccal sulcus for up to 13 months prior to successful reimplantation. It is stated to be important to try either to avoid, or at least to minimize, contact with the periosteum when the tooth is placed in the pouch if resorption is to be avoided.

SUPERNUMERARIES

The failure of one or more of the maxillary incisor teeth to erupt is most frequently due to either the presence of a supernumerary tooth or to lack of room in the arch, which is sometimes associated with early loss of a deciduous predecessor. Conversely, overlong retention of a deciduous tooth may also be associated with delayed eruption of its permanent successor. A complete failure of eruption may be seen in the presence of dilaceration (*see* p. 171). Supernumerary or extra teeth occur most frequently in the maxillary incisor region and in this area the vast majority of supernumeraries are found to lie on the palatal side of both the erupted standing teeth and the unerupted normal teeth (*Figs*. 6.8, 6.28, 6.29). Extra teeth are found less frequently in the premolar and third molar regions and in these sites there is a higher incidence of supernumeraries which closely resemble adjacent teeth and are often called 'supplemental teeth' (*Figs*. 6.1, 6.30–6.33). More than one supernumerary may be found in the maxillary incisor region, and in this site these extra teeth occur twice as frequently in males as in females and usually have abnormal forms, being either tuberculate or conical in shape. Tuberculate supernumeraries (*Figs*. 6.8*a* and *c*, 6.28) are seldom found to be inverted, and erupt only rarely. Conical supernumeraries (*Figs*. 6.3 and 6.8*b*) are not infrequently found to be inverted and often erupt. Unerupted tuberculate supernumeraries are almost invariably found to have incompletely formed roots

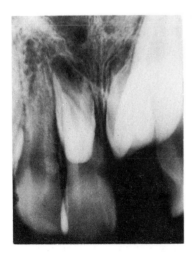

Fig. 6.28. Two supernumeraries in the maxillary incisor region.

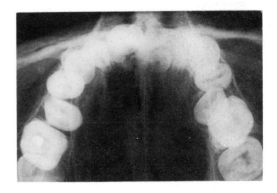

Fig. 6.29. Vertex occlusal radiograph in which a supernumerary can be seen lying on the palatal side of the unerupted central incisor.

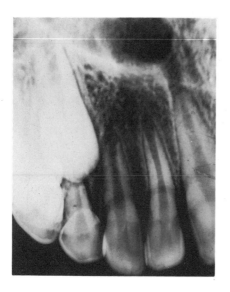

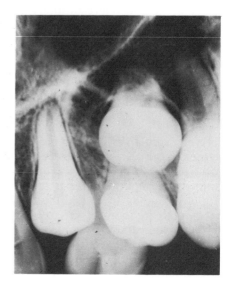

Fig. 6.30. Supplemental lateral incisor in dental arch.

Fig. 6.31. Supplemental tooth in maxillary premolar region.

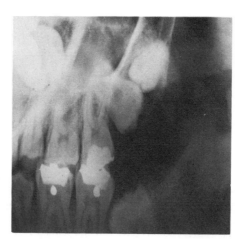

Fig. 6.32. A supplemental maxillary molar.

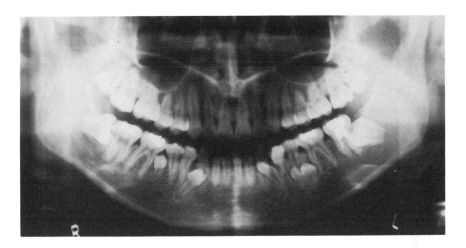

Fig. 6.33. Multiple supernumerary teeth in the mandibular premolar regions.

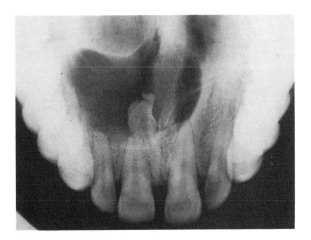

Fig. 6.34. Dentigerous cyst related to an inverted 'mesiodens'.

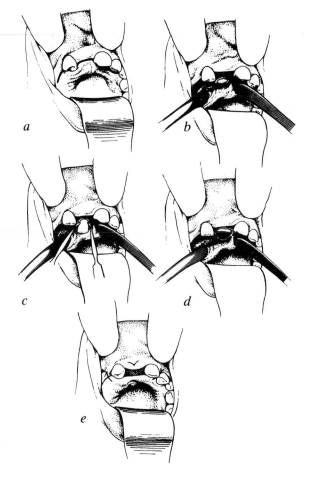

Fig. 6.35.   Removal of supernumerary tooth from the palate *(see* text for explanation).

and to lie on the palatal side of adjacent normal teeth, whilst conical supernumeraries are often found with completely formed roots and lying between the
upper central incisors (*Fig.* 6.3). Teeth of this type which lie in the midline of the
maxilla are frequently referred to as 'mesiodens'. This is a reasonable term
provided it is remembered that it refers to a particular form of supernumerary
tooth, the apex of which is seldom, if ever, found exactly in the midline. The
difference in root formation indicates that the tuberculate supernumerary forms
much later in development than either the conical form or the permanent upper
central incisor. For this reason it is believed by some that the tuberculate supernumerary is part of a third dentition, whilst the conical type is regarded as an extra
tooth in the second dentition.

   Whilst such factors as generalized or localized crowding in the arch, the type
and degree of central incisor displacement and root formation, and the relative
position of this tooth and the supernumerary are important predisposing causes of

delayed eruption of the permanent tooth, there can be little doubt that this condition is found to occur much more frequently in association with a tuberculate supernumerary than a conical one. It is therefore of great importance to differentiate between the two forms when treatment is considered. The tuberculate type must be removed as early as possible if the central incisor is to erupt in an acceptable time. Unless a conical supernumerary is causing either malpositioning or crowding of the central incisors it may sometimes be left in situ, especially if it is high up and away from the standing teeth. However, the dentist must not forget that inverted supernumeraries may migrate and cysts sometimes form in relation to a buried tooth when he makes the decision to put such a tooth 'on probation' (*Fig.* 6.34).

In almost every case supernumeraries should be removed as soon as it is possible to do so without damaging the adjacent teeth, and the technique employed to remove one from the incisor region is illustrated in *Fig.* 6.35.

The decision as to whether a palatal or labial approach should be employed is taken after a careful clinical and radiographic assessment of the case has been undertaken. In the majority of cases a palatal mucoperiosteal flap is raised after the palatal cervical margins have been incised from the second deciduous molar on one side to the second deciduous molar on the other side (*Fig.* 6.35*a*). When the flap is elevated from the bone it will be found to be tethered in the middle by the nerves and vessels passing through the incisive foramen. Whenever it is necessary to improve vision and surgical access, the flap should be freed by severing this neurovascular bundle close to the bone with a sharp scalpel. The brisk haemorrhage which results is easily controlled by applying pressure with a gauze pack soaked in hot saline (49 °C) to the area of the foramen for a few minutes.

The bone overlying the supernumerary teeth is removed with a sharp chisel, applied with hand pressure only (*Fig.* 6.35*b*). The bone in children is easily cut in this manner and mallets or burs should not be used if damage to other teeth is to be avoided. After the crown of the tooth has been widely exposed to facilitate positive identification of its morphological features (many supernumeraries are either conical or have crowns of abnormal form and exhibit dens invaginatus), the tooth is delivered by the use of a Warwick James elevator, utilizing bone as the fulcrum (*Fig.* 6.35*c*). Care should be taken to ensure that the easily detached dentine papilla is removed. After removal of any follicular remnants, bone fragments, or sharp edges (*Fig.* 6.35*d*), the flap is replaced and moulded to the palatal vault with a hot saline pack. Sutures are inserted buccolingually between the teeth and the knots tied on the labiobuccal side to avoid tongue worry (*Fig.* 6.35*e*). Healing is usually uneventful.

In some instances buried incisors can be exposed for orthodontic purposes at the same operation (*see* p. 161). Some operators prefer to either apply a cervical ligature to or cement a bracket onto the unerupted tooth at the time of surgery in order that orthodontic traction may be applied to it after healing of the soft tissues is complete.

DILACERATED TEETH

Although some authorities apply the term 'dilaceration' to any tooth with a hooked or bent root, others reserve the term for teeth which have the long axis of either the whole or part of the crown set at an angle to the root (*Fig.* 6.36). The condition is believed by many to be the result of trauma applied to the deciduous predecessor and transmitted to the forming permanent tooth. However, as the permanent incisors lie on the palatal side of the roots of their deciduous predecessors, trauma applied to the crown of the buried tooth in such a manner could not possibly move the incisal edge upwards and labially—the commonest type of deformity (*Figs.* 6.37*a*, 6.38)—unless the germ of the permanent tooth was already misplaced prior to the traumatic incident (*Fig.* 6.37*b*). Furthermore, if trauma was the sole aetiological factor a blow severe enough to cause dilaceration

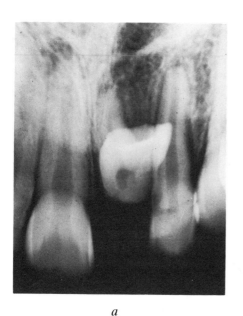

a

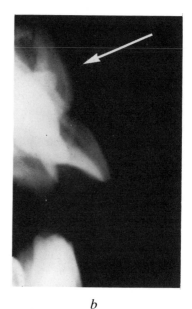

b

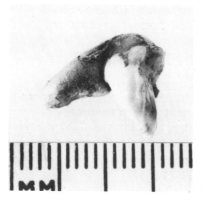

c

Fig. 6.36. Dilaceration of the left central incisor. *a*, Periapical radiograph. *b*, Lateral radiograph (arrow indicates the crown of the dilacerated tooth). *c*, Specimen.

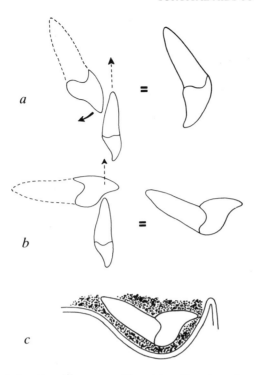

Fig. 6.37. The relationship of trauma to dilaceration. Note how the typical dilacerated incisor conforms to the contour of the alveolar ridge (*c*) (*see* text for explanation).

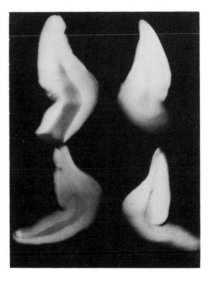

Fig. 6.38. Radiographs of sagittally sectioned dilacerated incisors.

would be likely on occasions to cause similar damage to the other central incisor. Such cases are extremely rare.

In one study dilacerated maxillary central incisors were found to occur six times more frequently in girls than in boys and neither macroscopic nor microscopic signs of mechanical injury could be detected in most of the specimens examined histologically. It appears likely that dilaceration is of developmental origin and is probably related to ectopic development of the tooth germ (*Fig.* 6.37c).

Dilacerated teeth are usually best removed via labial and palatal flaps. If the crown is divided from the root, each section can be delivered along its optimum line of withdrawal.

ABNORMAL FRENUM LABII

In some cases the upper central incisors are separated by a diastema, through which the labial frenum passes to gain attachment to the incisive papilla, which is seen to blanch when the lip and frenum are tensed (*see Fig.* 6.41a). A periapical radiograph often reveals a marked midline suture in these cases (*Fig.* 6.39). In the majority of patients the space between the central incisors closes as the permanent canines erupt, but an orthodontist may ask for the removal of the labial frenum as an adjunct to his appliance therapy. There is some evidence that in patients in whom there is a tendency towards spacing of the teeth, such as those with small teeth set in large jaws, the upper labial frenum may interfere with the formation of transeptal gingival, cervical and alveolar crest bundles of the periodontal ligaments between the central incisors. A midline diastema may also be associated with the presence of either diminutive lateral incisors or a supernumerary tooth in the mid line or both. On other occasions the lateral incisors are absent or an occlusal abnormality due to malpositioning of a lower incisor is present. There are great differences of opinion between orthodontists concerning the relationship of the frenum to the diastema and the indications and contra-indications for surgical treatment. Nevertheless, if the operation is performed at the optimum time in correctly assessed cases, the results are most gratifying. It is usual to delay frenectomy until the eruption of the lateral incisors and canines is complete and the diastema has failed to close naturally. The operation can be performed either before or after the central incisors have been approximated by appliance therapy.

The operation of *frenectomy* is designed to eliminate the fibrous tissue which is present in the midline suture between the roots of the maxillary central incisors and is an entirely different procedure to frenoplasty and frenotomy, which are operations designed to eliminate the fibrous band which raises the mucosa to form a frenum. *Frenoplasty* and *frenotomy* are undertaken to aid the prosthetist and are discussed on pp. 275 and 279.

The technique of frenectomy is illustrated in *Fig.* 6.40 and can often be performed under local anaesthesia with or without the use of premedication.

The upper lip is held out at right-angles to the anterior surface of the maxilla by an assistant throughout the operation (*Fig.* 6.40a). This not only tenses the frenum and facilitates dissection but aids haemostasis. An incision down to bone is made on either side of the frenum. When the palatal ends of these incisions are joined together the attachment of the underlying fibrous tissue to the bone is severed and the frenum springs upwards into the lip. The detached frenum and the

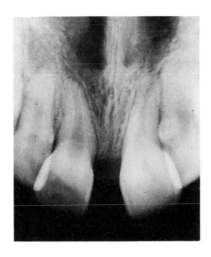

Fig. 6.39. Periapical radiograph of patient with abnormal frenum labii. A notch is present at the lower end of the median suture.

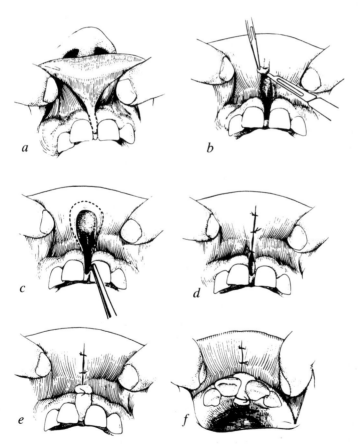

Fig. 6.40. Labial frenectomy (*see* text for explanation).

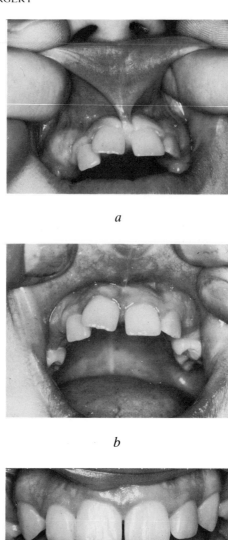

a

b

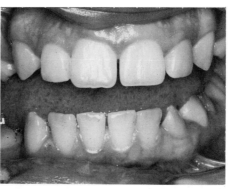

c

Fig. 6.41. Abnormal frenum labii. *a*, Before surgery. *b*, Two weeks after frenectomy. *c*, Two and a half years later following orthodontic treatment.

fibrous tissue underlying it are then dissected out of the undersurface of the lip, care being taken to preserve as much mucous membrane as is practicable (*Fig. 6.40b*). The median suture is then completely cleared of fibrous tissue by the use of either a Mitchell trimmer or a small rose-head bur (*Fig. 6.40c*). The mucosa on the undersurface of the lip is then undercut widely and approximated with interrupted sutures (*Fig. 6.40d*). The cover of a cotton-wool roll is impregnated with a paste composed of zinc oxide and oil of cloves, and sewn over the resultant gingival defect and left in situ for 2 weeks (*Fig. 6.40e, f*). Healing is uneventful and a typical result is illustrated in *Fig. 6.41b* and *c*.

SUBMERGED TEETH

A recent study revealed that almost 9% of children aged between 3 and 12 years had one or more of their primary molars in infra-occlusion, i.e. with the occlusal surface at a level lower than that of the neighbouring teeth. Such teeth are usually described as being submerged and the degree of abnormality may vary from being minimal to the complete disappearance of the tooth within the bone. The second deciduous molar is the tooth which is most frequently found to have become submerged and the condition is much more common in the mandible than in the maxilla. Wear facets are present on the occlusal surfaces of such teeth and indicate that at some time the tooth has been in occlusion. Amalgam restorations may be found in completely submerged teeth. An unexplained but localized deficiency in the vertical growth of the alveolar bone related to the affected tooth results in it becoming submerged as the adjacent teeth erupt normally. There is some evidence that infra-occlusion is much more common in some families and ethnic groups than in others.

Submerged teeth are often associated with absence of the permanent successor (*Fig. 6.42*). They are frequently the site of food stagnation, and the removal of such a tooth may be indicated either for orthodontic reasons or for the relief of

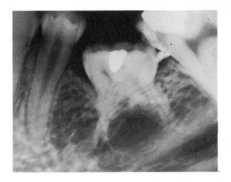 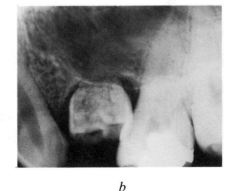

a	*b*

Fig. 6.42. Submerged second deciduous molars. The second premolars are absent. Note: *a*, Stagnation area between ⌐E6. *b*, Close relationship between ⌊E and antral floor.

pain. These teeth may become ankylosed and the roots may literally have to be drilled out. The removal of such a tooth should be preceded by the elevation of a large buccal mucoperiosteal flap. In the maxilla the creation of an oro-antral communication may complicate the extraction and the large flap facilitates the immediate repair of the defect (*see* p. 210).

ODONTOMES

Odontomes arise as a result of an aberration in the tissues responsible for the formation of teeth. Though regarded as tumours or hamartomas in the past they are now usually regarded as variations in development or malformations. In the 1971 World Health Organization classification they are broadly divided into complex and compound odontomes.

The complex odontome is a malformation in which all the dental tissues are represented, individual tissues being mainly well formed but occurring in a more or less disorderly pattern. They tend to occur in the posterior parts of the jaws, especially the mandible. Complex odontomes arise from an invagination of epithelium into the developing germ of a single tooth of a series or more rarely a supernumerary and so a normal structure is replaced by an anomalous one. The nature of the malformation depends upon the stage of development of the tooth germ and the degree of maturity and differentiation of its individual components at the time the invagination occurs and takes a variety of forms including the simple dens invaginatus (*Fig.* 6.12), dens in dente, dilated odontome (*Figs.* 6.43, 6.44), gemination (*Fig.* 6.45), and the deposition of all the dental tissues in a bizarre complex arrangement.

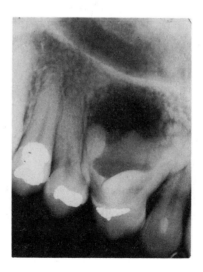

Fig. 6.43. Dilated odontome in the right maxillary canine region.

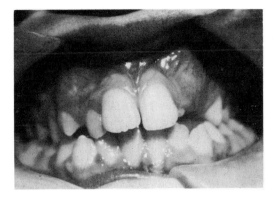

a

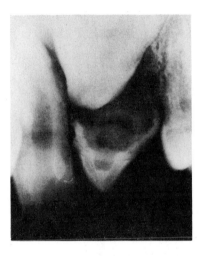

b

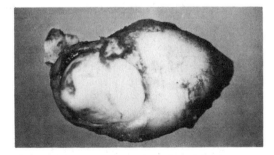

c

Fig. 6.44. Dilated odontome in the left maxillary lateral incisor region. *a*, Clinical appearance. *b*, Periapical radiograph. *c*, Surgical specimen.

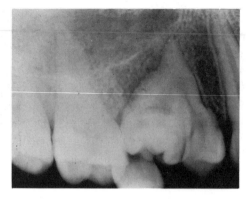

Fig. 6.45. Geminated odontome in the right maxillary premolar region.

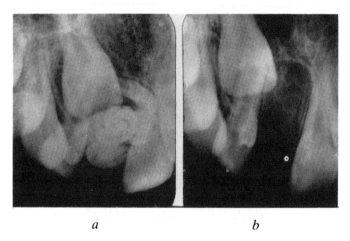

a   *b*

Fig. 6.46. *a*, Compound odontome in a patient aged 10 years. *b*, After the removal of the odontome the displacement of the central incisor is seen more clearly.

The compound odontome is a malformation in which all the dental tissues are represented in an orderly pattern so that the lesion consists of many tooth-like structures. It arises from an exorbitant proliferation of the dental lamina or its remnants and is thus a laminar odontome. The compound odontome is formed in addition to the normal teeth of a series and occurs most frequently in the anterior maxilla (*Figs.* 6.46, 6.47). Odontomes are often diagnosed in the second decade of life and are commonly associated with delayed eruption and gross displacement of related permanent teeth which is sometimes accompanied by retention of deciduous teeth and swelling or both. The increased use of routine radiographic examination has resulted in the presence of more of these lesions being discovered earlier before symptoms supervene (*Fig.* 6.48). Once detected, an odontome is usually best removed as soon as it is practicable to perform surgery without damaging adjacent teeth or tooth germs. The removal of compound odontomes is

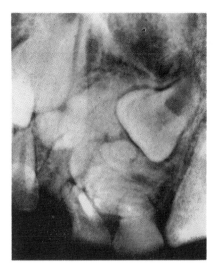

Fig. 6.47. Compound odontome in a 9-year-old patient.

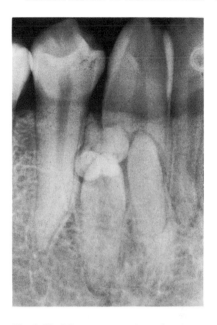

Fig. 6.48. The presence of this compound odontome and the two supernumerary teeth in the lower canine region was discovered during routine radiographic examination.

facilitated if the thin fibrous sac which encloses them can be preserved intact throughout the operation. The close apposition of the rough irregular surfaces of the larger complex odontomes and the investing bone makes their removal difficult unless associated chronic infection has caused some bone resorption. Both the surgical and the orthodontic treatment of such cases may be complicated and time-consuming and therefore it is usually best that they are undertaken in specialist centres.

CORTICOTOMY

Corticotomy is a surgical aid to orthodontics which can be utilized to shorten the duration of appliance therapy. It is of especial value in the treatment of young adults and can be used to facilitate the movement of one or more teeth in the anterior maxilla. An incision is made through both the labial and the palatal gingival crevices of the tooth or teeth to be moved and the teeth on either side. Flared vertical incisions are made at the buccal ends of the gingival margin incision and a broad based labial mucoperiosteal flap is elevated from the underlying bone. A large palatal flap is then reflected and the nerves and vessels emerging from the incisive foramen are divided to expose the palatal bone. A series of vertical cuts of predetermined width in the labial and palatal compact bone on

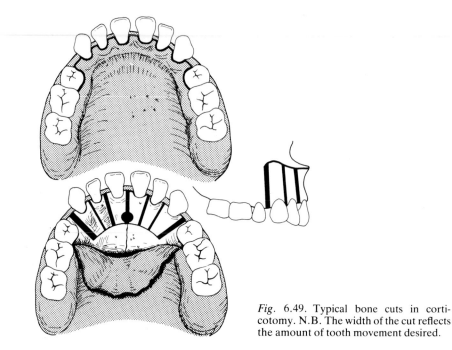

Fig. 6.49. Typical bone cuts in corticotomy. N.B. The width of the cut reflects
the amount of tooth movement desired.

each side of individual malaligned teeth are made with a bur (*Fig*. 6.49). The
apical ends of these cuts are joined by horizontal cuts through the compact bone
alone thus leaving the teeth to be aligned supported by cancellous bone only. The
mucoperiosteal flaps are then replaced and repaired with interrupted interdental
sutures. Orthodontic pressure, usually utilizing strong elastics, is applied to the
teeth and after a delay of a few days their alignment is rapidly effected. At the end
of the active phase of orthodontic treatment a retainer is fitted and is worn at all
times for the first month after surgery. After this it is usually only necessary to
wear the retainer at nights for the next 6 months. The excessive mobility of the
teeth being moved which sometimes complicates active orthodontic tooth
movement resolves rapidly during the period of retention.

Orthodontic surgery demands especial judgement, patience, precision, and
skill if worthwhile results are to be achieved. There are few branches of oral
surgery which offer more interest and satisfaction to the dental surgeon who takes
the trouble to master the techniques employed. In specialist centres, considerable
advances are being made in the use of surgery to remedy maxillary and mandibular
deformities which are too severe to respond to orthodontic therapy of a conventional nature. Proven techniques have been devised which enable the specialist
oral surgeon to alter the relationship between part of jaw and the remainder, of
one jaw to the other or of both jaws to the skull and the rest of the facial skeleton.
The dental surgeon should refer patients who both require and desire such
treatment for specialist opinion (*see* Chapter 16).

SUGGESTED READING

Adams C. P. (1954) Relation of spacing of the upper central incisors to abnormal fraenum labii and other features of the dento-facial complex. *Dent. Rec.* **74**, 72–86.

Andreason J. O. and Hjørting-Hansen E. (1966) Replantation of teeth I. *Acta Odontol. Scand.* **24**, 266–86.

Andreason J. O. and Hjørting-Hansen E. (1966) Replantation of teeth II. *Acta Odontol. Scand.* **24**, 287–305.

Barton P. R. and Rayne J. (1969) The role of alveolar surgery in the treatment of malocclusion. *Br. Dent. J.* **126**, 1–17.

Bergström K. and Jensen R. (1962) Central diastema and frenum labii. *Svensk. Tandläk.-Tidskr.* **55**, 70–72.

Brown I. D. (1981) Some further observations on submerging deciduous molars. *Br. J. Orthodont.* **8**, 99–107.

Budnick S. D. (1976) Compound and complex odontomas. *Oral Surg.* **42**, 501–6.

Cook R. M. (1972) The current status of autogenous transplantation as applied to the maxillary canine. *Int. Dent. J.* **22**, 286–300.

Di Biase D. D. (1969) Midline supernumeraries and eruption of the maxillary central incisor. *Dent. Pract.* **20**, 35–40.

Di Biase D. D. (1971) Mucous membrane and delayed eruption. *Dent. Pract.* **21**, 241–50.

Dixon D. A. (1963) Observations on submerging deciduous molars. *Dent. Pract.* **13**, 303–15.

Edlan A. and Subrtova I. (1967) *Corticotomy—Co-operation of the Oral Surgeon and the Orthodontist.* Proceedings of 2nd Int. Conference on Oral Surgery, Copenhagen. 1965. pp. 338–44.

Ferguson M. W. J. and Rix C. (1983) Pathogenesis of abnormal midline spacing of human central incisors. *Br. Dent. J.* **154**, 212–18.

Fordyce G. L. (1965) Surgical problems of orthodontic interest. *Dent. Pract.* **15**, 388–95.

Foster T. D. and Taylor G. S. (1969) Characteristics of supernumerary teeth in the upper central incisor region. *Dent. Prac.* **20**, 8–12.

Hitchin A. D. (1956) The impacted maxillary canine. *Br. Dent. J.* **100**, 1–12.

Hovell J. H. (1970) Surgical correction of facial deformity. *Ann R. Coll. Surg.* **46**, 92–107.

Howard R. D. (1970) The congenitally displaced maxillary incisor: a differential diagnosis. *Dent. Pract.* **20**, 361–70.

Joubert J. J. de V., Breytenbach H. S. and Staz J. (1981) Classification of odontomes with report of an invaginated odontome of complex type. *J. Dent. Assoc. S. Afr.* **36**, 823–7.

Kurol J. (1981) Infra-occlusion of primary molars, an epidemiological and familial study. *Common Dent. Oral Epidemiol.* **9**, 94–102.

McKay C. (1978) The unerupted maxillary canine. An assessment of the role of surgery in 2500 treated cases. *Br. Dent. J.* **145**, 207–10.

Moss J. P. (1968) Autogenous transplantation of maxillary canines. *J. Oral Surg.* **26**, 775–83.

Moss J. P. (1975) The indications for the transplantation of maxillary canines in the light of 100 cases. *Br. J. Oral Surg.* **12**, 268–74.

Reade P., Mansour A. and Bowker P. (1973) A clinical study of the autotransplantation of unerupted maxillary canines. *Aust. Dent. J.* **18**, 273–80.

Richardson A. and McKay C. (1965). The unerupted maxillary canine. The clinical level after surgical repositioning. *Br. Dent. J.* **118**, 123–6.

Stewart D. J. (1978) Dilacerate unerupted maxillary central incisors. *Br. Dent. J.* **145**, 229–33.

Thonner K. E. (1971) Autogenous transplantation of unerupted maxillary canines: a clinical and histological investigation over five years. *Dent. Pract.* **21**, 251–7.

Wilson H. E. (1960) The labial frenum. *Trans. Eur. Orthodont. Soc.* 34–40.

World Health Organization (1971) *Histologic Typing of Odontogenic Tumours.* Geneva, WHO. p. 30.

Chapter 7
The diagnosis and management of cysts of the jaws

A cyst may be defined as a pathological encapsulated collection of fluid. Several types of cyst occur in the jaws, most of which have an epithelial lining. Some of these are of dental origin whilst others are non-odontogenic. In one large series of odontogenic cysts, twice as many cysts were located in the maxilla as in the mandible.

SYMPTOMS

Not infrequently a cyst may be completely symptomless and the patient is quite unaware of the lesion until his attention is drawn to its existence by either his dental or medical adviser. In other cases the presence of a swelling or an intra-oral discharge causes the patient to seek professional advice. Although some patients describe the taste of an intra-oral discharge as being unpleasant, others may describe it as being either salty or sweet. In the latter case the discharge is frequently found to be purulent.

Acute infection of a cyst may cause the patient to present with a large acute abscess, whilst less severe infections may cause a dull throbbing pain. In large mandibular cysts this latter symptom may be accompanied by impairment of sensation in the lower lip on the affected side. In very rare instances pain and impairment of labial sensation may be caused by a non-infected cyst of the mandible and in these circumstances the symptoms are usually attributed to pressure. In completely or partially edentulous patients a cyst may be the cause of either discomfort under or difficulty in wearing dentures. Adjacent natural teeth may be either moved or tilted as the lesion expands.

SIGNS

Although some small cysts do not present any clinical signs and can only be detected by means of radiography, the vast majority of cysts are characterized by swelling (*Fig.* 7.1). Although the descriptive term 'egg-shell crackling' has long been associated with intra-bony cysts, palpation may reveal the swelling to be either frankly fluctuant or bony hard. In other cases the characteristic feeling of 'egg-shell crackling' may be noted, whilst on occasions the thin bone overlying the lesion is springy to the touch, a finding which has been well compared to the feeling experienced when a celluloid table-tennis ball is compressed between

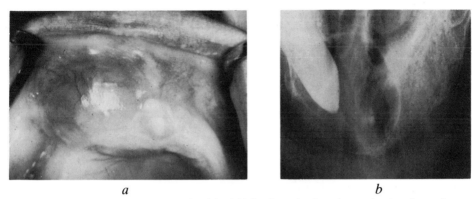

Fig. 7.1. *a*, Fluctuant swelling in right labial sulcus. *b*, Anterior occlusal radiograph showing dentigerous cyst related to buried right upper canine.

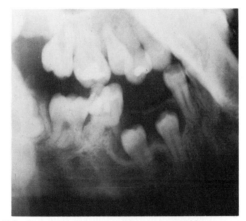

Fig. 7.2. Dentigerous cysts on two unerupted lower premolars.

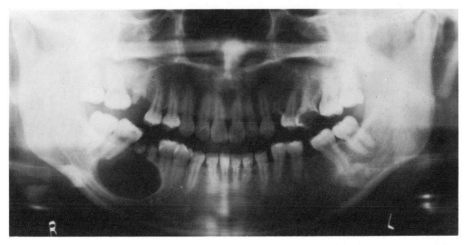

Fig. 7.3. A radicular cyst related to the pulpless root of the lower right first permanent molar.

finger and thumb. It must be emphasized that none of these findings on palpation is diagnostic of the presence of a cyst, for they are related solely to the thickness of the bone overlying the lesion at the site of examination. The findings vary from area to area in many larger lesions, and may be elicited in relationship to lesions other than cysts. The soft tissues overlying a cyst may be normal in colour, but when the lesion has perforated the enclosing bone the soft tissues often have a bluish tinge if the lesion is uninfected and are dark red if it is acutely infected. In the latter instance the tissues will be tender to touch.

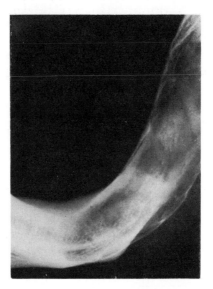

Fig. 7.4. The residual cyst has caused marked expansion of the buccal plate of the mandible but the lingual plate has not been affected to the same degree.

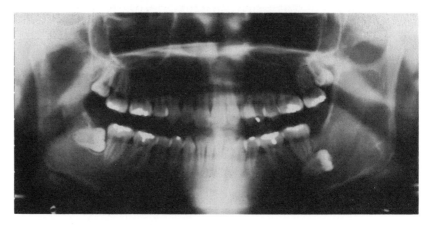

Fig. 7.5. This odontogenic keratocyst involving the left ascending ramus resembled a dentigerous cyst.

Whilst maxillary cysts may expand at the expense of either the labiobuccal or palatal plates of bone, mandibular cysts situated in the body of the lower jaw involve the labiobuccal plate and only rarely affect the lingual plate (*Fig.* 7.4). In fact so rarely is lingual expansion in the mandible due to the presence of a cyst, that many experienced clinicians regard the presence of lingual expansion of the body of the mandible as a sign which indicates the presence of a tumour until proved otherwise. This sign is occasionally associated with the presence of an odontogenic keratocyst (*see* p. 201 and *Fig.* 7.5).

The soft tissues related to a cyst should be carefully dried and examined for the presence of a sinus. Palpation may cause the discharge of a 'glairy' cholesterol-containing fluid or more frequently may produce a yellow purulent discharge in the presence of a sinus.

It is important to notate the erupted teeth present and to test their 'vitality', for whilst dentigerous cysts are related to the crown of an unerupted tooth, dental or radicular cysts are related to the apex of a pulpless tooth or root.

RADIOGRAPHIC APPEARANCES

The classic description of the radiographic appearances of an intra-bony cyst is an area of radiolucency surrounded by a radio-opaque line of condensed bone (*Figs.* 7.1, 7.6*a*). The characteristic margin may not be present when a cyst is either very large, or is infected, or when the contents are draining through a sinus (*Fig.* 7.6*b*). Despite this fact the diagnosis of a mandibular cyst seldom presents much difficulty. However, the radiographic differentiation between a maxillary cyst and the normal maxillary antrum may be extremely difficult on occasions, and when doubt arises the dental surgeon should employ a systematic approach whilst interpreting

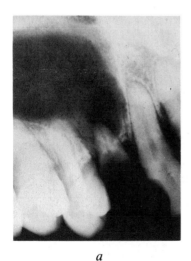
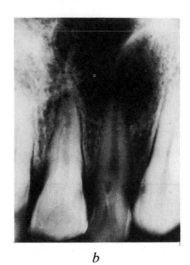

a   *b*

Fig. 7.6. *a*, Typical radiographic appearances of a dental cyst. *b*, Infected dental cyst related to pulpless lateral incisor of dens invaginatus type.

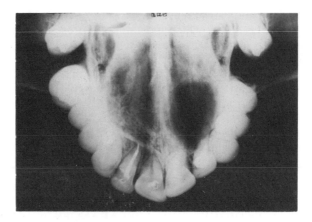

Fig. 7.7. Comparison of the two sides in this anterior occlusal radiograph confirms that the radiolucent area on the left is a cyst.

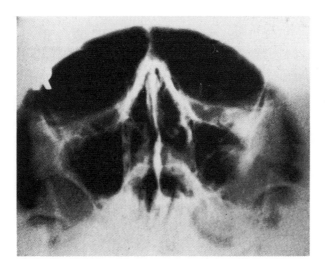

Fig. 7.8. Large dental cyst involving the left antrum.

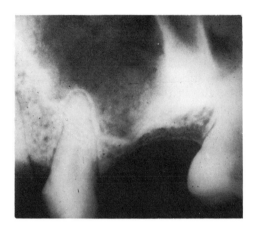

Fig. 7.9. Vascular channels in the wall of the antrum.

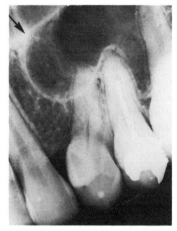

Fig. 7.10. The presence of the 'Y' sign of Ennis and vascular channels indicate that the radiolucent area related to this inadequately treated pulpless second premolar is the antrum.

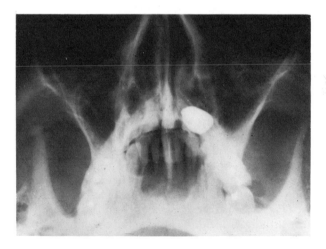

Fig. 7.11. Maxillary cyst filled with contrast medium.

the radiographs. Comparison between sides is a basic surgical principle and similar radiographic views of the identical area on the opposite side of the jaw should be available for inspection. In many instances comparison between the two sides resolves the difficulties (*Fig.* 7.7). An occipitomental view of the sinuses may prove of value in cases in which a large cyst is present (*Fig.* 7.8).

Vascular channels are often seen as branching radiolucent lines in the walls of the normal antrum (*Fig.* 7.9), whilst the differing levels of the normal antral and nasal floors create the so-called 'Y' sign of Ennis in the first premolar region (*Fig.* 7.10). The stem of the 'Y' is formed by the condensed bone of the floor of the nose, the lower arm is the anterior wall of the antrum below it, and the upper arm the anterior wall above it. This authority has also described a 'W' sign which is sometimes seen in the maxillary first molar region when a septum is present in the antrum. The use of these normal anatomical landmarks is often of great assistance when the interpretation of radiographs is undertaken. If doubt still persists the contents of the suspected cyst should be aspirated and examined for the presence of cholesterol crystals. It is essential to use a wide-bore needle as the cyst contents may be viscous. The presence of an odontogenic keratocyst may be detected preoperatively by either subjecting the aspirated liquid to electrophoretic examination or demonstrating the presence of keratinized squames in the cyst fluid (*see* p. 201). If desired, the aspirated fluid may be replaced with a thin contrast medium (e.g., neo-hydriol) and further radiographs taken to reveal the outline and extent of any cyst present (*Fig.* 7.11).

CLINICAL CLASSIFICATION OF CYSTS

Any detailed consideration of the pathological classification of cysts of the jaws is beyond the scope of this book, but certain clinical features of diagnostic value must now be mentioned.

Odontogenic cysts

Dentigerous or *follicular cysts* are related to the crown of an unerupted tooth (*see Figs.* 7.1, 7.2) and so, with the rare exception of the lesion related to a super-numerary tooth (*see Fig.* 6.34) inspection reveals the absence of a tooth from the dental arch (*see* p. 6). The presence of a pulpless tooth or root characterizes a *dental* or *radicular cyst* (*Fig.* 7.3), whilst when an odontogenic cyst is present in an edentulous area of a tooth-bearing portion of the jaws the term *residual cyst* is applied (*Figs.* 7.4, 7.12). Mothers sometimes bring their infants to a dentist for examination when they notice the presence of a pale-blue soft-tissue lesion on the children's gums (*Fig.* 7.13). These *cysts of eruption* overlie the crown of an unerupted tooth, usually a deciduous molar, are completely symptomless, and often burst spontaneously during mastication. If the lesion persists the soft tissue overlying it should be seized with toothed dissecting forceps and excised with a sharp scalpel. This simple manoeuvre can be readily performed under out-patient general anaesthesia and is usually followed by rapid eruption of the underlying tooth.

More rarely cysts are found in the periodontal membrane of an erupted vital tooth. These *lateral periodontal cysts* are usually of small size and are most commonly found in the lower canine, premolar, and third molar regions. Some authorities believe that these lesions may, on occasions, rupture into the gingival crevice and form the basis of an isolated deep periodontal pocket (p. 200 and *Fig.* 7.14). Another rare lesion, the *primordial cyst*, is discussed on p. 201.

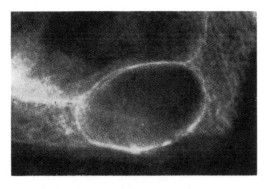

Fig. 7.12. Residual cyst in edentulous molar region which has elevated the antral floor. Note that whilst vascular channels are present in the wall of the antrum they are absent in the wall of the cyst.

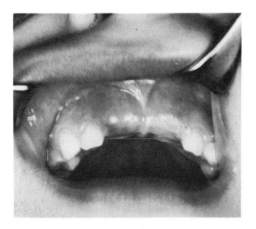

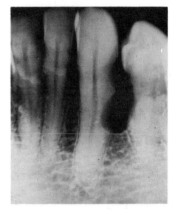

Fig. 7.13. Cyst of eruption related to right upper central incisor.

Fig. 7.14. Lateral periodontal cyst between the left lower canine and first premolar.

Non-odontogenic cysts

In addition to the odontogenic cysts already mentioned a number of non-odontogenic cysts may affect the jaws. The commonest of these is the *incisive canal cyst*, which is often described as being related to two vital central incisors and as appearing to be heart-shaped in radiographs (*Fig.* 7.15). This appearance is partly due to the presence of the anterior nasal spine and partly due to the projection of the cyst between the roots of the central incisors. In some instances and especially in edentulous patients, such a cyst may be either round or oval (*Figs*. 7.16, 7.26). It is sometimes difficult to differentiate on radiographic grounds between a large incisive foramen and an incisive canal cyst. The presence of a slit-like opening into the cyst alongside the incisive papilla may resolve the difficulty, whilst many dental surgeons regard the presence of any radiolucent area in the incisive canal region which has a diameter of 6 mm or more as being diagnostic of a cyst. Although many so-called *globulomaxillary cysts* are in fact dental or radicular cysts related to a pulpless lateral incisor often of the dens

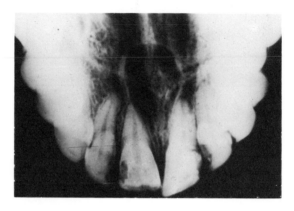

Fig. 7.15.   Incisive canal cyst.

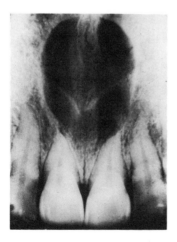

Fig. 7.16.   Large incisive canal cyst.

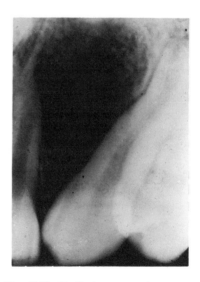

Fig. 7.17.   Radicular cyst related to a pulpless lateral incisor. Note the size and shape of the pulp canal in this tooth.

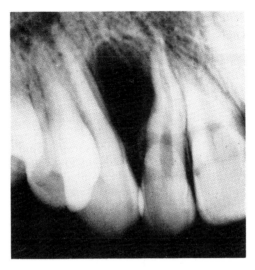

Fig. 7.18. Globulomaxillary cyst.

invaginatus type (*Fig.* 7.17), a true developmental cyst may undoubtedly occur in the region of the lateral incisors in a few very rare instances (*Fig.* 7.18). Marked tilting and displacement of the vital teeth adjacent to the lesion are characteristic of this type of cyst.

Radicular cysts

A radicular cyst arises from epithelial residues in the periodontal ligament, the epithelial cell rests of Malassez, as a result of inflammation which follows the death of the dental pulp. Radicular and residual cysts account for 55% of cystic lesions of the jaw. They are seldom seen in the first decade of life but otherwise have a wide age distribution. These lesions occur more frequently in males than in females, and may arise in any tooth-bearing area in the jaws with the anterior maxilla being the site most commonly involved. Radicular cysts are lined either in whole or in part by stratified squamous epithelium of variable thickness in which either mucous or ciliated cells and deposits of cholesterol crystals are frequently found (*Figs.* 7.3, 7.6 and 7.19).

THE TREATMENT OF CYSTS

All of the commonly used methods of treatment of cysts are modifications of two basic techniques: *total enucleation* and *marsupialization*. Total enucleation is the removal of the entire lining, whilst marsupialization is the conversion of the cyst into a pouch, the lining of which is continuous with the mucosa of the oral cavity. In the latter technique only a portion of the cyst lining is removed, the remainder being retained in situ to line the pouch. By means of marsupialization pressure within the cyst is eliminated and the cyst cavity is gradually obliterated by the regeneration of bone.

Both techniques have advantages and disadvantages, advocates and detractors. Enucleation has the advantage that no pathological tissue is retained. Whilst this is theoretically essential, neoplastic change in the lining of a marsupialized cyst appears to be an extremely rare phenomenon. The lining of a marsupialized cyst is indistinguishable from normal mucoperiosteum on histological grounds a few months after operation, although in one cytological study variable inflammatory changes were almost always present.

Following enucleation bone regeneration is more rapid than after marsupialization, whilst when primary closure of the wound is possible after enucleation the need for the construction of a cyst plug is avoided and both the importance and amount of postoperative care to be undertaken by the patient are reduced to a minimum. Marsupialization minimizes the danger of damage to adjacent structures such as the antrum, nose, the inferior dental nerve and vessels, and adjacent teeth and/or their nerve or blood supply. Although it may be a rather finicky procedure, it is a less severe operation and it is often possible for the occasional oral surgeon to treat a very extensive cyst under local anaesthesia and out-patient conditions by this means. After-pain and swelling are minimal after marsupialization.

Whilst the place of each form of treatment is largely a matter of personal opinion and preference, most authorities would advocate the enucleation of all cysts whenever this is possible without incurring the risk of damage to important structures adjacent to the lesion. The use of this technique undoubtedly causes the

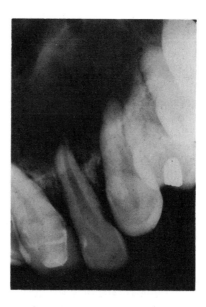

Fig. 7.19. This radicular cyst related to a pulpless lateral incisor of dens invaginatus type in a 14-year-old girl has enveloped the apices of adjacent vital teeth.

minimum postoperative inconvenience to both the dentist and his patient. Marsupialization is indicated when the age and general condition of the patient limit the amount of surgery to be undertaken, or in the treatment of infected cysts in which removal of all the lining cannot be assured due to the friability of the tissue. When the large size or infection of a cyst renders primary closure inadvisable, or the surgery is to be undertaken by an occasional oral surgeon, treatment by marsupialization is often to be preferred. The technique may also be employed to preserve the vitality of the pulps of adjacent teeth, the apices of which are in close relationship to the cyst lining (*Fig.* 7.19). Regardless of the method of treatment employed, the pulpal status of all teeth related to the lesion should be carefully determined both before surgery is undertaken and immediately postoperatively.

Splints should be constructed preoperatively if the size of the lesion makes fracture of the mandible a possibility.

THE TECHNIQUE OF ENUCLEATION

The creation of a large mucoperiosteal flap is an essential preliminary to enucleation of the cyst lining. If the incision is sited well in front of and well behind the lesion in situations in which bone has not been destroyed by the cyst (*Fig.* 7.20*b*), elevation of the soft tissues from the bone is facilitated, for the subperiosteal plane of dissection can be readily determined. The incision must be made down to bone through all layers of the gingiva. Then a periosteal elevator is carefully inserted under the margins of the flap and used to elevate the mucoperiosteum from the underlying bone until the margins of the bony defect are exposed. In this way any area in which the cyst lining is attached to the soft tissues overlying it is visualized. It is often possible to separate these soft-tissue layers without breaching the cyst lining by means of blunt dissection using a periosteal elevator covered in gauze (*Fig.* 7.20*c*). When difficulty is experienced in separating the cyst lining from either the antral or nasal lining on the inferior dental bundle, dissection may often be completed by packing ribbon gauze soaked in 10 vol hydrogen peroxide between the adherent soft tissues. After separating the bony margins of the defect from the cyst lining by means of blunt dissection, the thin bone overlying the lesion is removed with Rongeur forceps until the cyst sac is widely exposed. A plane of cleavage between the soft-tissue lining of the cyst and the enclosing bone is then utilized to deliver the cyst sac in one piece if this is practicable (*Figs.* 7.20*d*, 7.21).

Any tooth or root involved in the cyst is then either extracted or apicected as indicated and the edges of the bony cavity are smoothed. If the remaining bony cavity is small or can be saucerized by judicious bone removal, the wound can be closed by primary suture (*Fig.* 7.20*f*). It is much easier to reduce the size of the residual blood-clot by saucerization and collapsing the periosteum into the wound in the mandible than in the maxilla. Fortunately, organization of even large blood-clots resulting from the removal of cysts from the upper jaw usually proceeds uneventfully. Regardless of site, complete haemostasis must be obtained prior to closure of the wound if breakdown is to be avoided. After closure the cavity is filled with the blood-clot which results from postoperative

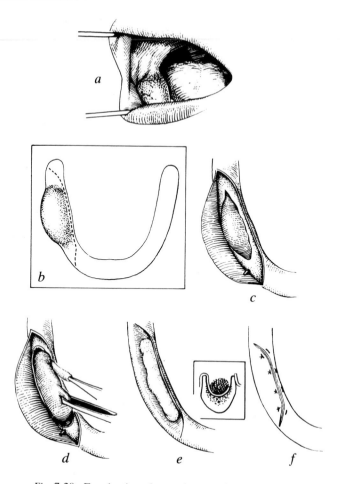

Fig. 7.20. Enucleation of a cyst (*see* text for explanation).

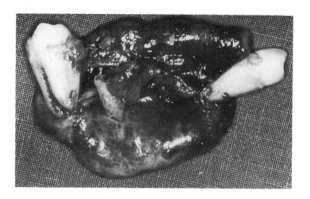

Fig. 7.21. An enucleated cyst sac with attached teeth and root.

oozing. In large infected cysts it is often preferable to turn the mucoperiosteal flap into the cavity and to hold it against the bony wall of the cavity by inserting a ribbon-gauze pack soaked in Whitehead's varnish (*Fig.* 7.20*e* and p. 78). This pack can be left in situ for 2 or 3 weeks postoperatively and when it is removed the bare bone will be seen to be covered with granulation tissue. It may be necessary to insert further packs into the wound until such time as the cavity is either obliterated or completely epithelialized.

It is sometimes possible to preserve ridge form by employing an osteoplastic flap during the enucleation of a cyst (*see* p. 268).

THE TECHNIQUE OF MARSUPIALIZATION

There can be no doubt that the poor opinion of this technique held by many authorities is due at least in part to the fact that in the past it has often been performed badly and that only an inadequate opening has been obtained. If the dentist makes only a small window in the lesion, rapid shrinkage of the annular scar surrounding the ostium occurs and is soon followed by recurrence of the cyst. For this reason any technique of marsupialization must be designed to ensure the patency of the ostium by producing an adequate opening surrounded by the minimum amount of scar tissue.

Before making an incision the dental surgeon must utilize all the clinical and radiographic evidence available to him to estimate the extent of the cyst. This assessment enables him to design a mucoperiosteal flap, the shape and size of which are related to the size of the ostium which will be left at the end of the operation (*Fig.* 7.22*b*). The soft tissues are then elevated to expose the bone overlying the lesion which is removed, by means of hand pressure on a sharp chisel or the use of Rongeur forceps, to expose the cystic sac which is maintained intact if practicable (*Fig.* 7.22*c, d*). Bone is excised until the cyst is as widely exposed as possible and the margins of the resultant bony defect are smoothed with a bone file. An incision shaped like a St. Andrew's cross is then made in the cyst lining (*Fig.* 7.22*e*), and the four triangular flaps which are thus created are turned outwards over the cut edges of the mucoperiosteum attached to the margins of the bony wound. These flaps are then sutured to the surrounding soft tissues, horizontal mattress sutures being used to suture the base of the mucoperiosteal flap to the cyst lining adjacent to it (*Fig.* 7.22*f*). The mucoperiosteal flap and excesses of the cyst lining are then removed and the latter sent for histological examination (*Fig.* 7.22*g*).

Any teeth involved in the lesion are either extracted or treated by means of apicectomy. Then the marsupialized cyst cavity is either packed with ribbon gauze soaked in bismuth iodoform paste or flavine emulsion, or a temporary cyst plug is made in black gutta-percha (*Fig.* 7.23*b*) and inserted. Whitehead's varnish is not favoured for this purpose as it occasionally sets hard and the pack may then be difficult to remove from undercuts. In some cases, and particularly in infected cysts, the excessive friability of the cyst lining makes the insertion of sutures at the margins of the cavity impracticable, and in these cases the ribbon-gauze pack can be used to hold the cyst lining and the cut surfaces of the mucoperiosteum at the edges of the wound together.

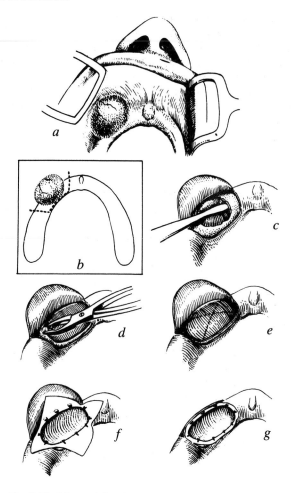

Fig. 7.22. Marsupialization of a cyst (*see* text for explanation).

One week after operation the pack and sutures are removed and either a cyst plug or an extension to an existing denture are made in black gutta-percha in order to keep the ostium of the cyst cavity patent. *Fig*. 7.23*b* shows how the plug is made to fit the ostium only and to exert no pressure on the remainder of the cyst cavity, whilst *Fig*. 7.23*c* shows how well-planned bone removal at operation makes it possible to utilize the flange of the denture to maintain the patency of the ostium without the use of a separate cyst plug (*Fig*. 7.23*d*).

If desired the black gutta-percha cyst plug can be replaced with one made of acrylic resin at a later date. At regular intervals the appliance should be reduced in depth but not in width, as it is essential to keep the ostium patent and minimize soiling of the cavity, whilst the defect fills up from its bottom and sides. The patient should be provided with a small syringe, such as that illustrated in *Fig*. 7.24, and instructed to use it after meals to cleanse the cyst cavity.

It must not be forgotten that unless an adequate ostium is secured and maintained the cyst will recur. On occasions it may be justifiable to use 'temporary' marsupialization for a period in order to reduce the size of the lesion and thus facilitate its enucleation at a later date. Many dental surgeons would employ such a procedure when treating a child who had a large cyst which involved the apices of a number of vital teeth. Enucleation of the lining of such a lesion might prejudice the retention of these teeth if performed immediately, while shrinkage of the marsupialized lesion might enhance the chances of retaining the involved teeth. Difficulty is sometimes experienced at the second operation in creating mucoperiosteal flaps of the size and shape required to obtain closure of the wound.

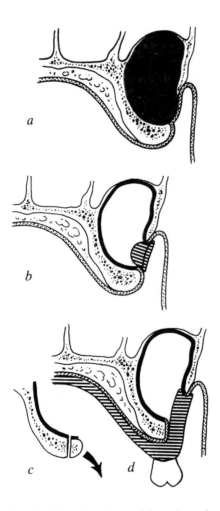

Fig. 7.23. Methods of maintaining the patency of the ostium of a marsupialized cyst (*see* text for explanation).

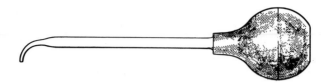

Fig. 7.24. Glass socket syringe with rubber bulb.

It is the practice of some ENT surgeons to marsupialize maxillary dental cysts into the antrum via a Caldwell–Luc operation, and then to perform an intranasal antrostomy. This technique has the disadvantage of leaving any existing deformity of the alveolar ridge, which may cause a prosthetic difficulty, whilst the removal of a tooth or root in relationship to the lesion may result in the creation of an oro-antral communication.

DIAGNOSTIC FEATURES AND TREATMENT OF OTHER TYPES OF ODONTOGENIC CYST

Cyst of eruption

This lesion is most commonly seen in the mouths of infants as a pale-blue fluctuant cyst overlying an unerupted tooth (*see Fig*. 7.13). The lesion is symptomless and often bursts spontaneously. If rupture does not occur in this manner, the soft tissues surmounting the lesion should be seized in toothed tweezers and excised with a scalpel.

Dentigerous (follicular) cyst

A dentigerous cyst contains the crown of an unerupted tooth, which may be either one of the normal series or a supernumerary (*see Fig*. 7.1). They represent about 17% of all jaw cysts, occur over a wide age range and are often related to an impacted tooth. Thus the mandibular third molar, maxillary permanent canine, mandibular premolars and the maxillary third molars are the teeth most frequently involved in that order. The lesions are believed to arise in the dental follicle which has been shown to have an important role in the resorption of bone. Dentigerous cysts appear to have a greater tendency than other simple jaw cysts to produce resorption of the roots of adjacent teeth. The radiographic appearances of a dentigerous cyst may be seen in the presence of other lesions such as an odontogenic keratocyst and so diagnosis must be confirmed histologically. In some patients below the age of 20 years it is possible to marsupialize the cyst and allow the tooth related to it to erupt into its normal position (*see Fig*. 7.2), but in the majority of cases the cyst should be enucleated and the related tooth extracted.

Lateral periodontal cyst

Any cyst occurring in the periodontal membrane between the base of the gingival crevice and the apex of the tooth is by definition a lateral periodontal cyst.

Although some of these lesions are related to an aberrant pulp canal of an adjacent pulpless tooth, it is customary to reserve the description 'lateral periodontal cyst' for the lesions related to vital teeth. These are most commonly seen in relationship to mandibular canines, premolars, and third molars (*see Fig.* 7.14). They are believed by some periodontists to play a role in the aetiology of isolated deep periodontal pockets, by becoming compound to the mouth via the gingival crevice. These lesions should be enucleated via a large mucoperiosteal flap without extraction of the related vital teeth, except in the case of mandibular third molars.

Primordial cyst

Approximately 11% of all jaw cysts are primordial cysts. They occur over a wide age range, especially in the second and third decades and in the older age groups. They are found more frequently in males than females and are believed to be due to cystic change occurring in either the dental lamina, the basal cells of the oral mucosa or the enamel organ before calcification commences and are most commonly seen in the ascending ramus of the mandible. The lesion may either replace a tooth from the normal dentition or arise from a supernumerary tooth bud. Primordial cysts often have thin friable linings and complete enucleation of them is a notoriously difficult undertaking. As they have a tendency to recur unless removal is complete, these operations are usually best undertaken by specialists working with full hospital facilities. Some authorities believe that primordial cysts may be the seat of neoplastic change if left untreated.

'Odontogenic keratocysts'

In recent years it has become apparent that some odontogenic cysts have a tendency to form daughter cysts and are more likely to recur after enucleation. Such lesions are called 'odontogenic keratocysts' and clinically resemble either dentigerous or residual cysts rather than radicular cysts. They do not appear to be of inflammatory origin and are regarded by many authorities as being primordial in origin. Histological examination of an odontogenic keratocyst reveals the presence of a lining of stratified squamous epithelium which is but a few cells thick and devoid of rete pegs. The basal layer is composed of columnar cells with either pyknotic or vesicular nuclei, whilst the surface is composed of either a keratinized or parakeratinized layer of cells. Keratinized squames may be present in the cyst fluid which is sometimes cheesy in consistency. If cyst fluid is aspirated from such a lesion and subjected to electrophoretic examination, it is found to have a very low content of soluble proteins in comparison with the patient's serum (*Fig.* 7.25A). As fluids from simple dental cysts contain albumin in amounts similar to that found in blood serum, this difference is of diagnostic significance. Determination of the total soluble protein content of the cyst fluid (*Fig.* 7.25B) may also be of great value, for as far as is known at present odontogenic keratocysts exhibit no characteristic signs and symptoms, and great difficulty is often experienced in differentiating them from either simple cysts or ameloblastomata (*see below*). A preoperative diagnosis of odontogenic keratocyst forewarns the oral surgeon that wide excision of the lesion, including the removal of any soft tissue and cancellous bone immediately related to it, is indicated.

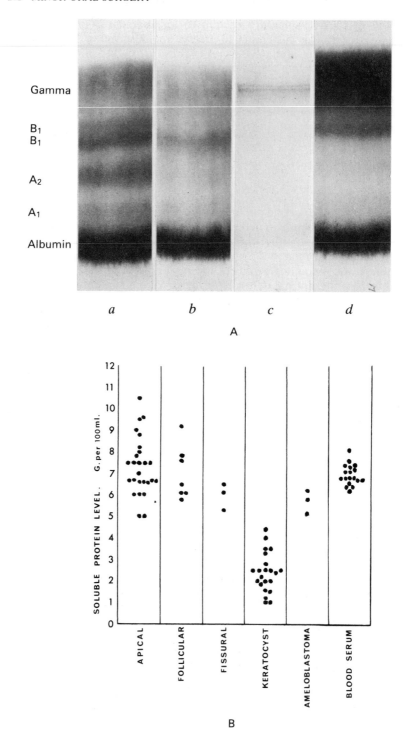

Fig. 7.25. A, A series of four electrophoretograms, the cathodic pole above, the anode below. *a,* Normal serum control showing typical protein bands of albumin, alpha-, beta-, and gammaglobulins. *b,* Typical apical or dentigerous cyst fluid showing absence or diminution of the larger moleculed globulins. *c,* Fluid from a keratocyst showing absence of soluble proteins. *d,* Fluid from an uninfected apical cyst showing typical diminution of alpha-globulins but with a high concentration of gammaglobulin. This raised gammaglobulin (immunoglobulin) level is frequently seen, and may represent the presence of a local immune reaction to the cyst and its contents. B, Chart showing measured levels of total soluble proteins from various types of cysts of the jaws and sera. A soluble protein level below 4·0 g/100 ml may strongly suggest keratocyst, while levels above 5·0 g/100 ml suggest other types of cyst.

THE DIAGNOSIS AND TREATMENT OF NON-ODONTOGENIC CYSTS OF THE JAWS

Incisive canal cysts

These lesions, which are sometimes called nasopalatine duct cysts, account for approximately 12% of all jaw cysts. Males are affected most frequently and the presence of the cyst is usually detected in the fourth, fifth or sixth decades of life. Incisive canal cysts have extremely variable epithelial linings and are thought to arise from vestigial epithelial-lined structures found in the nasopalatine canal. Such cysts may create difficulties in diagnosis, especially when appearing in radiographs to be related to pulpless central incisors. The lesion is classically described as being heart-shaped. This appearance is due to the shadows cast by the anterior nasal spine and the roots of the central incisors (*see Fig.* 7.15). Incisive canal cysts may be round in shape when present in an edentulous maxilla (*Fig.* 7.26).

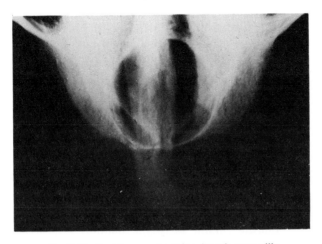

Fig. 7.26. Incisive canal cyst in edentulous maxilla.

These lesions are often symptomless and are discovered by accident when radiographs are taken for some other purpose. On other occasions the patient may complain of pain in the region of the incisive papilla or of a salty-tasting discharge from this area. In these circumstances examination may reveal the presence of either a tender inflammatory swelling or a slit-like sinus at the side of the incisive papilla, through which a probe can be passed into the lesion.

It is frequently difficult to decide on radiographic findings alone whether a large incisive canal or an incisive canal cyst is present. As a matter of convenience it is usual to regard all lesions more than 6 mm in diameter as cysts and to put smaller lesions 'on probation'.

Incisive canal cysts should be carefully enucleated, an operation made difficult by the friability of the cyst sac, its adhesion to the overlying mucoperiosteum, and the projection of the lining up the incisive canal which is often present. Removal is facilitated if a large palatal flap is raised after the gingival crevices from first premolar to first premolar have been incised vertically.

Globulomaxillary cysts

Although many of the lesions described as globulomaxillary cysts are in reality radicular cysts in relationship to a pulpless lateral incisor (*see Fig*. 7.17), developmental cysts in the maxillary lateral incisor region occasionally occur (*see Fig*. 7.18). The vitality of all the related teeth should be tested prior to operation and it will be found that many teeth, whose roots appear on radiography to be hopelessly involved, will give a normal response. Whilst it may be possible to preserve the vitality of such teeth by the use of marsupialization, the resultant cyst cavity seldom fills up completely and enucleation should be performed when the size of the marsupialized cyst has decreased sufficiently to permit this to be undertaken without prejudicing the vitality of the related teeth.

AMELOBLASTOMA

This lesion was once called a 'multilocular cyst' and is often included in lists of odontogenic cysts. It is in fact a locally malignant tumour of dental origin which rarely, if ever, metastasizes and may occur in either a cystic or a solid form, or as a combination of both. As both the prognosis and treatment of the ameloblastoma vary markedly from those of simple cysts the dental surgeon must ensure that his diagnosis of a cystic lesion in the jaw is correct. Whilst the ameloblastoma may affect either jaw it is most frequently found in the ascending ramus and posterior part of the body of the mandible. Simple cysts rarely cause expansion of the lingual plate of the body of the mandible and the presence of this sign should be taken as an indication of the presence of tumour until proved otherwise. Whilst in the radiographs the roots of teeth adjacent to either lesion may be seen to be resorbed, the resorption tends to be sharply defined in the presence of a cyst (*Fig*. 7.27) whilst in the ameloblastoma it is often ragged. The classic 'soap bubble' sign (*Fig*. 7.28) is unfortunately not present in all cases of ameloblastoma.

A definitive diagnosis cannot be made without biopsy examination (*see* p. 332) and it is imperative that an adequate specimen be obtained if the presence of tumour is to be detected. Ameloblastoma is treated by wide local excision.

If the general dental practitioner suspects the presence of either an extensive cyst or an ameloblastoma he should refer the patient to a colleague who possesses both the skill and facilities to investigate thoroughly and treat effectively such a lesion.

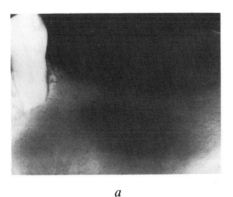
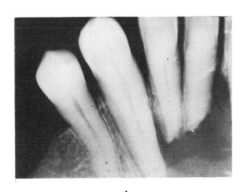

a   *b*

Fig. 7.27. Resorption of vital teeth adjacent to, *a*, radicular cyst and, *b*, ameloblastoma.

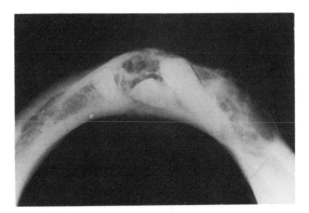

Fig. 7.28. 'Soap-bubble' radiographic appearance of an ameloblastoma.

SUGGESTED READING

Browne R. M. (1970) The odontogenic keratocyst. Clinical aspects. *Br. Dent. J.* **128**, 225–31.
Cabrini R. L., Barros R. E. and Albano H. (1970) Cysts of the jaws: a statistical analysis. *J. Oral Surg.* **28**, 485–9.
Ten Cate A. R. (1972) The epithelial cell rests of Malassez and the genesis of the dental cyst. *Oral Surg.* **34**, 956–64.
Chuong R., Donoff R. B. and Guralnick W. (1982) The odontogenic keratocyst. *J. Oral Maxillofac. Surg.* **40**, 797–802.

Fickling B. W. (1965) Cysts of the jaw: a long-term survey of types and treatment. *Proc. R. Soc. Med.* **58**, 847–54.

Fordyce G. L. (1956) Probable nature of so-called haemorrhagic cysts of the mandible. *Br. Dent. J.* **101**, 40–2.

Hopper F. E. (1982) Bilateral cysts of the mandible. *Br. Dent. J.* **153**, 306–7.

Howe G. L. (1965) Haemorrhagic cysts of the mandible. *Br. J. Oral Surg.* **3**, 55–91.

Killey H. C., Kay L. W. and Seward G. R. (1977) *Benign Cystic Lesions of the Jaws, their Diagnosis and Treatment*, 3rd ed. Edinburgh, Churchill.

Kramer I. R. H. (1963) Ameloblastoma: a clinico-pathological appraisal. *Br. J. Oral Surg.* **1**, 13–28.

Rud J. and Pindborg J. J. (1969) Odontogenic keratocysts: a follow-up study of 21 cases. *J. Oral Surg.* **27**, 323–30.

Schulz P., von Skerst H., Rummel H. H. et al. (1981) Cytological findings in cases of marsupialised odontogenic cysts. *J. Max. Fac. Surg.* **9**, 35–41.

Seward G. R. (1965) Dermoid cysts of the floor of the mouth. *Br. J. Oral Surg.* **3**, 36–47.

Toller P. A. (1967) Origin and growth of cysts of the jaws. *Ann. R. Coll. Surg.* **40**, 306–66.

Toller P. A. (1970) Protein substances in odontogenic cyst fluids. *Br. Dent. J.* **128**, 317–22.

Toller P. A. (1970) The osmolality of fluids from cysts of the jaws. *Br. Dent. J.* **129**, 275–8.

Voorsmit R. A. C. A., Stoelinga P. J. W. and van Haelst J. G. M. (1981) The management of keratocysts. *J. Max. Fac. Surg.* **9**, 228–36.

Wilkinson F. C. (1952) Adamantinoma: a review of twelve cases. *Med. Press* **228**, 90–8.

Chapter 8

Extractions and the maxillary antrum

The maxillary air sinus, or antrum, is a pyramid-shaped cavity situated within the maxilla. It is of importance in the practice of dentistry for not only must antral disease, such as inflammation and neoplasia, be considered during the differential diagnosis of dental disease but the air sinus may be involved during oral surgical procedures.

The nerves and blood vessels which supply the teeth pass between the bony wall and antral lining to enter the apices of the tooth roots. Pathological lesions occurring in the antrum may involve these nerves and cause symptoms in and around the teeth (*see* p. 221). Great difficulty may be experienced in differentiating between a maxillary cyst and the antral cavity during the interpretation of radiographs (*see* p. 187).

Dental infections may involve the antrum either by direct spread or via the lymphatic system and cause maxillary sinusitis. It has been claimed that as many as 20% of all cases of sinusitis are of dental origin. Patients afflicted with such a condition frequently complain of an offensive odour in the nose which is not detectable to others.

ANTRAL INVOLVEMENT DURING TOOTH EXTRACTION

The size of the maxillary antrum varies between individuals and the right and left antra are not uncommonly found to be of different sizes in the same patient.

The roots of all the upper cheek teeth from the first premolar to the maxillary third molar may be in close relationship to the antrum. In some instances as much as one-half of the length of the roots of these teeth may form part of the wall of the antrum and may only be separated from the cavity of the air sinus by paper-thin bone and the mucosal lining of the antrum (*Fig.* 8.1). The thin bone enclosing the roots may exhibit deficiencies in some patients whilst in others it is destroyed by pathological processes related to the apices of the teeth (*Figs.* 8.2, 8.3). In a minority of cases acute and chronic maxillary sinusitis may complicate dental infections.

During the extraction of a tooth related to the air sinus, an oro-antral communication may be created and either the whole tooth or a root be displaced into the antrum. Whilst the basic cause of both these complications is the presence of a large air sinus, fewer roots would be pushed into antra if the following precautionary measures were taken more frequently.

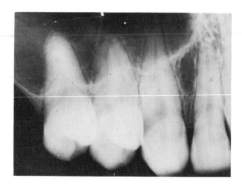

Fig. 8.1. Periapical radiograph showing an abnormally large antrum extending forwards to the lateral incisor area.

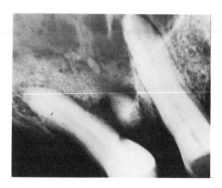

Fig. 8.2. Loss of antral floor due to chronic inflammation associated with 4| root.

The dental surgeon should never attempt to apply forceps to a maxillary cheek tooth, or root, unless a sufficient amount of both its palatal and buccal surfaces are exposed to permit the blades to be applied under direct vision (*see* p. 97 and *Fig.* 4.16).

As a general rule it is better to leave in situ the apical one-third of the palatal root of a vital maxillary molar if it is fractured during forceps extraction, unless there is a positive indication for its removal. Successful 'transalveolar' removal of such root fragments necessitates the sacrifice of a large amount of alveolar bone and in most instances it is good practice to put the fragment 'on probation'. Palatal root fragments of vital teeth seldom cause symptoms and can always be removed if and when they do so. The patient should be informed that a root fragment has been left and told the reason for this decision. A note must be made in the patient's case records that a root has been retained and should include such details as size and site.

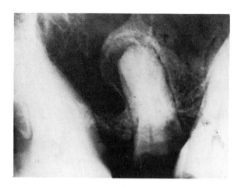

Fig. 8.3. Periapical granuloma on premolar root eroding bony floor of antrum.

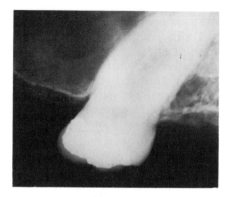

Fig. 8.4. The alveolar bone enclosing this isolated maxillary molar is weakened by an extension of the antrum.

If a patient requests the removal of an isolated maxillary molar tooth or gives a history of antral involvement complicating previous extractions, the removal of the tooth should not be undertaken until a pre-extraction radiograph has been carefully studied. A history of antral involvement complicating previous extractions probably indicates the presence of a large maxillary air sinus and a thin antral floor. The alveolar bone supporting an isolated maxillary molar is often weakened by an extension of the antral cavity into it and the extraction of such a tooth with forceps may be complicated by either the creation of an oro-antral communication, the displacement of a root into the sinus, or fracture of the maxillary tuberosity (*Fig.* 8.4).

The operator should never attempt to deliver fractured maxillary roots by passing an elevator or Coupland's chisel up the socket. When removal of any maxillary root is indicated it should be preceded by accurate localization based upon a thorough clinical investigation and the careful interpretation of good radiographs (*see* p. 103). A 'transalveolar' approach should be employed to remove such a root.

THE REMOVAL OF TOOTH ROOTS FROM THE ANTRAL FLOOR

The removal of maxillary roots or teeth by dissection should be performed under direct vision. After a large mucoperiosteal flap has been raised, sufficient bone

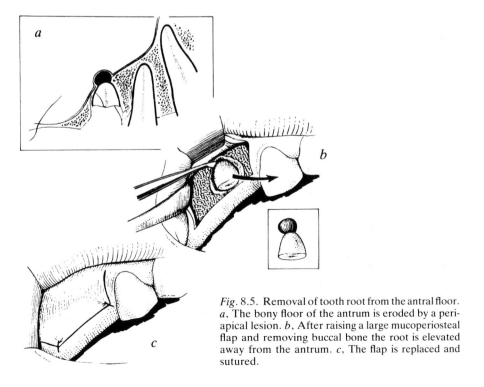

Fig. 8.5. Removal of tooth root from the antral floor. *a*, The bony floor of the antrum is eroded by a peri-apical lesion. *b*, After raising a large mucoperiosteal flap and removing buccal bone the root is elevated away from the antrum. *c*, The flap is replaced and sutured.

should be removed to permit the insertion of an elevator above the broken surface of the root. Force can then be applied in such a manner that the root is moved away from the antrum (*Fig.* 8.5*b*). If the extraction is complicated by the creation of an oro-antral communication the large buccal mucoperiosteal flap should be used to repair it as described below.

ORO-ANTRAL COMMUNICATIONS

Despite every care being exercised, oro-antral openings will sometimes be created during the extraction of maxillary cheek teeth from patients with large antra. If promptly diagnosed and correctly treated they usually heal without incident.

If the operator suspects that the antrum has been opened he should attempt to confirm his suspicions by means of the 'nose-blowing' test, in which the patient attempts to blow through his occluded nares with his mouth open. In the presence of an oro-antral communication, air will be heard to pass through the defect, and will displace a wisp of cotton-wool held over the socket, whilst any blood present in the socket will be seen to bubble. Examination of the fragment of bone attached to the tooth will reveal that its upper surface is composed of smooth condensed bone if the antral floor has been breached (*see Fig.* 8.19*b*).

Whilst the nose-blowing test is not always positive in the presence of an oro-antral communication it is seldom, if ever, necessary to pass instruments or silver probes into the *freshly opened* antrum and *never* necessary to squirt fluid into the air sinus to confirm the diagnosis. Such manoeuvres carry the risk of contaminating the antrum with oral micro-organisms. Unless the suspicion that the antrum has been opened can be disproved, the case should be treated as if an oro-antral opening is present.

TREATMENT OF THE NEWLY CREATED ORO-ANTRAL COMMUNICATION

The factors which cause an oro-antral communication to persist are the size of the bony defect and the presence of infection in the maxillary antrum, and treatment must be planned with these factors in mind. As a newly created opening heals by organization of a blood clot, the dental surgeon must try to provide support for this blood clot and to prevent the ingress of organisms into the air sinus. The patient must not be allowed to rinse the mouth until the defect is repaired or the antrum will be contaminated with oral flora, some of which may become pathogenic in their new environment and cause infection. If circumstances permit, the bony defect should then be covered with a mucoperiosteal flap. Various methods of achieving this aim are available for use, and the choice of technique to be employed should be governed by the surgical experience of the operator and the facilities and operating time at his disposal when the complication occurs. In cases of doubt specialist aid should be enlisted (*see* Chapter 16).

The simplest method is illustrated in *Fig.* 8.6 and requires the minimum time, surgical skill, and facilities. Mucoperiosteal flaps, obtained by reducing the height of the bony socket, are loosely sutured over the defect. The use of a suitably trimmed piece of chemically treated lyophilized sterilized collagen sheeting

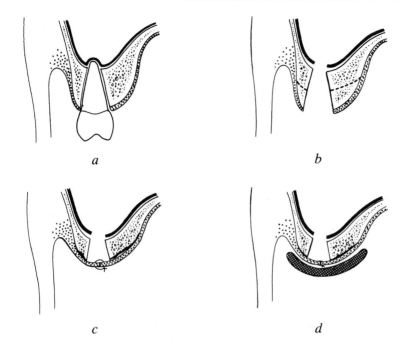

Fig. 8.6. The treatment of a newly created oro-antral communication (*see* text for explanation).

prepared from porcine dermis to cover the bony defect has recently been advocated. After trimming the material to shape with scissors, buccal and palatal extensions of it are placed under the adjacent buccal and palatal mucoperiosteum, the edges of which are sutured together to provide support.

Whenever conditions permit, it is better to use an undercut buccal flap lined with periosteum as illustrated in *Fig.* 8.7. A broad-based buccal flap is raised by means of subperiosteal dissection, which is carried out well above the reflection of the mucous membrane (*Fig.* 8.7*a*). A horizontal cut is then made through the periosteum alone above the reflection (*Fig.* 8.7*b, c*) and the inherent elasticity of the mucous membrane then permits the mucosa to be advanced and sutured to the palatal mucoperiosteum without tension (*Fig.* 8.7*d, e*). It is convenient to incise the periosteum with a No. 12 scalpel blade (*see Fig.* 3.11). This incision is often complicated by a brisk haemorrhage which should be arrested by means of pressure exerted upon a hot saline pack (49 °C) before the undercut flap is sutured into place. Horizontal mattress sutures should be employed for this purpose and left in situ for 2 weeks. This is an excellent method of repair which, however, requires more operating time and surgical skill than the method previously described, and is often accompanied by some postoperative haematoma formation and loss of depth in the buccal sulcus (*Fig.* 8.8*b*). Uneventful primary repair at the 2-month follow-up appointment can be interpreted as a permanent repair, whilst any loss of sulcus depth present at that time is likely to persist.

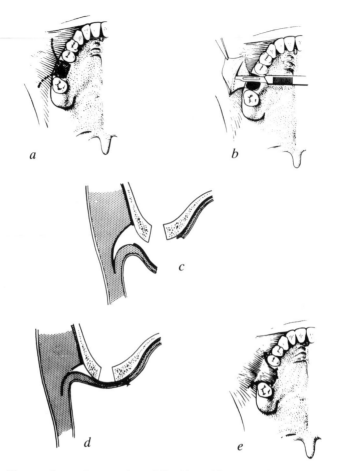

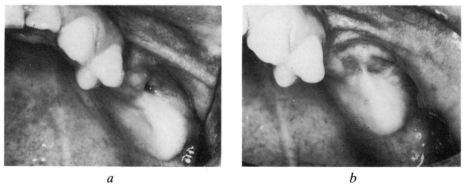

Fig. 8.7. The use of an undercut periosteal-lined buccal flap to repair an oro-antral opening. The cross-hatched area must be excised when a chronic oro-antral fistula is treated (*see* text for explanation).

Fig. 8.8. A large oro-antral fistula in ⌊6 region (*a*) has been soundly repaired with a buccal flap, but some loss of sulcus depth has occurred (*b*).

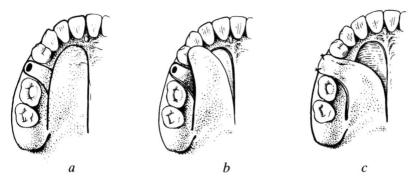

Fig. 8.9. The use of a palatal flap to repair an oro-antral fistula situated high up in the buccal sulcus.

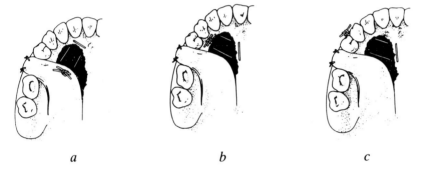

Fig. 8.10. Suturing a pack over a bare area of the palate. *a*, Incorrect, *b* and *c*, Correct (*see* text for explanation).

It is not always possible to cover oro-antral communications situated high up in the sulcus with a buccal flap, even when the soft tissues lying either behind or in front of the defect are utilized. In such cases it is often better to use a palatal mucoperiosteal flap based upon its blood supply (*Fig.* 8.9). Palatal flaps tend to shrink when elevated from the bone and their thickness and consistency make them more difficult to reposition than buccal flaps. The bare bony base of the resultant palatal defect may be covered by a pack, composed of Whitehead's varnish on ribbon gauze, held in position by means of mattress sutures inserted into the margins of the attached mucoperiosteum. Sutures passed through the flap itself for this purpose may pull it away from its new position towards the donor area and so these retaining sutures should be inserted only into the attached mucoperiosteum (*Fig.* 8.10*b* and *c*).

Whichever method is utilized to cover the bony defect, additional support for the repair should be provided by covering the area with either an acrylic extension to a denture, a shellac base-plate, a thin sheet of black gutta-percha or composition, or the outer covering of a cotton-wool roll impregnated with zinc oxide and oil of cloves paste. The cover may be either ligated to adjacent teeth if any are present or sutured to the gum in edentulous regions.

The patient should be instructed to blow his nose only when he is forced to do so, and then to blow it *without* first occluding the nares by pinching his nose between finger and thumb. Decongestant nose drops and inhalations should be prescribed and the patient should be carefully instructed in the method of using them.

NOSE DROPS AND INHALATIONS

The ostium of the maxillary antrum is situated high up on the wall of the sinus (*Fig.* 8.11) and decongestant nose drops and inhalations should be prescribed for use by the patient whenever it is essential to ensure the patency of this natural opening. This is necessary in the presence of maxillary sinusitis and during the post-operative period after the repair of an oro-antral communication. Ephedrine nasal drops BPC contain ephedrine hydrochloride 1% and chlorbutol 0·5% in normal saline, and if used in combination with either benzoin inhalation BPC or Karvol inhalant capsules are ideal for this purpose if correctly used. As many patients appear to believe that the floor of the nose goes vertically upwards rather than backwards, it is essential to detail carefully the method of use of nose drops or inhalations whenever they are prescribed.

When using the nose drops the patient should lie across a bed or couch, with his head hanging over the edge at a lower level than his trunk. His face should be turned so that the side on which the affected antrum is situated is in the most

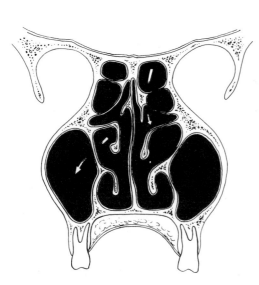

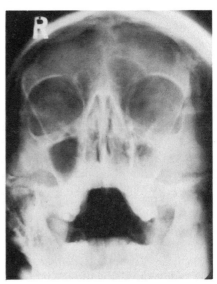

Fig. 8.11. Diagrammatic transverse section of the maxilla. The ostium of the antrum is arrowed and opens into the middle meatus of the lateral nasal wall.

Fig. 8.12. Occipitomental radiograph of a patient with an acute infection of the left antrum.

dependent position. Three drops of the solution are then placed in the appropriate nostril and allowed to trickle backwards until they are tasted by the patient. Nose drops should be used in this way twice or three times daily and if possible the patient should take an inhalation immediately after inserting the nose drops. If Tinct. Benzoin. Co. inhalations are prescribed the patient should be warned that, as the substance is messy, only a receptable which can either be cleansed or discarded at the end of the course of treatment should be used for this purpose. An old pudding basin is an excellent receptacle for the purpose, and after a pint of boiling water has been placed in it 1 teaspoonful of the inhalant should be floated on the surface of the water. The patient then sits with his nose above the resultant solution, covers his head with a towel, and takes 40 good sniffs.

This regime should be instituted whenever a freshly created oro-antral opening has been repaired and should be continued until healing is complete. In such cases it is usual to leave intra-oral sutures in situ for 2 weeks, unless they become either loose or infected.

Although most patients with acute maxillary sinusitis quickly obtain relief from their symptoms by using decongestant nose drops and inhalations, it is sometimes necessary to supplement this treatment with antibiotic therapy (*see* *Fig*. 8.12 and p. 249).

In the vast majority of patients the measures described above lead to spontaneous healing of the oro-antral communication. If a fistula persists the patient should be referred for a second opinion. A fistula is usually defined as an abnormal communication between the lumen of one viscus and either the lumen of another or a body surface. It is customary to apply the term oro-antral fistula to any persistent communication between the antrum and the mouth which has become either wholly or partially epithelialized.

CHRONIC ORO-ANTRAL FISTULAE

Most patients afflicted with a chronic oro-antral fistula are best treated in specialist oral surgery centres to which they should be referred by the general dental practitioner (*see* p. 398).

The first aim of treatment is to eliminate any coexisting antral infection (*Figs*. 8.12, 8.13). Oro-antral reflux can be prevented by the insertion of a well-fitting acrylic base-plate, which covers the defect without entering it. The antrum is washed out with warm normal saline, usually via the fistula, twice weekly until a clean return is obtained. Decongestant nose drops and inhalations are prescribed for use by the patient and antibiotic therapy is sometimes required. When selecting the antibiotic to be employed it must be remembered that in one study of paranasal sinusitis a pure culture of anaerobic organisms was obtained in 12% of the patients and a mixed culture of aerobic and anaerobic organisms in 21% of cases (*see* p. 255).

When treatment of this nature is employed most oro-antral fistulae shrink in size and may even heal spontaneously, especially if any epithelium lining the track is removed either by cauterizing the track with a silver-nitrate solution or trichloracetic acid, or by freshening the edges of the fistulous track with a barbed broach. Persistent oro-antral fistulae can be closed with either an undercut periosteal-lined buccal flap or a palatal mucoperiosteal flap (*see Figs*. 8.7, 8.9). Whenever it

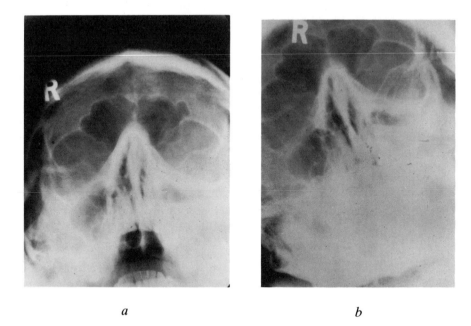

a   b

Fig. 8.13. Occipitomental radiograph of a patient with a left-sided chronic sinusitis. N.B. The fluid level seen in (*a*) moves when the head is tilted (*b*).

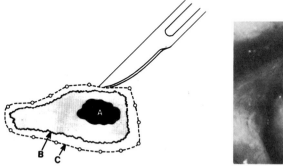

Fig. 8.14. Determining the correct line of incision prior to the repair of an oro-antral fistula (*see* text for explanation).

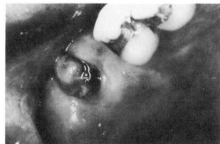

Fig. 8.15. Polypoid tissue prolapsing through an oro-antral fistula.

is possible the dentist should design this flap in such a way as to ensure that its margins are supported by bone during the postoperative period. To this end it is helpful to determine the precise extent of the bony defect by the use of a sharp probe before incising the soft tissues. *Fig*. 8.14 illustrates that the soft-tissue defect (A) provides no indication whatsoever of the precise size and shape of the underlying bony defect (B). The line of incision is shown at (C). Until the bony defect is outlined in this way at operation it may not be possible to make the correct choice of donor area in some cases. In the presence of persistent chronic infection of the air sinus either an intra-nasal or extra-nasal antrostomy may be required if successful closure of the fistula is to be achieved. However, all therapeutic measures designed to combat the infection should be employed before such radical surgery is undertaken for it may be associated with such postoperative complaints as headache and neuralgia.

The antral lining is sometimes said to prolapse through any defect in the bony wall of the maxillary air sinus (*Fig*. 8.15). Although it has been believed that such a prolapse is composed of healthy intact antral lining, experience reveals that these soft-tissue projections are usually polypoid in nature. In the vast majority of instances careful examination will reveal the presence of an oro-antral fistula and a chronically infected antrum.

It is imperative that such lesions should be biopsied and sent for histological examination at the earliest opportunity. In the absence of tumour the condition may be treated in the manner outlined above.

DISPLACEMENT OF A TOOTH OR ROOT INTO THE ANTRUM

This complication of tooth extraction is most likely to occur when the bony floor of the antrum has been eroded by a periapical lesion (*see Figs*. 8.2 and 8.3). Isolation of a maxillary cheek tooth predisposes to this accident, for the antral cavity tends to invade the surrounding edentulous areas whilst the supporting alveolar bone is often condensed in response to the increased occlusal load, thus rendering fracture of a root during extraction more likely. For this reason it is better to remove such teeth by dissection. The incidence of this mishap, in which the root displaced is most frequently that of a first permanent molar, could be greatly reduced if the simple precautions outlined on p. 208 were observed.

If a tooth or root is displaced into the antrum whilst a patient is under endotracheal anaesthesia, it should be removed via a Caldwell–Luc approach via the canine fossa, suitably modified to permit an adequate closure of the concomitant oro-antral communication. This technique is a form of extra-nasal antrostomy.

However, in most instances the patient is an out-patient being treated under either local or nitrous-oxide anaesthesia. In these circumstances the dental surgeon should perform a simple repair of the oro-antral opening (*see Fig*. 8.6) and make no attempt to recover the root, either by the passing of instruments or snares into the antrum via the socket or by enlarging the bony defect. He should then refer the patient to either a specialist oral surgeon or an ENT specialist for treatment (*see* Chapter 16). Foreign bodies should be removed from the maxillary air sinus as soon as is practicable, for their presence may be associated with chronic infection, rhinolith formation, or both of these undesirable sequelae.

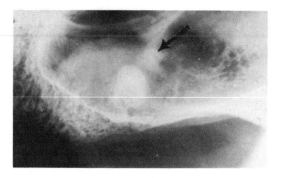

Fig. 8.16. At operation the arrowed root fragment was found to be lying loosely in the left maxillary sinus, whilst the lower root was in the palatal socket.

It is often difficult to tell whether a root is in the antral cavity proper or is lying outside the antral lining (*Fig.* 8.16). The 'head-shaking test' though helpful is by no means infallible. The procedure is performed as follows. Intra-oral periapical radiographs are taken to show the position of the root. Identical views are taken after the patient has bent forwards and shaken his head from side to side. If the root is revealed to have changed position it is said to be within the antral cavity proper, whilst if it maintains its position it is probably lying between the antral lining and the bony wall of the antrum. Unfortunately, some roots lying inside the antral cavity proper are stuck to the lining by means of blood clot or granulation tissue and fail to move.

Experience shows that whilst the buccal roots of molars are not uncommonly pushed up between the antral lining and the bony wall of the air sinus, it is rare for palatal roots to be so displaced. Palatal roots are sometimes pushed into the thick soft tissues covering the palate, where unfortunately they cannot be located by means of palpation.

The roots of vital teeth may for practical purposes be regarded as sterile, and if such a root is outside the lining it may be left in situ and put 'on probation', if in the opinion of the surgeon circumstances warrant this. All other roots should be removed via an extra-nasal antrostomy.

The use of antibiotics is indicated if the root fragment is infected, there is pre-existing disease of the air sinus, the antrum was either washed out from below or otherwise infected during the operation, or acute maxillary sinusitis complicates the healing period. Many surgeons use antibiotics routinely in these cases (*see* p. 249).

FRACTURE OF THE MAXILLARY TUBEROSITY

Occasionally during the extraction of an upper molar the supporting bone and maxillary tuberosity are felt to move with the tooth. This mishap is due to the invasion of the tuberosity by the antrum, which is common when an isolated maxillary molar is present, especially if the tooth has divergent or hyper-cementosed roots or is over-erupted (*see Fig.* 8.4). Pathological gemination

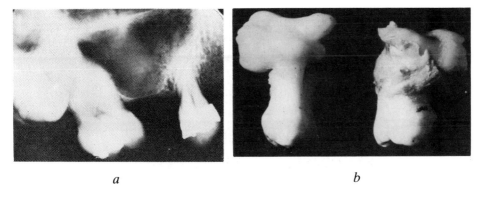

a   *b*

Fig. 8.17. *a*, Radiograph and, *b*, specimens of a case of bilateral concrescence.

between an upper second molar and an erupted or semi-erupted third molar is a rare predisposing cause (*Fig.* 8.17).

When fracture of the maxillary tuberosity occurs the forceps should be discarded and a large buccal mucoperiosteal flap raised (*Fig.* 8.18*a*, *b*). The bony fragment and the tooth should then be freed from the palatal soft tissues by blunt dissection and lifted from the wound (*Fig.* 8.18*c*). The soft-tissue flaps are then apposed with mattress sutures (*Fig.* 8.18*d*), which evert the margins and are left in situ for at least 10 days.

Some authorities advocate splinting of the fragment until union occurs and the tooth can be removed by dissection. Whilst this method works well in the treatment of other types of alveolar fracture, it is not favoured for the treatment of fracture of the maxillary tuberosity complicating tooth extraction for a variety of reasons. As the tooth is usually being extracted for the relief of pain due to either caries or periodontal disease, the symptom will not be relieved if the tooth is retained. Firm bony union is seldom obtained under these circumstances and the tuberosity may become detached again when extraction is reattempted. The method is laborious, the construction of cast silver cap splints is often required, and the results of treatment are no better than when the fractured tuberosity is dissected out. Following removal of the tuberosity, new bone is usually laid down in the area and provides a firm base for the denture (*Figs.* 8.18*e*, 8.19).

If a pre-extraction radiograph reveals the presence of a large antrum, an attempt to prevent fracture of the tuberosity should be made by dissecting the tooth from its attachments and sectioning it if necessary.

If either antral involvement or tuberosity fracture complicates the extraction of teeth from one maxilla, it is sound practice to radiograph the teeth on the opposite side before removing them, as the other antrum may also be enlarged. Prior knowledge of the condition enables the operator to make arrangements to either avoid the complication or deal with it effectively if it occurs.

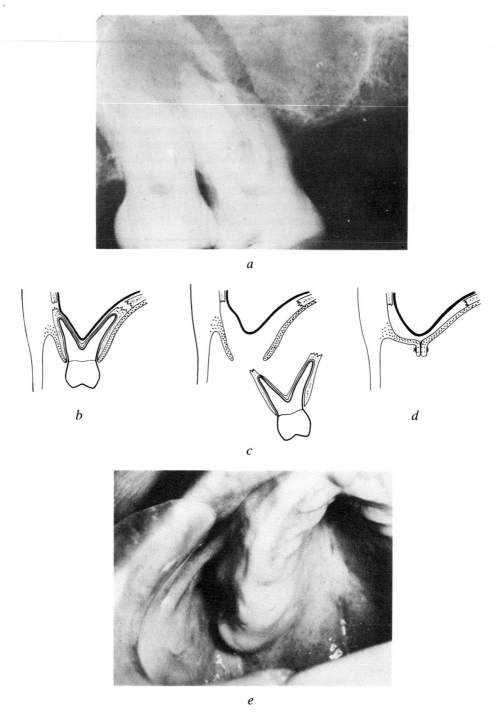

Fig. 8.18. The surgical treatment of a fractured tuberosity (*see* text for explanation).

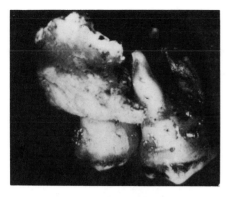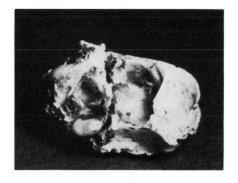

a   *b*

Fig. 8.19. Fractured tuberosity viewed from (*a*) side; (*b*) above. N.B. Smooth compact bone forming the antral wall (*see Fig.* 8.18).

MALIGNANT DISEASE OF THE SUPERIOR MAXILLA

The dentist has a duty always to keep the possibility of cancer in his mind when diagnosing and treating patients. By promptly referring those cases in whom the presence of malignant disease is suspected to either a surgical or radiotherapy centre, he will facilitate early diagnosis and prompt treatment and improve the chances of cure to a significant degree. Patients afflicted with malignant disease of the maxilla may present in the dentist's surgery in the first instance, and the dental surgeon should always bear the condition in mind when dealing with a patient complaining of either maxillary pain, for which no dental cause can be found, or a swelling of the cheek, in whom neither a dental inflammatory cause nor a skin infection can be detected. Other suspicious symptoms are epistaxis, the loosening of a cheek tooth without demonstrable cause, excessive bleeding after dental extractions, and the failure of a maxillary socket to heal normally, especially if proliferation of the soft tissues is present in the affected area. Examination may reveal narrowing of the palpebral fissure and depression of the corner of the mouth on the involved side (*Fig.* 8.20*a*). Intra-orally a swelling in the buccal sulcus may be present. Such a swelling may either be ulcerated or have many thin-walled blood vessels on its surface (*Fig.* 8.20*b*).

Radiographs may reveal erosion of either the compact bony wall of the air sinus or the roots of the maxillary cheek teeth (*Fig.* 8.21).

In the later stages of the disease proptosis may occur and the patient may complain of nasal obstruction and discharge on the affected side, diplopia, and unexplained weight loss in addition to the symptoms already mentioned.

Whenever the dentist is unable to make a diagnosis or suspects the presence of neoplasia he should obtain a second opinion (*see* Chapter 16).

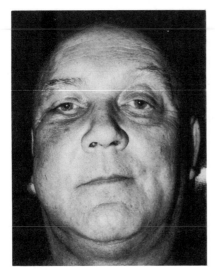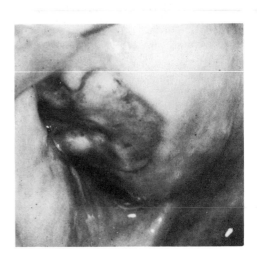

a   b

Fig. 8.20. Carcinoma of the right antum. *a*, The palpebral fissure is narrowed and the corner of the mouth is depressed on the affected side. *b*, Intra-oral inspection revealed the presence of an ulcerated swelling in the right maxillary buccal sulcus.

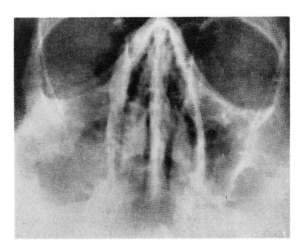

Fig. 8.21. The lower parts of both the inner and the outer walls of the right antrum have been eroded by a carcinoma.

SUGGESTED READING

Ehrl P. A. (1980) Oro-antral communications. *Int. J. Oral Surg.* **9**, 351–8.

Fickling B. W. (1957) Oral surgery involving the maxillary sinus. *Br. Dent. J.* **103**, 199–214; *Ann. R. Coll. Surg.* **20**, 13–35.

Jones E. H. and Steel J. S. (1969) Roots in the maxillary sinus. *Aust. Dent. J.* **14**, 8–11.

Mitchell R. and Lamb J. (1983) Immediate closure of oro-antral communications with a collagen implant. *Br. Dent. J.* **154**, 171–4.

Norman J. E. and Cannon P. D. (1967) Fracture of the maxillary tuberosity. *Oral Surg.* **24**, 459–67.

Van Cauwenberge P., Kluyskens P. and van Renterghem L. (1975) The importance of the anaerobic bacteria in paranasal sinusitis. *Rhinology* **13**, 141–5.

Wilson C. P. (1954) Malignant disease of the superior maxilla. *Ann. R. Coll. Surg.* **14**, 285–302.

Chapter 9
Orofacial infections and their management

THE SPREAD OF INFECTION

Dental disease is the underlying cause of most of the inflammatory swellings which occur either in or around the jaws. Inflammation may commence at either the root apices or gingival margins of erupted teeth, or in the soft tissues which surround and overlie the crown of an unerupted or partially erupted tooth (*see* p. 238). Inflammation around the apices of the tooth roots may result in the formation of pus which, taking the line of least resistance, bursts through the enclosing bone and involves the surrounding soft tissues. Once an infection enters the tissues it may resolve, become localized, or spread.

Many factors may play a part in determining the progress of each individual inflammatory process and for purposes of discussion they can be conveniently divided into those factors relating to the invading organism, those relating to the host, and anatomical factors. For the sake of clarity, each of these groups will be considered separately, but the dental surgeon must always remember that factors included in more than one group may be operative in a particular case.

Factors relating to the organism
Whilst the natural defence mechanisms of the host may be able to deal effectively with a few bacteria, they may be overwhelmed by the introduction into the tissues of a large number of micro-organisms. Thus the number of bacteria invading the tissues may have an important role in determining the progress of an infection. Some organisms have much more ability to damage the host than others and these are described as being more virulent. The virulence of the invading micro-organisms plays a very important part in determining the progress of an inflammatory process. The systemic reaction of an infected patient may reflect the degree of virulence of the causative organisms and this finding may be of assistance to the clinician when he attempts to assess the case. In some instances it is believed that different bacteria aid and abet each other in causing disease, and they are then said to act in symbiosis.

Certain micro-organisms produce spreading factors and spreading infections whilst others produce localizing factors and localized infections. Thus some streptococci produce hyaluronidase, an enzyme which dissolves the intercellular cement substance, and fibrinolysin which breaks down fibrin. The presence of these substances in the infected tissues facilitates the spread of the inflammatory process. On the other hand, some staphylococci produce a substance called coagulase, which produces fibrin from plasma, which tends to localize the inflammatory lesion. The vast majority of oral infections are caused by streptococci or staphylococci whilst such gram-negative bacteria as *Escherichia coli*, klebsiella and pseudomonas are involved less frequently. Both the nature of any discharge and the presence of signs of either localization or spread of infection may assist the dental surgeon during diagnosis.

Factors related to the host

General bodily resistance to disease varies greatly between individuals and also at different times in the same person. It is altered by many factors including age, the presence of a debilitating disease such as diabetes mellitus or chronic nephritis, chronic alcoholism, drug addiction or the immunity of the patient. Immunity may be inborn (species-immunity) or may be acquired either by having the disease or by artificial means. Undernourished individuals have a low resistance to infection and vitamin deficiencies are believed by some authorities to be of particular importance in this respect.

The site of entry of the infecting organisms may also affect the progress of an infection, for not only does the physical texture of the involved tissue and its content of histiocytes and lymphocytes govern both the amount and rate of extension of the inflammatory process, but movement of the part aids the flow of tissue fluid and lymph, and thus disseminates infection. It is believed that certain inflammatory processes cause the liberation of a 'leucocytosis-promoting factor' and 'leucotaxine'. The former substance is said to act on the bone marrow and encourage leucocytosis, thus producing more granulocytes to be attracted to the site of the inflammation by the leucotaxine. Such a stimulus to the natural defences of the body would aid the localization or resolution of an infective process.

Anatomical factors

Infections tend to spread along and be limited by muscle and fascial planes, especially when pus is present. Pus resulting from dental infections is often formed within bone which it must perforate before entering the soft tissues. In most cases pus tracks along the line of least resistance and perforates the bone at the site where it is thinnest and weakest. The points of weakness vary in differing areas of the jaws and some of the directions in which pus, formed in a periapical lesion, may spread into the surrounding soft tissues are illustrated in *Fig. 9.1*.

Infections may also spread along blood vessels or via the lymphatic system. Although it is not unusual for more than one anatomical factor to be of importance in the spread of a particular infection it is convenient to consider them separately.

When pus bursts through either the maxillary and mandibular labial and buccal plates its spread is largely dependent upon the insertions of the muscles of facial expression. The *buccinator muscle* arises from a horseshoe-shaped line which begins and ends on the alveolar process buccally to the upper and lower first permanent molars. The posterior end of the muscle is inserted into the pterygo-mandibular raphe. Thus, when pus arising from an infection on a molar perforates either the maxillary or mandibular buccal plate, it presents intra-orally if it is inside the attachment of the buccinator muscle to the jawbone and extra-orally if it is outside this muscle attachment. In adults the muscle attachment is usually above

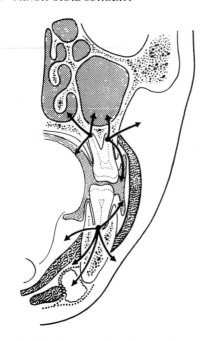

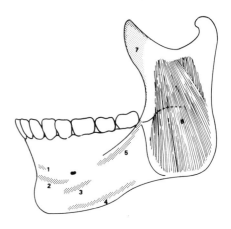

Fig. 9.2. Muscle attachments on the labiobuccal surface of the mandible. 1, Mentalis. 2, Depressor labii inferioris. 3, Depressor anguli oris. 4, Platysma. 5, Buccinator. 6, Masseter. 7, Temporalis.

Fig. 9.1. Directions in which pus, formed in a periapical lesion, may track (*see* text for explanation).

the apices of the upper molar roots but in a child they are often above the line of attachment and inflammatory swellings may present in the cheek rather than being confined to the buccal sulcus. Abscesses related to the anterior molars tend to track around the anterior edge of the buccinator attachment into the cheek and may present under the skin of the cheek at the lower border of the mandible. Infection from the posterior lower molars may present in the cheek and often tends to spread posteriorly.

Abscesses originating in relation to the lower premolars which burst through the buccal cortical plate are confined to the buccal sulcus by the *depressor muscles of the lower lip and the angle of the mouth* which have their origins below the apices of these teeth (*Fig.* 9.2).

The levators of the upper lip and the angle of the mouth are attached high up on the maxilla and so abscesses on the upper anterior teeth tend to be confined to the labial sulcus. Due to the thickness of the labial plate of the socket of the lateral incisor, abscesses on this tooth often burst into the palatal tissues. The *levator anguli oris muscle* has its origin in the canine fossa just below the infra-orbital foramen. On occasions the root apex of the maxillary canine is situated above this attachment and so infection on this tooth can cause a swelling deep to the *levator labii superioris muscle* and near to the inner canthus of the eye. From this position the infection may spread into the loose connective tissue of the lower eyelid or via the angular vein into the cavernous sinus. Infection spreading from the root apices of either the upper and lower premolars rarely forms a swelling in the cheek (*Figs*. 9.2 and 9.3).

In the lower molar region the buccal bone becomes progressively thicker towards the third molar region and so the risk of pus bursting through the lingual plate increases. However, the lingual plate in this area is composed of very dense bone and so lingual perforation in infections related to the second and third lower molars is rare and in many instances the pus forces its way along the periodontal membrane, destroys inter-radicular bone and discharges in the gingival crevice, usually on the buccal side due to the lingual tilt of lower molars. This is fortunate as deeply situated infections are of more serious import than superficial ones.

When a mandibular infection bursts lingually, it presents intra-orally if the apices of the involved teeth lie above the attachment of the mylohyoid muscle, as is usually the case with the incisors, canines and premolars, and extra-orally if they lie below the attachment of that muscle, as the apices of the second and third molars often do (*Fig*. 9.4). The apices of the first lower molar have a variable relationship with the origin of the *mylohyoid muscle* which is usually only

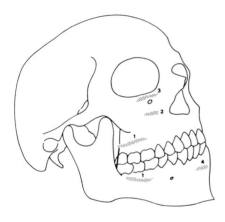

Fig. 9.3. Origins of the muscles of facial expression. 1, Buccinator. 2, Levator anguli oris. 3, Levator labii superioris. 4, Mentalis.

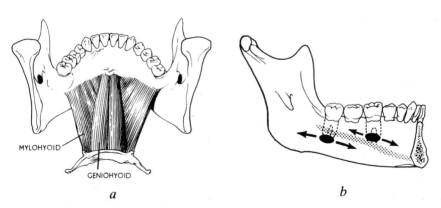

a

b

Fig. 9.4. *a*, Muscles of the floor of the mouth. *b*, Spread of pus, from apical infections on lower molars, which tracks lingually.

continuous in the molar region. Anteriorly the muscle usually arises by a series of slips between which lymphatics and blood vessels pass.

Infections arising from the apices of the lower anterior teeth may present in the labial sulcus. More commonly the attachment of the *mentalis muscle* directs the spread of infection either downwards and forwards towards the skin or downwards and backwards into the submental fascial space. The skin may be perforated in the midline of the chin between the points of insertion of the two mentalis muscles to form a sinus.

Planes of fascia are normally bound together by loose connective tissue and when these attachments are destroyed by a spreading infection it is convenient to refer to the resultant area as a fascial space. Although it must be emphasized that these spaces are potential rather than actual spaces and that they intercommunicate and it is unusual to see a patient with an infection completely limited to such a fascial space, it is useful for purposes of description to know the boundaries and contents of these entities.

The *submental space* referred to above lies below the mylohyoid muscle between the anterior bellies of the two digastric muscles.

The *superficial sublingual space* lies between the oral mucosa of the floor of the mouth and the underlying mylohyoid muscle, whilst the *deep sublingual space* lies between the mylohyoid muscle and the layer of deep cervical fascia which separates that muscle from the submandibular salivary gland. Both spaces are bounded laterally by the inner surface of the mandible and medially by the genioglossus, the geniohyoid and the hyoglossus muscles. They communicate posteriorly with the submandibular and pharyngeal regions. Thus, infections may track along the hyoglossus muscle to reach the opening of the larynx and may cause oedema of the loose connective tissue in this area with resultant closure of the opening. The two sublingual spaces intercommunicate with one another and with the submandibular space via the gaps in the anterior part of the mylohyoid muscle and also around its posterior border. The *submandibular space* contains the submandibular salivary gland and is enclosed by the two layers of deep fascia which are derived from the investing layer of the cervical fascia below and are attached to the inner surface and the lower border of the mandible above. The submandibular space communicates with the pharyngeal spaces and the infratemporal region. An abscess in the submandibular region rarely reaches the skin surface from which it is separated by the investing layer of the cervical fascia. Instead it usually spreads locally and may involve the submandibular gland and the submental triangle to present as a swelling of the whole area.

Infection spreading posteriorly from the mandibular molar region may pass either buccally or lingually to the ascending ramus. If it passes buccally it may either spread between the masseter muscle and the skin and superficial fascia overlying it, or extend subperiosteally beneath the masseteric attachment into the so-called *submasseteric space*. Infection passing backwards on the inner side of the ascending ramus involves the *lateral pharyngeal space*, which is bounded anteriorly by the pterygomandibular raphe and posteriorly by the styloid process and its attached muscles. The outer wall of the space comprises the medial pterygoid muscle, the ascending ramus of the mandible, and the deep surface of the parotid salivary gland, whilst the medial wall is formed by the cervical fascia covering the outer surface of the superior contrictor muscle and is continuous with that forming the carotid sheath (*Fig.* 9.5). Infection originating from pericoronitis (*see*

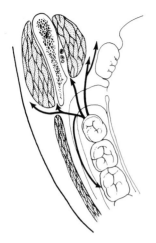

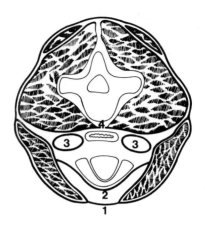

Fig. 9.5. Directions in which pus may track backwards from the mandibular molar region (*see* text for explanation).

Fig. 9.6. The fascial planes of the neck. 1, Investing layer. 2, Pretracheal fascia. 3, Carotid sheath. 4, Prevertebral fascia.

p. 238) related to the lower third molar may pass between the pharyngeal mucosa and the superior constrictor pharyngeus muscle to form a swelling around the lower pole of the tonsil.

A pericoronal abscess related to a distally inclined lower third molar may burst into the tissues lying behind, and thus outside the buccinator muscle and the pterygomandibular raphe. It may then spread backwards into the submasseteric space or more rarely into the *infratemporal region*. From there it may spread upwards into the temporal region between the zygomatic arch and the temporalis muscle or backwards into the lateral pharyngeal space.

Many of the spreading infections affecting the deeper structures are characterized by an increase in temperature and trismus (*see* p. 233) rather than swelling.

The *fascial planes of the neck* are best regarded as a series of vertical cylinders, an arrangement which permits infection to spread either upwards to the base of the skull or downwards as far as the thorax.

Fig. 9.6 illustrates how the investing layer of the deep cervical fascia splits to enclose the sternomastoid and trapezius muscles. It is attached to the base of the skull, the hyoid bone and the mandible above and to the sternum and the clavicle below. The fascia divides to enclose the parotid gland and the layer deep to the gland blends with the periosteum on the lateral surface of the ascending ramus to form the outer boundary of the *masticator space*. The ascending ramus of the mandible and the temporomandibular joint are contained within this space which is bounded internally by the pterygoid muscles. The carotid sheath surrounds the carotid arteries, the jugular veins and the vagus nerve whilst the prevertebral fascia lies in front of the prevertebral muscles. A potential space, the *retropharyngeal space* therefore exists behind the pharynx. The pretracheal fascia envelops the thyroid gland.

As there are no horizontal layers of cervical fascia an infection may spread from the floor of the mouth, over the posterior border of the mylohyoid muscle, and down the neck to interfere with deglutition and respiration.

The arrangement of the fascia which clothes the walls of the lateral pharyngeal space is such that infections may spread upwards to the base of the skull, downwards to the glottis, or into the mediastinum. Cavernous sinus thrombosis may result from an ascending infection via the pterygoid plexus or the foramina in the base of the skull and either oedema of the glottis or mediastinitis may complicate a descending infection. It is these dangerous complications which make infection of the lateral pharyngeal space one of the most serious conditions seen in dental practice. It may complicate an infection around the second and third mandibular molars or be secondary to a submandibular space infection. On rare occasions pus forming within the parotid salivary gland may rupture the thinner medial layer of the fascia enclosing the gland and invade the lateral pharyngeal space. Patients with infections in this area complain of difficulty in swallowing (dysphagia) and may speak with the so-called 'hot potato' voice.

Infections may spread via the bloodstream causing the serious complications of bacteraemia or infection of the cranial venous sinuses.

Periapical infections arising in relation to the maxillary incisor, canine and first premolar teeth may spread into the upper lip and canine fossa. If the infection gains entry into the superior labial venous plexus it may spread via the facial and angular veins and enter the cranium, causing the serious complication of cavernous sinus thrombosis. Acute infections of the soft tissues in the infra-orbital region of the cheek may rapidly become dangerous unless effective treatment is instituted promptly.

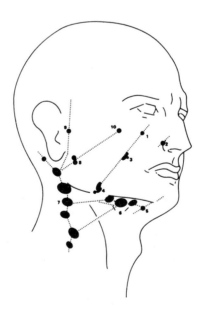

Fig. 9.7. Lymph nodes of the face and neck. 1, Infra-orbital. 2, Nasogenial. 3, Buccinator. 4, Facial. 5, Submental. 6, Submaxillary. 7, Deep cervical (jugulodigastric). 8, Parotid. 9, Pre-auricular. 10, Malar.

Infection may also reach the cranial cavity by haematogenous spread from the infratemporal region or the lateral pharyngeal space via the pterygoid plexus of veins.

It is fortunate that spread of infection from the oral cavity to the cranial cavity is rare for it is an extremely serious complication.

Infection may also spread via the lymphatic system. Most of the lymph vessels from the teeth drain into the submandibular lymph nodes (*Fig.* 9.7). The only exceptions are those of the mandibular incisors which drain into the submental lymph nodes and the lymphatics from the third molars which drain directly into the jugulodigastric group of deep cervical lymph nodes. Thus these lymph nodes are often enlarged, palpable and tender in the presence of oral infections and may be the site of abscess formation.

The facial group of lymph nodes is situated just in front of the border of the lower attachment of the masseter muscle. In younger patients particularly, they may become enlarged and tender as a result of a dental infection, often related to a deciduous molar tooth (*see Fig.* 1.6). When such involvement occurs, these nodes may become tethered either to the overlying skin or to the periosteum adjacent to them. This fact and the tendency of these nodes to break down and form an abscess of the cheek may be the cause of considerable diagnostic difficulty.

The lymph vessels from the maxillary teeth run under the mucous membrane lining the maxillary antrum towards either the posterior superior alveolar foramina or the infra-orbital foramen. Infection spreading along them may cause a maxillary sinusitis.

Lymph vessels from the lower premolars and molars run through the mandibular canal to leave the mandible via the mandibular foramen. It is probable that infection from the lower teeth can spread backwards along these vessels.

DIAGNOSIS OF OROFACIAL INFECTIONS

Unless each patient presenting with an orofacial infection is thoroughly investigated and meticulously assessed before treatment is given, avoidable mishaps will occur. All relevant details in the case history must be elicited and a clinical examination performed, supplemented where necessary by such special methods of examination as radiography. A patient afflicted with an acute infection looks ill and may have either a flushed, dry, and hot skin or a pale, cold, and clammy appearance. Examination of the first kind of patient usually reveals elevation of the temperature, pulse, and respiration rate. In the second type of case the temperature may be normal, or even on occasions subnormal, and the patient's eyes appear dull. This type of patient is exhibiting a poor resistance to the infection and is often referred to as being 'toxic'. Despite the absence of a febrile reaction antibiotic therapy should be initiated immediately for all such patients if deterioration in their condition is to be avoided. These patients, together with those in whom the presence of either submandibular cellulitis, respiratory obstruction, or cavernous sinus thrombosis is suspected, should be referred to hospital as emergency cases for specialist treatment.

During diagnosis the dental surgeon should attempt to determine the general medical history, health and resistance to infection of the patient, the cause, location, extent, type and stage of the infection, and whether pus is present in the tissues. A localized rise in temperature in the soft tissues overlying pus can often be demonstrated if the technique of examination illustrated in *Fig*. 1.4 is employed. Fluctuation may be elicited by either of the methods illustrated in *Figs*. 1.2 and 1.3. Pressure is applied with one finger, whilst any fluid thrill present is detected by a 'watching finger' which is held still. The examination should always be performed in two planes at right-angles to each other. Only after the dentist has obtained this information is he able to make an accurate clinical assessment and formulate an effective treatment plan.

TREATMENT OF INFECTIONS OF DENTAL ORIGIN

Treatment should be initiated without delay after diagnosis, for procrastination undermines the chances of success. During treatment the condition and progress of the patient should be kept under review. Should the patient fail to respond to treatment the case must be reassessed and if necessary the therapy modified. For purposes of discussion it is convenient to divide therapy into general and local measures, but in practice it is necessary to combine both kinds of treatment in most cases. The relative importance of each measure varies from patient to patient and treatment planning may require considerable clinical judgement.

General measures

General measures may be either supportive or curative in nature. As has been mentioned above, movement of a part facilitates spread of infection and so rest of the affected part is a logical way of combating infection. Whilst it is difficult to put the oral tissues at rest, a patient with a severe dental infection will undoubtedly benefit from a period of bed-rest combined with good nursing. This is best provided under hospital conditions and the dental surgeon should not hesitate to refer the patient for such treatment if in his opinion it is indicated. Unfortunately it is often difficult to persuade out-patients of the value of rest.

Oral infections may make mastication difficult and swallowing painful, and so a nourishing but soft diet should be given. A daily fluid intake of at least 3 litres should be prescribed in order to prevent the onset of dehydration. The use of analgesic drugs to control pain does much to speed the patient's recovery (*see* p. 84).

Antibiotic therapy

Although the introduction of antibiotic therapy has revolutionized the treatment of inflammatory conditions, an antibiotic should only be employed if there is a positive indication for its use. Such indications include 'toxicity', the presence of a debilitating disease or valvular lesion of the heart, the severity of an infection, the presence of inflammation in a dangerous site, or failure of an infection to respond to local treatment. In theory an antibiotic should only be prescribed after *in vitro* tests have shown that the infecting organism is sensitive to it. On most occasions, however, either the condition or circumstances of the patient make it necessary to initiate antibiotic therapy before the organism can be cultured and its sensitivity to antibiotics determined in the bacteriological laboratory. In these circumstances the clinician is forced to rely on his clinical experience when choosing an antibiotic.

Having prescribed one antibiotic, the dental surgeon should normally only change to another if, in the presence of adequate surgical drainage (*see* p. 234), the treatment has no effect after 72 hours. However, if the condition of a seriously ill patient shows no sign of improvement after 48 hours of antibiotic therapy the possibility of changing the therapeutic regime should be given careful consideration. On occasions *in vitro* tests show that organisms cultured from specimens taken from a patient being treated with an antibiotic are either resistant or insensitive to that drug. In this situation the clinician must be guided by the response of the patient to treatment up to that time when deciding whether to either modify or alter the antibiotic therapy. When the patient is responding to treatment he should continue to receive the antibiotic first chosen until the full course of treatment prescribed is completed. Clinical experience shows that the sensitivity of organisms to antibiotics *in vivo* often differs from that *in vitro*.

The antibiotic of choice in dental practice is penicillin, unless the patient has a history of hypersensitivity to the drug. When prescribing an antibiotic the dental surgeon must ensure that an adequate dosage is given, for a sufficiently long period, by a route that guarantees that the drug is absorbed and reaches the site of the inflammation. Penicillin given by the oral route is of great value when children are being treated. Clinical experience shows it to be less effective in adults. As the drug should only be given when there is a positive indication for its use, and in these circumstances maximum effectiveness is the aim, the intramuscular route is usually indicated. Those patients who are sensitive to penicillin should be treated with other antibiotics (*see* p. 255). Antibiotic therapy must be continued until the infection is overcome, and patients should be impressed with the importance of adhering to the therapeutic regime advocated and not to discontinue or vary therapy at their own discretion. A course of antibiotic therapy should last for at least 3 days (*see* p. 255).

Local measures

Many dental infections can be controlled by local treatment alone. The most important local measures available are drainage of pus and removal of the cause, and these should be employed whenever this is practicable. In many dental infections pus is trapped between the alveolar bone and the roots of the involved tooth, and extraction of the offending tooth attains both objectives and is followed by speedy resolution. Many abscessed teeth are loose and are easily picked out of their sockets, but in some cases trismus, which may be defined as limitation of opening of the mouth due to muscle spasm, limits access to the involved tooth. In these circumstances it is bad practice to force the jaws apart whilst the patient is under general anaesthesia, for this breaks down the natural defensive barriers to infection and so spreads the infection. Surgical drainage should be obtained and antibiotic therapy initiated. As the infection subsides trismus is relieved and the tooth can then be extracted with ease. There is no purpose in removing the tooth if it is not the cause of the infection, and indeed the extraction of a mandibular third molar which is the site of acute pericoronitis may serve only to convert a soft-tissue infection into a more serious one, involving both hard and soft tissues (*see* p. 243).

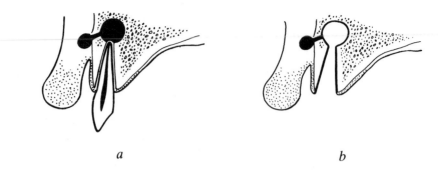

a   *b*

Fig. 9.8. Sagittal section of an abscessed incisor. *a*, The pus has tracked into the labial sulcus. *b*, The removal of the tooth drains the intra-bony lesion but not the pus in the soft tissues.

It has been shown that antibiotics do not enter closed collections of pus and that the use of such drugs is not a substitute for surgical drainage. As soon as fluctuation is present in an inflammatory area the pus should be drained. Drainage must be adequate and when practicable should be dependent. If fluctuation is present in the soft tissues, removal of the tooth alone, or the institution of drainage through its pulp canal, never provides adequate drainage, even if pus comes down the socket or the canal (*Fig.* 9.8). Adequate incision of the soft tissues is indicated.

When attempting to save abscessed pulpless teeth, an intra-oral incision should be made in the labial sulcus whenever fluctuation, induration, or tenderness is present in that site. It is much better practice to make an occasional intra-oral incision unnecessarily in such circumstances than to lose the involved tooth due to failure to obtain adequate drainage. Such an intra-oral incision should be made through the mucous membrane only, parallel to the surface of the alveolar bone and at least half an inch in length. The closed blades of a pair of sinus forceps are thrust through the incision and into the abscess, and then opened, liberating the pus (*Fig.* 9.9). This method of opening an abscess ensures that no blood vessel or nerve is damaged and is called Hilton's method. The conscientious postoperative

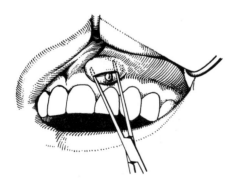

Fig. 9.9. Hilton's method of draining an abscess.

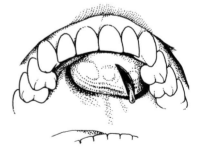

Fig. 9.10. The drainage of a palatal abscess.

use of hot saline mouth-baths usually ensures that the incision stays open as long as drainage is required (*see* p. 86).

When palatal abscesses are opened the incisions should be made antero-posteriorly parallel to the nerves and blood vessels in an attempt to minimize the risk of damage to these structures. In many instances it is best to remove an ellipse of tissue in order to ensure that the incision line is not sealed as the tongue moulds the elevated mucoperiosteum back to the palatal vault (*Fig.* 9.10).

When pus is deeply situated in the tissues an attempt should be made to localize the infection prior to instituting drainage. In most instances this can be done by the use of hot saline mouth-baths, and intra-oral drainage is instituted as soon as fluctuation can be elicited. The patient should be instructed to add half a tea-spoonful of salt to a tumblerful of hot water, and to take the resultant solution into the mouth as hot as is possible without incurring the risk of sustaining a scald. The hot saline is then held in the mouth over the inflamed area for as long as possible. Mouth-bathing should be practised for as long a period as possible and repeated as frequently as is practicable.

Although intra-oral drainage has the advantage of avoiding external scarring, when a dental infection has spread into tissues outside the buccinator or mylohyoid muscles, it can usually only be dealt with effectively by means of extra-oral drainage. Localization may be obtained by the application of heat to the facial skin overlying the inflammation, by the use of either kaolin poultice BP or short-wave diathermy. By carefully positioning the heat it is often possible to localize the inflammation in such a way that the skin incision may be sited in a submandibular skin crease, where the resultant scar will cause minimal disfigurement. After cleansing the skin with ½–1% cetrimide in surgical spirit, extra-oral drainage should be established by the use of Hilton's method. The operator should resist the temptation to incise over the most fluctuant part of the mass and should make

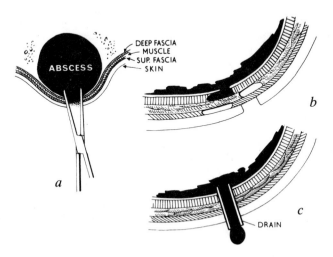

Fig. 9.11. *a*, Although drainage has been established, it will not be maintained, for movement of the overlying tissues tends to seal off the opening (*b*). *c*, The insertion of a drain aligns the holes in the different tissue planes and pus drains either through or around the drain.

the incision either in or parallel to a skin crease at the side of the fluctuant area, thus ensuring that the resultant scar will be neither depressed nor retracted.

When the pus has to pass through two or more tissue planes, a drain should be inserted to ensure that dependent drainage is maintained (*Fig.* 9.11). Either a corrugated or tubed rubber or a polythene drain may be used for this purpose, and the end of the drain should be inserted through the incision and into the abscess cavity with sinus forceps. The portion of the drain which extrudes from the wound should be both sutured to the skin and transfixed by a safety-pin, in order to prevent the entire drain passing into the soft tissues. A sterile thick gauze dressing is then placed over the wound and held in place with adhesive strapping. It is usual to leave a drain in situ for 2–5 days and to remove it as soon as pus stops discharging along it. Face masks should be worn and a 'no touch' technique employed whenever dressings are changed and drains are either inspected, cleansed, shortened, or removed. After removal of the drain a hygroscopic agent, such as magnesium sulphate (Morris's paste), may be applied to the wound for a few days in order to encourage the drainage of any residual pus.

In most instances the more severe and extensive dental infections are best treated by oral surgeons working with the benefit of all the hospital facilities which may be required. When pus is present both above and below the mylohyoid or buccinator muscles, 'through-and-through' drainage should be instituted (*Fig.* 9.12). In this technique a rubber-tube drain is inserted, which passes through the oral mucosa and underlying tissues and out of the skin. Despite its appearance the drain is stated by most patients to be very comfortable and particularly so when inserted on the lingual side of the mandible. In this situation when the infection

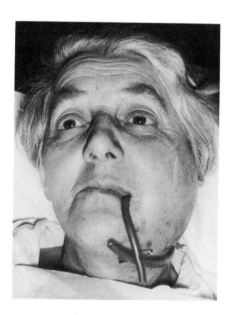

Fig. 9.12. 'Through-and-through' drainage of a large abscess related to retained third molar roots in an 80-year-old patient. The dressing has been removed for purpose of illustration.

and swelling in the tissues of the floor of the mouth begin to subside, the intra-oral end of other types of drain becomes more exposed and tends to irritate the undersurface of the tongue. Small holes can be cut in the tubing prior to the insertion of a 'through-and-through' drain, thus allowing the wound to be irrigated with ease if so desired. Slight rotation of such a drain through the wound will often relieve an obstruction to the drainage of pus. When the inflammation subsides the intra-oral portion of the drain is removed first, thus allowing the mucosal wound to seal off. A day or two later the resultant dependent extra-oral drain is removed and a dressing applied.

Drainage of a *submasseteric abscess* can often be obtained via an intra-oral incision made parallel and slightly lateral to the external oblique ridge. Care should be taken to avoid damage to Stensen's duct. However, it is sometimes preferable to obtain dependent drainage by means of an extra-oral incision made below and behind the angle of the mandible.

Infections of the *lateral pharyngeal space* are best drained through an intra-oral incision, made in the lateral wall of the pharynx whilst the patient is under general anaesthesia.

Difficulty in obtaining satisfactory anaesthesia is a common problem encountered during the treatment of orofacial infections. Local analgesia can only be employed if it can be obtained without the need to inject into acutely inflamed tissues. Infection in the floor of the mouth is a positive contra-indication to out-patient general anaesthesia owing to the risk of oedema of the glottis. All such patients should be sent as emergencies to hospital for treatment. Very fluctuant areas in the buccal and labial sulci can often be incised very satisfactorily under refrigeration anaesthesia. The infected area is isolated by the insertion of gauze packs, and ethyl chloride is sprayed on to the most fluctuant part until frosting

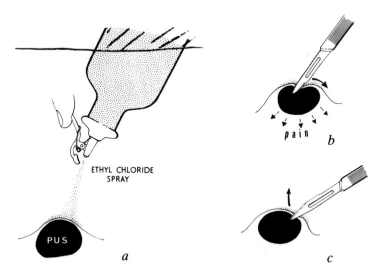

ETHYL CHLORIDE
SPRAY

PUS

pain

a

b

c

Fig. 9.13. *a*, When used to produce refrigeration anaesthesia, ethyl chloride spray anaesthetizes only the overlying tissues, which are covered with 'snow'. *b*, Downwards pressure with a No. 15 blade therefore causes pain by increasing pressure within the abscess. *c*, Pain can be avoided by using a No. 11 blade with an outwards motion.

occurs. An incision is then made through this site to liberate the contained pus. The dental surgeon using this technique must remember that as only the superficial tissues are anaesthetized, any pressure on the lesion during incision will cause pain. For this reason a triangular No. 11 blade should be used in the manner illustrated in *Fig*. 9.13. Some operators prefer to make such an incision using electrosurgery without anaesthesia.

Any instrument used during the extraction of an abscessed tooth or the drainage of an abscess must not be used again when working in a non-infected area of the same patient. If a virulent acute infection is present it is best to limit the amount of surgery to that required to deal with the infection.

PERICORONITIS

Pericoronitis may be defined as an infection involving the soft tissues surrounding the crown of a partially erupted tooth. The resulting inflammation may be acute, subacute, or chronic in nature, whilst ulcerative gingivitis may occur in some cases.

Although theoretically any tooth may be involved in such an inflammatory process, in practice the mandibular third molar is affected in the vast majority of cases.

A potential space, the 'follicle', exists between the hood of gum overlying the partially erupted tooth and the crown of the tooth. The follicle communicates with the oral cavity proper by means of a sinus passing through the soft tissues which is almost invariably demonstrable during clinical examination (*Fig*. 9.14). If a probe is passed along the sinus the unerupted tooth may be felt lying at the bottom of it. Inflammation probably begins in the follicle and then extends into the overlying soft tissues, thus producing the clinical entity to be described. Pericoronitis is a very common condition which affects both sexes equally and the incidence of

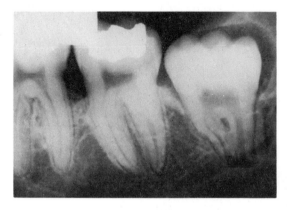

Fig. 9.14. The follicular space surrounds the crown of this unerupted third molar and is enclosed by a layer of condensed bone. At the mesial end of the crown the bony capsule is deficient. N.B. The interdental septum between the first and second molars has been affected by periodontal disease.

which appears to be increasing. It may affect patients of any age but it is most frequently seen in patients between 16 and 30 years of age, with the peak incidence in the 20–25-year-old age-group. The incidence varies with the season and is highest in the spring and autumn. The condition is seen most frequently in members of the more highly educated sections of the community—a finding which is perhaps due to the early loss of mandibular molars which occurs more frequently in the less dentally conscious members of society.

Amongst conditions which are believed to predispose to pericoronitis are upper respiratory infections, emotional stress, fatigue and pregnancy, in which it most commonly complicates the second trimester. There is no evidence to support the suggestion that menstruation plays any part in the causation of some cases of pericoronitis. The presence of an impinging maxillary tooth is a common finding in patients suffering from pericoronitis and, although it is not known whether such a tooth can initiate an attack of pericoronitis, there can be no doubt that by crushing the hood of gum overlying the tooth, which is often referred to as the operculum, it can both intensify and prolong such an attack.

Clinical classification of pericoronitis

Although it is not possible to correlate clinical findings with specific bacterial agents, it is both convenient and useful during treatment planning to divide cases of pericoronitis into acute, subacute, and chronic on the basis of the history.

Acute pericoronitis

This is characterized by a severe throbbing intermittent pain which is exacerbated

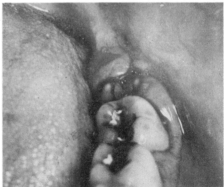

Fig. 9.16. Acute pericoronitis of left lower third molar.

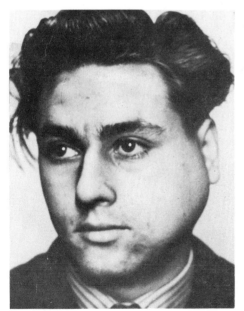

Fig. 9.15. Facial swelling due to acute pericoronitis related to an impacted left lower third molar.

by chewing, interferes with sleep, and frequently radiates into adjacent areas. Some degree of trismus is also present and the patient may complain of extra-oral swelling and discomfort during swallowing (*Fig.* 9.15).

Examination reveals an ill patient and the temperature, pulse, and respiration rate may be increased. The submandibular lymph-nodes are enlarged and tender to palpation, and a foetor oris may be noted. The affected gum flap is swollen and tender, and gentle pressure may cause a discharge of pus from beneath it (*Fig.* 9.16). Sloughing or ulceration may be present in the area of the operculum, which may show signs of indentation related to the cusps of an impinging maxillary tooth. There is often evidence of cheek biting in the affected molar area.

Subacute pericoronitis

This is characterized by a continuous dull ache which only radiates infrequently. The patient often complains of some stiffness of the jaw, intra-oral swelling, and an unpleasant taste.

Subacute pericoronitis causes less systemic upset than the acute variety and pyrexia is rarely a feature of the condition, but enlargement and tenderness of the submandibular lymph nodes are almost invariable findings. Intra-oral examination reveals the presence of an oedematous gum flap overlying the tooth. Gentle pressure on this operculum expresses a discharge from beneath the gum flap in many cases. More rarely the gum overlying the tooth is either ulcerated or indented due to pressure from an upper tooth. Cheek biting complicates the condition in a significant number of patients, whilst a foetor oris is noticeable in a few patients. In a minority of cases fluctuation may be elicited in either the pericoronal region or in the buccal sulcus (*Fig.* 9.17). Sometimes pus tracks from the third molar region and presents in the buccal sulcus alongside the first molar, a condition known as 'migratory abscess of the buccal sulcus' (*Fig.* 9.18).

Pus is formed as a result of subacute pericoronitis and tracks submucosally along the inclined gutter formed by the body of the mandible and those fibres of the buccinator muscle which are attached to the sloping external oblique ridge.

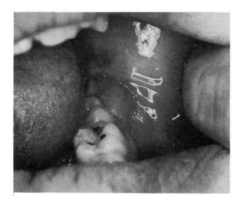 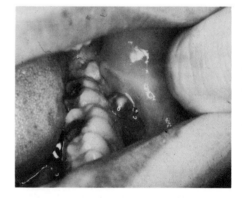

Fig. 9.17. Acute pericoronal abscess which had extended anteriorly to involve the buccal gingiva of the second molar.

Fig. 9.18. Migratory abscess of the buccal sulcus with sinus formation.

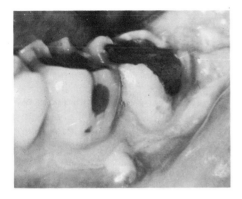

Fig. 9.19. Chronic sinus alongside first lower molar due to pericoronitis on lower third molar.

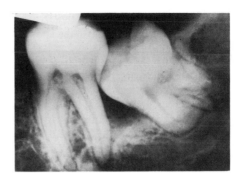

Fig. 9.20. 'Crater-like' defect seen in chronic pericoronitis.

The pus then pools in the loose connective tissue lining the undersurface of the mucosal reflection alongside the first molar. In those cases where treatment is delayed an intra-oral sinus may be present (*Figs.* 9.18 and 9.19).

Chronic pericoronitis

This is characterized by a dull pain or mild discomfort lasting for only a day or so and interspersed with remissions lasting many months. The patients almost invariably complain of an unpleasant taste. A crater-like defect may be seen in radiographs of the area (*Figs.* 9.20, 9.21).

It is very rare for a patient to present with *bilateral concurrent* pericoronitis even when there is a history of dual pericoronal infection, and in the presence of such a condition the dentist should carefully exclude all other possibilities (e.g., ulcerative gingivitis, blood dyscrasias) before making such a diagnosis.

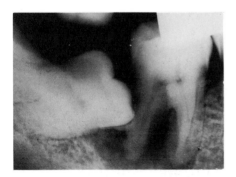

Fig. 9.21. Advanced case of chronic pericoronitis, with tartar formation and destruction of the supporting tissues of the second molar.

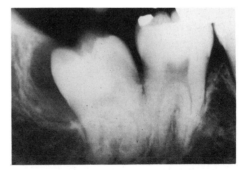

Fig. 9.22. The follicle extends deeply down the distal surface of the third molar. The margin of the bone enclosing the follicle is irregular due to chronic inflammatory changes.

The management of pericoronitis

History

Each case should be thoroughly investigated along classic lines and many important points may be noted during history-taking. The age of the patient and his home address and occupation may influence the type of treatment which should be employed in a particular case. When dealing with younger patients in whom growth of the jaws is incomplete, a conservative policy may be indicated, whilst in older patients it is usually better to remove the tooth after controlling the inflammation by conservative measures. If the patient finds it difficult to attend for treatment due to either the distance involved or his employment, the treatment plans may have to be modified accordingly. Careful note should be taken of the type, duration, and periodicity of pain so that other causes of pain may be eliminated and the type of pericoronitis determined (*see* p. 239).

Swelling may be confined to the soft tissues in the third molar area or it may spread into either the lower part of the face or the floor of the mouth. If acute infection spreads either distally or buccally the patient may complain of trismus. Patients afflicted with subacute pericoronitis often complain of some 'stiffness of the jaw'.

When teeth are lying in lingual obliquity (*see* p. 122), the lingual bony plate may be thinned or even perforated and infection may spread readily from the 'follicle' into the soft tissues of the floor of the mouth (*see Fig.* 5.15*b*). If such an inflammatory process extends posteriorly, the patient may complain of difficulty in swallowing (dysphagia) in contradistinction to difficulty in mastication. Any patient who presents complaining of dysphagia should be referred to a specialist oral surgeon without delay, for oedema of the glottis and asphyxia may result unless intensive treatment is instituted promptly. The frequency and nature of previous attacks of pericoronitis should be determined and taken into consideration when a decision is made whether to extract or retain a mandibular third molar. Inquiries should be made concerning the patient's past and present general health. The importance of determining the patient's general condition before treatment is commenced cannot be overemphasized (*see* Chapter 2).

Clinical examination

Examination should begin with the recording of the patient's axillary temperature, pulse, and respiration rate. During history-taking the general condition of the patient will have been noted, particular attention being paid to whether the patient looks healthy or ill, 'toxic' or 'non-toxic'. The presence, extent, and consistency of an extra-oral swelling are determined, and the submandibular and cervical areas palpated to detect the presence of enlarged and/or tender lymph nodes (*see Fig.* 1.5). The degree of trismus is measured by placing fingers between the jaws in the incisor region and estimating the amount of opening in fingerbreadths. If the patient's fingers are used for this purpose, errors introduced by variations in the width of the fingers of differing dental surgeons may be avoided.

The mandibular third molar region is then examined and the presence of swelling, tenderness, pus, or ulceration noted. The amount of the tooth which is visible is recorded or, if only a sinus can be detected, a blunt probe should be inserted into it and the buried tooth felt with its tip. In many cases the operculum, overlying the tooth, is crushed between the partially erupted lower tooth and an impinging maxillary molar when the jaws are closed together. This trauma causes the inflammation to persist until the presence of the impinging upper molar is diagnosed and remedied. A straight dental probe held on its side is placed distal to the occlusal surface of the upper third molar. The patient is asked to close the teeth together and the probe is drawn forwards gently. Any resistance to the movement of the probe is an indication that the upper tooth is impinging upon the operculum. The buccal sulcus should be examined and any swelling present there tested for fluctuation.

Both sides of the floor of the mouth should be examined and the presence of either tenderness or induration noted. Even in the presence of marked trismus a finger or a mirror handle can usually be gently inserted between the teeth for this purpose, if time is taken and the confidence and co-operation of the patient obtained. The caries and periodontal status of the patient must also be noted, particular attention being paid to the molar teeth on the affected side.

Special methods of examination

If required to confirm the diagnosis, or a suspicion that a very deep pocket is present distal to the third molar, intra-oral or extra-oral radiographs may be taken (*Fig.* 9.22). However, if the diagnosis can be made with confidence after completion of the clinical examination, more accurate positioning of the intra-oral film packet is possible if the radiographic examination is deferred until infection is controlled and trismus relieved, thus resulting in better definition and an absence of distortion in the radiograph (*see* p. 116). Whilst pericoronal infections of short duration do not produce changes in bone which can be demonstrated radiographically, a chronic pericoronal infection may cause a crater-like defect (*see Figs.* 9.20, 9.21).

Other special methods of examination, such as total and differential counts of the white blood corpuscles and bacteriological examination, are indicated if the infection is severe (*see* Chapter 13 and p. 247).

Treatment of pericoronitis

Once a definitive diagnosis has been made it is possible to both plan and institute treatment. This should be done without delay, for procrastination merely serves to prolong the duration of treatment and allows complications to occur. General and local measures are available for the treatment of pericoronitis and the relative value of and indications for the use of each varies in individual cases. For the sake of clarity these measures will be discussed separately before a treatment programme is advocated for each clinical variety of pericoronitis.

General treatment

This includes taking as much rest as possible—bed-rest should be ordered for toxic patients—and the provision of a soft and nourishing diet. An analgesic may be prescribed for the relief of pain (*see* p. 84), whilst antibiotic therapy should be instituted if the patient has either a congenital or rheumatic heart lesion, is suffering from a debilitating disease such as diabetes or nephritis, or appears 'toxic'. The presence of tenderness and/or induration in the floor of the mouth is another positive indication for the systemic use of antibiotics (*see* p. 255).

Local measures

These alone suffice to effect a cure in most cases. If an impinging maxillary molar is non-functional and over-erupted it should be extracted, and local anaesthesia may be used for this purpose if desired. If the partially erupted tooth is to be retained and the impinging tooth either is, or is likely to be, functional, the appropriate sharp cusps of the maxillary molar should be ground down with a mounted stone. If pus is present in the buccal sulcus, drainage must be instituted under either refrigeration anaesthesia or general anaesthesia, and it is possible to extract an impinging tooth, if so desired, during the same period of general anaesthesia. If fluctuation or tenderness is present in the floor of the mouth, the use of general anaesthesia in the dentist's surgery is contra-indicated owing to the danger of oedema of the glottis, and the patient should be referred to a specialist oral surgeon without delay. The presence of pus outside the buccinator is an indication for extra-oral drainage and in most instances these patients are best referred for specialist care, for such complications as submasseteric abscess, cellulitis, or peritonsillar infection may occur.

The application of caustics to the 'follicular' space is of great value in relieving pain. After ensuring that all necessary materials and instruments are ready, the affected mandibular molar region is isolated with cotton-wool rolls and dried. A

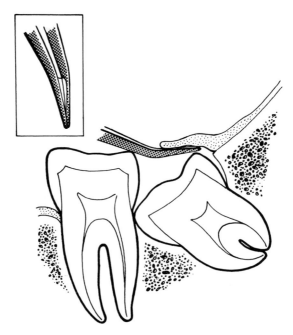

Fig. 9.23. A *small* amount of caustic solution is conveyed between the beaks of tweezers to the follicle.

small amount of the caustic solution is conveyed between the beaks of a pair of college tweezers to the area. The closed beaks of the tweezers are inserted under the flap and opened, thus allowing the caustic to flow by means of gravity and capillary attraction into the deeper crevices of the follicle (*Fig.* 9.23).

The caustic solution used for this purpose is dictated by the personal preferences of the operator, and chromic acid, phenol liquefactum, trichloracetic acid, and Howe's ammoniacal solution of silver nitrate are the solutions most frequently employed. Other dental surgeons prefer to use crystals of silver nitrate fused on to the end of a silver probe for the purpose. Whichever form of caustic is employed, any excess of it must be dealt with. Hydrogen peroxide is utilized for this purpose when chromic acid has been used, whilst excess silver nitrate is neutralized by the application of oil of cloves on a pledget of cotton-wool. This produces a black precipitate in the treated area. When other caustics have been employed it is usual to paint the area with glycerin in order to limit the flow of the caustic. The cotton-wool rolls are then promptly removed and the patient encouraged to use liberal amounts of a bland mouthwash. Despite the undoubted efficacy of caustics employed in this way, some authorities prefer to avoid using them and use either a 1% solution of cetrimide or a 0·05% solution of chlorhexidine to irrigate under the flap. Tweezers are then used in the manner previously described to instil one drop of an astringent solution into the follicle (*Fig.* 9.23). Talbot's solution of iodine may be used for this purpose and is made up as follows:

Iodine   183 gr (12 g)
Zinc iodide   110 gr (7 g)
Water   82 minims (4·5 ml)
Glycerin to 1 fl oz (28·4 ml)

Frequent hot saline mouth-baths should always be prescribed, and care taken to stress the need for taking hot, but not scalding, saline into the mouth at frequent intervals and holding the solution over the infected area for as long as is possible. This simple local measure is of great value in combating pain and speeding resolution in pericoronitis. Heat should never be applied to the skin of the cheek by means of poultices or hot-water bottles unless the use of external drainage is obligatory.

The involved tooth plays only a passive role in the aetiology of pericoronitis and it is usual to delay the extraction of it until the acute infection is controlled. Removal of the tooth in the presence of acute inflammation predisposes to osteitis and acute osteomyelitis, especially if the patient has acute ulcerative gingivitis.

Once an erupting tooth has been the seat of pericoronitis the condition tends to recur, unless the tooth either erupts or is extracted. The removal of lower third molars for pericoronal inflammation is followed by a significant incidence of 'dry sockets', even when such an extraction is delayed for at least 2 weeks after any clinical evidence of inflammation can be detected. The frequency with which this unpleasant complication occurs can be markedly reduced by removing the tooth under antibiotic cover. When the operation is being performed under regional anaesthesia and out-patient conditions, a single intramuscular injection of 1·3 ml of Triplopen, given 30 min prior to surgery, suffices for this purpose (*see* p. 252). However, the use of systemic penicillin for this purpose has not found widespread favour amongst oral surgeons. The prophylactic administration of Metronidazole Tablets BP (Flagyl) in a dosage of 200 mg 8-hourly for 3 days starting on the day of extraction appears to be just as effective in reducing the incidence of 'dry sockets'.

Treatment of acute pericoronitis

Whenever possible antibiotics should be employed in the treatment of acute pericoronitis, for they give rapid control of the infection, lessen the risk of serious complications, and shorten the treatment period. However, once an abscess has formed it should be incised, for the exhibition of antibiotics does not obviate the necessity for surgical drainage. A daily intramuscular injection of 2 ml of procaine penicillin injection fortified BP for 3 days suffices in most instances, although more severe cases may require treatment for 6 days. Patients who are allergic to penicillin may be given either Erythromycin estolate 250–500 g or Metronidazole Tablets BP (Flagyl) 200 mg 6-hourly for 5 days. Patients who fail to respond to such a regime should be referred to hospital. Even when antibiotics are employed the value of local measures should not be underestimated. If the patient uses hot saline mouth-baths conscientiously, they are a most effective therapeutic measure. The elimination of the impinging cusps of a maxillary molar, by either the extraction or grinding of the upper tooth, speeds resolution and eases pain. The application of a caustic below the gum flap also eases the pain and the prescription of suitable analgesic tablets is also of value in this respect.

Once the infection is controlled a decision with regard to the fate of the tooth should be made, for procrastination tends to be followed by a recurrence of pericoronitis. Removal of the gum flap overlying the mandibular third molar is only of value when orthodontic exposure of the tooth is both justified and technically possible. Thus in most cases the involved tooth should be extracted soon after the infection has been controlled.

Treatment of subacute pericoronitis

Subacute pericoronitis usually responds to the local measures previously detailed and antibiotic therapy is required only infrequently. At the first visit it is often possible to extract an impinging maxillary molar, cauterize the follicular space,

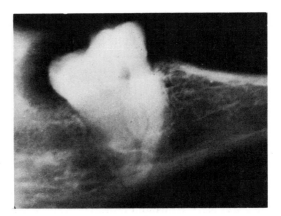

Fig. 9.24. A deep follicle which was the site of recurrent attacks of subacute pericoronitis. N.B. The margin of the follicle is no longer sharply defined owing to resorption of the condensed layer of the bone as a result of inflammation.

and instruct the patient in the use of hot saline mouth-baths. An appointment at which the involved tooth will be extracted is then arranged in 7–14 days' time, and the patient is discharged with instructions to return at once if the local inflammatory reaction fails to subside. Antibiotics are prescribed if the general condition of the patient necessitates their use (e.g., presence of debilitating disease, valvular heart disease, etc.). If fluctuation is present drainage of the pus should be instituted via an intra-oral incision.

In some cases of subacute pericoronitis radiographs reveal the presence of a large deep follicular shadow in relationship to the crown of the involved tooth (*Figs*. 5.12, 9.24). Experience shows that in such cases the use of local therapy alone controls the infection only slowly, whilst in many instances thick creamy pus can be expressed when pressure is applied to the operculum several days after the disappearance of pain and tenderness. In these 'deep pocket' cases the involved tooth is usually either a disto-angular or a vertical impaction (*see Fig*. 9.22). When subacute pericoronitis supervenes it usually responds quickly to a 3-day course of procaine penicillin injection fortified BP, and the involved tooth can be extracted on the third day on which the antibiotic is administered.

Treatment of chronic pericoronitis
Chronic pericoronitis responds to the local measures already described and the use of antibiotics is seldom required.

After infection has been controlled the dental surgeon must plan his treatment promptly if recurrence is to be avoided. When doing this, he is often faced with the problem of what to advise the patient who also has a completely uninfected, partially erupted contralateral mandibular third molar. The likelihood that such a tooth will become the seat of pericoronitis, if it is retained when the other third molar is extracted as a result of pericoronal infection, is so great that it is good practice to advise the prophylactic extraction of the uninfected impacted tooth in the vast majority of instances.

OBTAINING SPECIMENS FOR BACTERIOLOGICAL EXAMINATION

The bacteriologist can be of great assistance to the dental surgeon undertaking the treatment of infections of dental origin, for not only can pathogenic micro-organisms be isolated but their sensitivity to various antibiotics can be determined by means of *in vitro* tests. Therefore the dental surgeon should lose no opportunity of enlisting the aid of an experienced bacteriologist. Especial care should be taken during the collection of samples for bacteriological examination, in order to ensure that the specimen reaches the laboratory in optimum condition. Different bacteriological laboratories favour differing methods of collection, packaging, and disposal of specimens, and the dental surgeon should ensure that he is fully conversant with, and observes, the requirements of the particular laboratory which serves him. Containers and swabs should be obtained from the bacteriological laboratory so that they are available when they are required.

Whenever possible, samples of pus should be obtained by means of aspiration. After cleansing the skin or mucosa overlying the collection of pus with ½–1% cetrimide in surgical spirit, the tissues are punctured with a sterile large-bore needle (e.g., size No. 1). Pus is then obtained by means of aspiration into a sterile syringe, transferred to a sterile, labelled, round screw-capped bottle of appropriate size, and sent immediately to the bacteriological laboratory. Fluid specimens should never be put into test-tubes plugged with cotton-wool. Such a practice is dangerous, for specimens may be split and hands, clothing, or other articles may become infected. A sterile screw-capped bottle of such a size that it need never be more than two-thirds full should be used for the purpose.

All specimens sent for examination should be accompanied by a request form detailing the examination desired and summary of the case history. Particular reference should be made to the type, amount, and timing of any antibiotic therapy which may have been given. It is of great importance that the bacteriologist should be provided with adequate clinical notes, not only because these may help in the interpretation of laboratory findings, but also because they may suggest the use of special culture methods for the isolation of particular organisms.

When pus is less plentiful, swabs should be taken at the time drainage is instituted. When an extra-oral incision is made, the type of swab illustrated in *Fig.* 9.25*a* may be employed. It consists of a thin wooden stick, around one end of which some cotton-wool is twisted. The whole is enclosed in a long test-tube, the mouth of which is closed with a cotton-wool plug. The swab and its container are sterilized prior to use. It is most convenient if an assistant takes a swab of the pus which is liberated when the operator opens the blades of the sinus forceps. The sterile swab is removed from its container just before the sinus forceps are inserted, and inoculated from inside the incision as indicated by the dentist. The swab is then withdrawn, care being taken to ensure that it does not touch any other site before being replaced in the container. It is then dispatched to the laboratory together with the necessary details listed above.

It is sometimes difficult to obtain a swab of pus exuding from an intra-oral incision without contamination, if the standard swab is used. In these circumstances a West's nasopharyngeal swab should be used (*Fig.* 9.25*b*). This is a long flexible wire, with a swab at one end, contained within a curved glass-tube, both ends of which are plugged with cotton-wool. The swab and its container are sterilized prior to use. When it is desired to take a swab of pus from an intra-oral site the plugs are removed and the tube is inserted into the mouth, the curved portion being directed towards the area from which the swab is to be taken. The

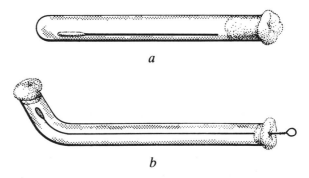

a

b

Fig. 9.25. Bacteriological swabs.

swab is then pushed out of the curved end of the tube and inoculated with pus. It is then withdrawn into the glass-tube which is removed from the mouth. The swab is protected by the glass-tube and oral contamination is thus avoided. The ends of the tube are plugged with cotton-wool and the swab dispatched to the laboratory as previously described.

Whenever a diagnosis of actinomycosis is considered to be a possibility, as much pus as can be obtained should be sent to the laboratory together with a specific request that a search be made for this particular organism. Special anaerobic methods of culture must be utilized if *Actinomyces israelii* is to be isolated. When little or no pus is present, and attempts at aspiration appear to be unsuccessful, the needle should be placed in a sterile tube and sent to the laboratory for culture of the contents of its lumen.

ANTIBIOTIC PREPARATIONS

As a result of intensive research, a host of antimicrobial drugs are available for use in the practice of medicine and surgery, and the number is constantly increasing. An *antibiotic* is defined as a substance produced naturally by a living micro-organism which is active in either preventing or inhibiting the growth or survival of another organism. Many of the antibacterial agents now in use are either partially or wholly produced by synthetic means and so are more properly called *chemotherapeutic agents*. However, they are often called antibiotics by clinicians. These drugs may either inhibit the multiplication of micro-organisms, in which case they are described as being *bacteriostatic*, or they may kill organisms, when they are described as being *bactericidal*. This classification is not absolute, for bactericidal drugs are also bacteriostatic and some bacteriostatic agents exhibit bactericidal activity when used in high concentrations.

As many bactericidal drugs, especially penicillins, can only kill rapidly multiplying micro-organisms, their lethal effect may be lessened in the presence of bacteriostatic agents such as the tetracyclines. Such antibacterial drugs as the penicillins and sulphonamides are extensively bound to plasma proteins in the bloodstream, only a fraction being unbound and in free solution. The pharmacological activity of these drugs is dependent upon this unbound component which is free to enter the interstitial and cerebrospinal fluids, the body cells, body cavities, and joint spaces. A particular agent can only be safely and usefully employed if the person prescribing it is familiar with the indications for and contra-indications to its use, in addition to the possible side-effects, the available preparations, and the recommended dosages. The dental surgeon is fortunate in that relatively few antibiotic preparations are required for the efficient practice of oral surgery.

Penicillin

The penicillins are bactericidal antibiotics which appear to act by interfering with the biosynthesis of the cell walls of susceptible micro-organisms. Most of them, such as benzylpenicillin, do not kill gram-negative bacteria and have a comparatively narrow spectrum of antibacterial activity. Naturally-occurring resistant strains are found even amongst susceptible organisms and some of these produce penicillinase, an enzyme which breaks down penicillin. Fortunately, clinical experience has revealed that most acute oral infections are caused by gram-positive cocci and respond to penicillin therapy and in the absence of a history of hypersensitivity to the drug, systemic penicillin therapy remains the antibiotic treatment of choice in the practice of oral surgery. A number of penicillin preparations are available for use by the dental surgeon.

Benzylpenicillin injection BP

This is supplied in vials containing the crystalline sodium salt of benzylpenicillin together with pyrogen-free water for injection, which is packed separately (*Fig*. 9.26). In the unopened vial the material will retain its potency for at least 3 years at room temperature.

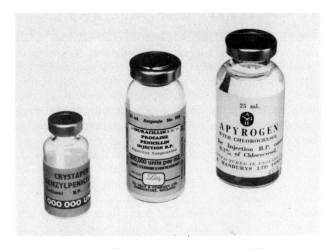

Fig. 9.26. Crystalline and procaine penicillins.

Penicillin is extremely soluble and 150 mg (250000 units) will dissolve in 1 ml of water. As injection of this hypertonic solution may give pain, solutions containing 60–120 mg (100000–200000 units) per ml are often employed. If kept at a temperature of between 2 and 10 °C, a solution may be used for up to 7 days after preparation. It is usual to keep penicillin solutions in a refrigerator and to add a buffer salt (e.g., 0·6% sodium citrate solution) if it is desired to keep the solution.

The individual dose is 150–600 mg (250000–1000000 units) intramuscularly. The peak concentration of the drug in the blood is reached about half an hour after injection and falls away rapidly thereafter and so at least 300 mg (500000 units) should be given every 4–6 hours in order to maintain a satisfactory blood concentration.

Procaine penicillin injection BP

This is a suspension of the relatively insoluble procaine salt (*see Fig*. 9.26). Each millilitre of the suspension contains 300 mg (300000 units) of procaine penicillin.

The dosage usually varies from 600 mg (600 000 units) to 1200 mg (1 200 000 units) daily by intramuscular injection. A depot is established by injection into the muscle and, from this, small quantities of soluble penicillin are released slowly. Reasonably effective blood levels are then maintained for up to 24 hours, though the high concentrations associated with benzylpenicillin are never attained. The suspension should be kept in a cool place and protected from light.

Procaine penicillin injection fortified BP

This is a suspension containing 300 mg (300 000 units) of procaine penicillin and 60 mg (100 000 units) of benzylpenicillin per ml (*Fig.* 9.27). It thus produces an initial high blood concentration combined with a sustained effect. It is usually

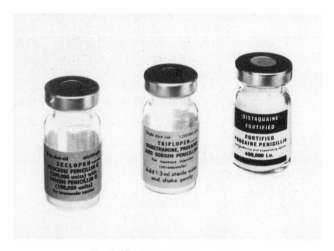

Fig. 9.27. Long-acting penicillins.

given in doses of 2–3 ml by intramuscular injection. The drug should be kept in a refrigerator and should be used within 7 days after preparation of the suspension if kept during this period at a temperature of between 2 and 10 °C.

Intramuscular injections of suspensions of penicillin tend to cause more afterpain than aqueous solutions of the drug.

Benzylpenicillin tablets BP

These are supplied in two strengths: 125 mg (200 000 units) and 250 mg (400 000 units). They should be kept in a cool dry place and are given in doses of between 125 and 500 mg every 4 hours. Blood levels may be inadequate after this preparation has been taken by mouth, for unfortunately benzylpenicillin is unstable in an acid medium and so a considerable portion of the drug ingested is rendered inactive by the acidity of the gastric contents.

Phenoxymethylpenicillin tablets BP (penicillin V tablets) and Phenoxymethyl-penicillin capsules BP (penicillin V capsules)

These can be obtained in three strengths: 60, 125, and 20 mg. They should be kept in a cool dry place and administered in doses of between 125 mg (200000 units) and 250 mg (400000 units) every 6 hours, before food. Phenoxymethylpenicillin resists destruction in gastric juice and is claimed to be more dependable than benzylpenicillin when given orally, though its behaviour in this respect is far from consistent. As the presence of food in the stomach and duodenum interferes with the absorption of penicillin V, the drug should be taken no later than 30 min before a meal and no sooner than 2–3 hours after the ingestion of food.

Amoxycillin (Amoxil)

This is a penicillinase-susceptible penicillin which is stable in the presence of gastric acid and which is readily absorbed from the gut to produce high serum levels. It is only 17% protein-bound in serum as compared to 59% for penicillin G and so is a highly effective bactericidal antibiotic against most gram-positive and many gram-negative micro-organisms when given in an adult oral dosage of 250–500 mg every 8 hours. In severe infections it can also be given by either intramuscular or intravenous injection. It should not be given to pregnant women.

Cloxacillin (Orbenin)

This is not destroyed by either bacterial penicillinase or gastric acid and so its use is reserved for the treatment of penicillin-resistant staphylococcal infection. It is supplied in both 250-mg capsules and an injectable solution. The dose is 500 mg by mouth or 250 mg by intramuscular injection 6-hourly.

Triplopen

This is another proprietary antibiotic preparation which has been found to be of value in the practice of oral surgery (*Fig.* 9.27). Each single dose vial of this preparation contains: benethamine penicillin G, 500000 units; procaine penicillin G, 250000 units; sodium penicillin G, 500000 units; together with buffering and suspending agents. The addition of 1·3 ml of pyrogen-free water forms a suspension which, when given intramuscularly, quickly provides a high bactericidal level in the blood, followed by therapeutic levels which are maintained for 3–4 days. In practice, a single intramuscular injection of triplopen 30 min before surgery has been found to reduce markedly the incidence of 'dry socket' following the removal of mandibular third molars which have previously been the seat of pericoronitis.

Erythromycin

Erythromycin is classified as one of the macrolide antibiotics, all of which possess a macrocyclic lactone ring, and is believed to act by inhibiting protein synthesis within the bacterial cell. It has a narrow spectrum of antibacterial activity similar to that of benzylpenicillin and so forms a useful alternative drug for use in patients who are hypersensitive to penicillin. Erythromycin is bacteriostatic in low concentrations, can also exhibit bactericidal activity in high concentrations, and has been found to be especially suitable for the treatment of acute pyogenic infections of the oral soft tissues. The most useful preparation in dental practice is erythromycin estolate (Isolone) which is acid stable and is supplied in 250-mg capsules. Gastro-intestinal upsets such as nausea, vomiting, epigastric discomfort and diarrhoea not infrequently complicate the use of the drug. The much more rare, and serious symptoms of jaundice, fever and abdominal pain indicate the onset of a drug-induced hepatitis, and if the therapy is stopped immediately these symptoms quickly regress. Erythromycin should not be given to such a patient again.

Most oral infections will respond to an oral dose of 250–500 mg 6-hourly given for 5 days. Erythromycin is also used for prophylactic purposes in patients requiring antibiotic cover (*see* p. 257).

Cephalosporins

Cephaloridine (Ceporan) is active against many gram-positive and gram-negative bacteria. As absorption after oral administration is not satisfactory it must be given intramuscularly. It is usually given in doses of 500 mg–1 g 6-hourly for either serious infections or prophylaxis as an alternative to penicillin. Cephaloridine should be used with caution in patients who exhibit hypersensitivity to penicillin for the possibility of cross-sensitivity exists.

Cephalexin monohydrate capsules or tablets (Keflex) in a dosage of 250–500 mg 8-hourly are a useful, if costly, alternative to erythromycin.

Clindamycin

Clindamycin (Dalacin C) is a much superior chemical modification of lincomycin, and is a narrow-spectrum antibiotic mainly active against gram-positive cocci. Like erythromycin it acts by inhibiting protein synthesis within the bacterial cell. Although it is bactericidal it is less potent and more costly than penicillin which has a wider antibacterial spectrum. Bacterial resistance to it develops rapidly. Clindamycin is one of the very few antibiotics which is selectively secreted by the salivary glands and so is especially useful in treating infections in those glands. It also appears to become concentrated in infected bone and so its use is indicated in the treatment of osteomyelitis. As it has been shown to be especially effective in the treatment of bacteroides infection it has been suggested that the good response obtained in treating dental infections is due to this property rather than its good penetration of bone.

When taken orally its absorption is not affected by the presence of food in the stomach but it may produce diarrhoea. As pseudomembranous colitis has occurred during therapy clindamycin should be used only for the treatment of serious oral infections caused by organisms known to be sensitive to it. It is available in capsules or as Dalacin C phosphate injection and is given in an adult dosage of 150–300 mg every 6 hours.

Metronidazole

Metronidazole (Flagyl) is a nitroimidazole chemotherapeutic agent which is active against anaerobic micro-organisms, especially bacteroides, clostridia and anaerobic streptococci. It is also anti-trichomonal, anti-amoebic and anti-parasitic but both aerobic and facultative anaerobic bacteria are usually resistant to it. Metronidazole taken orally is well absorbed even in the presence of food and may be used to treat oral infections known to be due to anaerobic micro-organisms and acute ulcerative gingivitis and to both treat and reduce the incidence of 'dry sockets'. The usual adult dosage is 200–400 mg t.d.s. for 5 days. The drug should not be administered to pregnant women or to patients with monilial infection. All patients must be warned to avoid drinking alcohol whilst taking metronidazole and for 3 days after completing the course of treatment if the unpleasant side effects of nausea and vomiting are to be avoided. Metronidazole has no effect against aerobic organisms, therefore in mixed infections appropriate anti-aerobic antibiotics must also be used. No antagonistic reactions with other antibiotics have been noted.

Tetracycline

Tetracycline (Achromycin) is active against many gram-positive and gram-negative bacteria and was thus often called a 'broad-spectrum' antibiotic. Its action was predominantly bacteriostatic rather than bactericidal. It is available either in the form of *tetracycline tablets BP* or *tetracycline capsules BP*, in the strengths of 50, 100, or 250 mg. The drug should be kept in a cool place. Unfortunately its effectiveness in the treatment of oral infections has declined over the years to such a degree that it is now unusual to isolate a *Streptococcus viridans* which is sensitive to tetracycline from such an infection. This chemotherapeutic agent is no longer dependable in the treatment of staphylococcal infections but is still very effective in the treatment of infections caused by gram-negative bacteria. Tetracyline is best reserved for use in combating those infections which fail to respond to penicillin therapy. The dose is 1–3 g daily, in divided doses taken at 6- or 8-hourly intervals.

Tetracyclines are incorporated into any tissue which is calcifying at the time they are ingested and may produce permanent discoloration of the teeth. For this reason they should not be prescribed for pregnant women or young children. Other side-effects include pruritus ani, nausea, vomiting, abdominal pain, flatulence and diarrhoea which are common, whilst less often soreness of the tongue may develop. Formerly it was believed that these gastro-intestinal disturbances were due to the action of the antibiotic upon vitamin synthesis by intestinal flora and absorption in the gut. Thus it was customary to prescribe vitamins, and *vitamin capsules BPC* were often used for this purpose. Each capsule contains: vitamin A activity 2500 units; aneurine hydrochloride, 1 mg; riboflavine, 0·5 mg; nicotinamide, 7·5 mg; ascorbic acid, 15 mg; and antirachitic activity (vitamin D), 300 units; and the patient was instructed to take a vitamin capsule each time a dose of tetracycline was taken. These vitamin capsules should be kept in a cool place and protected from light.

More recent work has indicated that the gastro-intestinal complications of tetracycline therapy may be due either to a direct action of the antibiotic on the mucosa or to infection with monilia, and so it is now customary to prescribe *nystatin tablets BP* with tetracycline. One 500000-unit tablet is taken with each dose of tetracycline.

Mysteclin capsules, each of which contains tetracycline hydrochloride 250 mg and nystatin 250000 units, provide a convenient form of therapy. Yet another approach to this problem is the use of bacterial replacement therapy by prescribing a commercial preparation of antibiotic-resistant *Lactobacillus acidophilus*. Yoghurt is a simple and inexpensive alternative to this preparation.

It has been shown that when iron preparations and tetracycline are given by mouth they interact, and in these circumstances neither may be absorbed. For this reason iron by mouth should not be prescribed whilst a patient is receiving a tetracycline.

Chloramphenicol

This antibiotic should not be prescribed by dental practitioners, for aplastic anaemia may complicate its use, and safer alternatives are available.

Choice of antibiotic preparation

It is notoriously difficult to compare the results of different bacteriological investigations because of the variety of methods and materials employed. However, there is strong evidence that the microbiology of oral pyogenic infections is changing and that the proportion of infections due to aerobic gram-negative bacilli is increasing. Nevertheless there is still wide agreement that penicillin remains the antibiotic of choice in the treatment of pyogenic infections of dental origin except in those patients who are allergic to penicillin in whom erythromycin is the antibiotic of choice.

Under hospital conditions severe infections of dental origin should be treated with 4-hourly intramuscular injections of 600 mg (1000000 units) of benzylpenicillin until the infection is overcome. When severe soft-tissue infections are being treated antibiotic therapy is usually continued for 48 hours after the symptoms have subsided. Infections involving salivary glands and lymph nodes often require antibiotics for at least 10 days, whilst osteomyelitis is an indication for at least 1 month's antibiotic therapy. Such a regime is usually impossible to maintain under out-patient conditions and is not required when less dangerous infections are being treated. In these circumstances treatment should be initiated with an intramuscular injection of 2–3 ml of procaine penicillin injection fortified BP. It can then be continued with either daily injections of a similar nature or twice-daily intramuscular injections of 2 ml procaine penicillin injection BP. In less severe cases treatment may be maintained orally—phenoxymethylpenicillin tablets, for example, in a dose of 250 mg every 6 hours. A clinical response should be observed within 72 hours, in which case treatment should be continued for a further period which should not exceed 7 days. If there is no response after 72 hours another antibiotic should be substituted, preferably on a basis of bacteriological findings.

The only important side-effect of the penicillins is hypersensitivity which may complicate the use of any form of the antibiotic. As cross-hypersensitivity probably exists between all the penicillins in a susceptible patient, an alternative antibiotic must be used whenever there is a history of an allergic reaction complicating the use of any form of penicillin. The vast majority of cases of antibiotic allergy are due to penicillin and its derivatives, skin rashes being the most frequent manifestation and anaphylactic shock the most serious. Administration of the antibiotic should be discontinued and treatment instituted immediately (*see* p. 263). Erythromycin estolate given in an oral dose of 250–500 mg 6-hourly for 5 days effectively combats most oral infections.

Tetracyclines should not be used in the treatment of severe infections as their effectiveness in the treatment of pyogenic infections of dental origin has declined markedly over the years.

Combinations of antibiotics are seldom required in the practice of oral surgery. However, on those rare occasions when it is necessary, penicillin and streptomycin, both of which are bactericidal when present in sufficient concentration, may be given together and appear to potentiate each other. Most of the other antibiotics in common use are bacteriostatic and in combination give simple additive effects. The combination of penicillin with a bacteriostatic agent such as tetracycline may actually decrease the effectiveness of the penicillin therapy and may increase the risk of untoward effects occurring (*see* p. 249).

ANTIBIOTIC COVER

There is a considerable debate concerning which patients should be given antibiotic cover when undergoing dental treatment and great difficulty may be experienced in identifying those at risk especially as 40% of patients afflicted with infective endocarditis have no history of previously recognized heart disease. Nevertheless, the importance of a carefully taken and detailed medical history cannot be over-emphasized in this regard. Whenever a patient who has a history of either congenital or rheumatic heart disease, cardiac surgery or the insertion of a prosthetic valve or a cardiac pacemaker requires any dental treatment in which bleeding may occur the dental surgeon should contact the patient's physician and enlist his co-operation in the management of the case. It is important to appreciate that patients with asymptomatic heart lesions are just as much at risk from infection as those with disabling disease. In these circumstances no such patient should ever be allowed to undergo either an oral surgical procedure or scaling of the teeth without antibiotic prophylaxis.

In the absence of a history of hypersensitivity to the drug, an adult dose of 2 ml of procaine penicillin injection fortified BP, containing 600 mg (600000 units) of procaine penicillin and 120 mg (200000 units) of benzylpenicillin, should be given intramuscularly 30 min before the dental operation is undertaken. The dose is repeated daily on each of the following 3 days if practicable. In other circumstances penicillin V may be substituted in an oral dosage of 500 mg 6-hourly.

Some authorities have claimed that such a regimen is neither acceptable nor practicable in general dental practice and point out that injections, however well performed, may be counter-productive as patients may deliberately suppress a relevant history in an endeavour to avoid them. They go on to state that a single dose of 3 g of amoxycillin, taken as a draught prepared from a fruit flavoured sachet, 1 hour prior to the dental procedure being performed is equally as effective as regimes utilizing injections. A second similar dose should be taken 8–10 hours after the first. If such a regime is utilized *the first dose must be taken in the presence of either the dentist or a nurse in order to ensure that the instructions have been complied with.* If amoxycillin in 3-g sachets is not available sugar-free Amoxil dispersable tablets (500 mg) can be used (3 g can be suspended in 30 ml water).

Patients who have a history of hypersensitivity to penicillin should be given a course of erythromycin estolate (Isolone). Two 250-mg capsules should be taken 2 hours before operation followed by one capsule 3 times a day. If 250 mg are given every 8 hours, the time at which the doses are taken can be arranged so as to ensure that the patient gets almost 8 hours' sleep; one dose being taken before retiring and one on waking. This treatment should be continued for 5 days. An alternative regimen is to give a loading dose of 1·5 g erythromycin 1 hour before treatment followed by from one to eight 6-hourly doses of 500 mg as desired. However, a loading dose of this size produces nausea and vomiting in some patients. In such circumstances a different erythromycin preparation should be tried rather than the dose being reduced. If gastro-intestinal symptoms continue to be experienced Cephalexin may be used despite the slight risk of cross-sensitivity with penicillin.

In an attempt to prevent a recrudescence of rheumatic fever some young patients are given prophylactic antibiotic therapy for very long periods. Penicillin is often employed for this purpose, and it has been demonstrated that such patients may risk an attack of bacterial endocarditis unless another antibiotic is given when dental extractions or other forms of oral surgery are undertaken. It has been claimed that the viridans streptococci found in such patients are only relatively resistant to penicillin and are killed by moderately increased doses of penicillin or a single very large dose of either amoxycillin or erythromycin stearate 1·5 g orally given under supervision 1–2 hours before treatment followed by a second dose of 500 mg 6 hours later.

If circumstances permit an attempt should be made to assess the sensitivity of the oral flora to antibiotics by culturing a mouth swab and performing *in vitro* tests. However, in practice this is not always possible, and so either cephaloridine or erythromycin are used for this purpose after consultation with the patient's physician. Cephaloridine has the advantage that it can be given without interrupting the course of prophylactic penicillin therapy since the two drugs do not interfere with the action of each other. Cephaloridine (0·5 g) is usually given intramuscularly 20 min before surgery, and this dose is repeated 6 hours postoperatively. Injections of cephaloridine 250 mg are then given 6-hourly for 3 days. Many practitioners avoid the need for repeated intramuscular injections in children by giving erythromycin estolate 250–500 mg by mouth 6-hourly for 3 days postoperatively after giving the first two injections of cephaloridine. As the onset of bacterial endocarditis may be insidious, patients should be advised to report any untoward symptoms or signs to their medical practitioner.

If the patient is to be treated under general anaesthesia the stomach should be empty. In these circumstances antibiotics should be given either parenterally or at least 3–4 hours preoperatively. Intramuscular injections of amoxycillin may be painful and so adults at risk who are to have a general anaesthetic should be given amoxycillin 1 g in 2·5 ml of 1% lignocaine hydrochloride before induction and a further 500 mg by mouth 6 hours later. These dosages should be halved in children under ten years of age.

Patients who have had one or more attacks of endocarditis on whom a dental procedure is to be performed under antibiotic cover should be treated in hospital. Those who are to be given a general anaesthetic and have either a prosthetic valve or an allergy to the penicillins or have been given penicillin in the previous month should also be referred for specialist care.

Antibiotic cover is also employed when surgery is undertaken for patients afflicted with a debilitating disease on prolonged steroid therapy, or those who have had therapeutic irradiation of the site of operation. Some authorities also advise its use when surgery or scaling is performed on patients who have suffered a cardiac infarction which may have damaged the endocardium.

Paediatric dosage of antibiotics

No one likes being given intramuscular injections and, when small children are being treated, repeated injections may become an ordeal for the patient, the parents and the clinician. Fortunately oral administration of antibiotics is both practicable and effective in children and intramuscular injections are seldom required in these cases. In many instances small children will take the drug when it is prepared as a syrup, whilst refusing to swallow tablets or capsules. Dosage is usually related to body-weight and *Table* 9.1 will be found useful when antibiotic therapy is to be prescribed for a child.

For the purposes of antibiotic cover children aged from 5 to 10 years can be given a single dose of 1·5 g amoxycillin, or 1 g of erythromycin 1 hour before treatment is commenced. Those under 5 years of age can be given half this dose. Erythromycin can conveniently by given to children in the form of erythromycin ethylsuccinate (100 mg in 5 ml).

Table 9.1. Average Oral Paediatric Doses of Antibiotics (mg)

Age	Birth	6 Months	1 Year	2 Years	5 Years	10 Years	
Average weight	7 lb (3·2 kg)	17 lb (8 kg)	22 lb (10 kg)	28 lb (13 kg)	40 lb (18 kg)	65 lb (30 kg)	*Available as*
Penicillin G							Tablets: 250 and 125 mg Syrup: 125 mg in 5 ml
	62·5	62·5	125	125	125	250	Tablets: 250, 125, and 60 mg Liquid: 62·5 mg in 5 ml and 125 mg in 5 ml
Penicillin V							
Tetracycline							Tablets: 250, 100, and 50 mg Suspensions: 25 mg in 1 ml
	25	75	100	125	150	200	
Erythromycin							Tablets: 250 and 100 mg Liquid: 20 mg in 1 ml

Notes: 1. Dose to be repeated 6-hourly four times a day.

2. Where small doses of liquid result it is suggested that syrup simplex BP is added to a final volume of 5 ml (1 teaspoonful).

INTRAMUSCULAR INJECTIONS

As has been stated previously, penicillin is the antibiotic of choice in the practice of dental surgery. When the use of this drug is indicated, administration of it by means of an intramuscular injection has several advantages over the oral route. The surgeon can be certain that the prescribed dose has been administered at the correct time and that the blood level of the drug will not be affected by such variable factors as the gastric acidity or the level of absorption from the gut. Disadvantages of the technique include the need for injection and a certain amount of inconvenience for both the operator and his patient when administration is undertaken on an out-patient basis. Nevertheless, when penicillin therapy is indicated, the intramuscular route is usually the most desirable and effective method of administration and every dental surgeon should be able to give the antibiotic by this means.

Intramuscular injections have certain advantages when compared with ordinary hypodermic injections. Fluids which are too irritant to be deposited under the skin can be injected into a muscle with perfect safety. A larger volume of drug can be deposited in muscles, and the vascularity of these structures ensures that the drug enters the bloodstream rapidly and acts more quickly than when an ordinary hypodermic injection is used.

As intramuscular injections are made more deeply than hypodermic injections, the risk of damaging important structures such as vessels and nerves is correspondingly increased and every precaution must be taken to guard against such mishaps.

Selecting an injection site

Great care must be taken to ensure that a safe site is chosen for the injection. Although the sciatic nerve runs beneath the inner and lower parts of the buttock, most authorities favour the gluteal muscles as the site of intramuscular injections. Difficulties sometimes arise due to a nurse confusing the layman's conception of the buttock with that of the anatomist (*Fig. 9.28*). Anatomically speaking, the buttock is bounded above by the iliac crest and is roughly circular in shape. Intramuscular injections should always be given into the upper outer quadrant of the buttock, avoiding those parts close to the iliac crest. Accurate localization is facilitated if the palm of the left hand is placed across the lower half of the buttock and kept in situ throughout the injection. In most instances injections into the gluteal muscles are given whilst the patient is lying face downwards on a bed. However, a minority of doctors prefer to give the injection with the patient sitting on either a bed or a stool, and claim that it is impossible for the sciatic nerve to be damaged if this position is used.

Other authorities favour either the front or the outer aspect of the thigh as the site for intramuscular injections. The needle is inserted either into the outer aspect, one hand's width below the great trochanter, or into the front of the thigh, half-way between the groin and the knee. When using the latter site care must be taken not to inject at too high a level or the femoral canal may be entered. Most ambulatory patients seem to experience more pain when the muscles of the thigh are used as the site for intramuscular injections than when the gluteal muscles are utilized for the purpose.

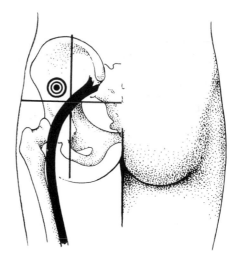

Fig. 9.28. Anatomist's buttock (left); Layman's buttock (right) (*see* text for explanation).

Fluid can only be deposited in a muscle without causing pain and damage if there is room for it between the muscle fibres. The muscles of the lower limb are concerned with locomotion and posture, and are composed of coarse fibres. On the other hand, the muscles of the arm are concerned with relatively fine movement and therefore have much finer fibres. The fibres of which the deltoid muscle is composed are coarser than those of the other arm muscles, and this muscle has been used as the site for intramuscular injections. However, as it has a much smaller bulk than the gluteal and thigh muscles and overlies important motor nerves, it should only be employed for the purpose when the more desirable sites are not available for use.

Technique of intramuscular injection

The equipment, drugs, and materials needed to make the injection should be placed on a tray and covered with a sterile towel until required for use. Although individual preferences govern the choice of items, the contents of a typical tray are illustrated in *Fig.* 9.29. The operator should have spotlessly clean hands and take care to ensure that he does not touch either the needle or any part of the syringe which will come into contact with the drug to be administered.

Penicillin is unstable in water and is supplied in rubber-capped vials, to which sterile, pyrogen-free water has to be added. The manufacturer's instructions should always be carefully followed. The pyrogen-free water is first measured by drawing it into the syringe and then added to the penicillin. The resultant fluid is then drawn into the syringe.

When a rubber-capped multi-dose vial is being used it should be well shaken until all sediment has disappeared prior to use. The rubber cap is cleansed with ½–1% cetrimide in spirit before the needle is inserted through it. Suspensions must be well shaken before use. An equivalent volume of air should be introduced

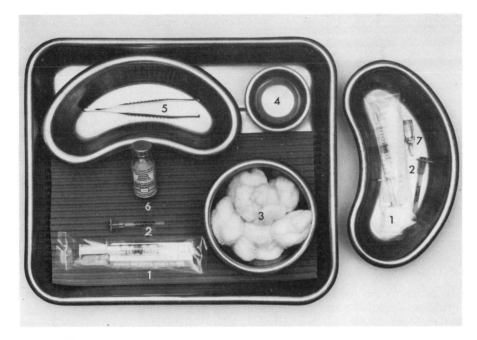

Fig. 9.29. Contents of an injection tray. 1, Disposable 2-ml syringe; 2, Disposable needle; 3, Cotton-wool swabs; 4, Cetrimide in spirit; 5, Tweezers; 6, Penicillin; 7, 1 in 1000 adrenaline solution.

with the syringe before withdrawing the drug or, alternatively, a second needle may be thrust through the cap to admit air as the fluid is withdrawn. Bubbles of air must be expelled from the syringe after filling it. To do this the syringe should be held vertically with the needle upwards. The side of the barrel should be gently tapped to dislodge bubbles adhering to it, and then the large bubble above the medicament should be expelled by gently pressing the plunger. If this is not done the quantity of fluid in the syringe cannot be measured accurately against the graduations, and air is likely to be injected with the drug.

A sterile disposal syringe, fitted with a 5-cm (2-inch) size No. 1 needle (*Fig.* 9.30), is usually employed when intramuscular injections are given. It is filled as described above, care being taken to avoid blunting the needle by bringing its point into contact with the glass wall of the container. The skin covering the selected site is cleansed with ½–1% cetrimide in spirit and made taut with the fingers of the left hand. The syringe is held in the right hand like a pen with the tip of the middle finger resting upon the needle mount. The needle should be introduced vertically to the skin surface with a sharp dart-like thrust and should be plunged deep into muscle. If the ulnar border of the operator's right hand meets the skin at the precise moment that the needle enters the tissues the prick is hardly felt. When a needle breaks the fracture almost always occurs at the junction between the shaft and the hub. For this reason a needle should never be inserted for its full length or great difficulty may be experienced in grasping and withdrawing a broken fragment from the tissues.

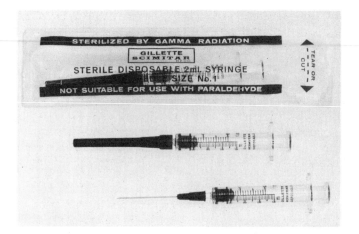

Fig. 9.30. Sterile disposable 2-ml syringes and size No. 1 needles.

In order to ensure that the needle has not entered a vessel the plunger is withdrawn slightly before the injection is given. Should blood enter the syringe, the needle must be withdrawn and another site selected for the injection. The fluid should be injected quite slowly and firm counter-pressure applied with an antiseptic swab whilst the needle is withdrawn, in order to prevent escape of the irritant solution into the subcutaneous tissues.

An alternative technique

A sharp 5-cm (2-inch) size No. 1 needle is held by the hub and introduced vertically to the skin surface with a quick dart-like thrust and plunged into the muscle. Once the needle is in position the previously filled syringe is connected to it. If the needle has entered a vessel blood will usually flow from its hub before the syringe is connected. Nevertheless, the aspiration test should always be performed before the injection is completed.

Safety precautions

Every precaution must be taken to ensure that the correct dose of the correct strength of the right drug is given by the desired route to the right patient. After the identity of the patient has been confirmed, the label on the container of the drug and the dosage drawn up for injection should be checked by someone other than the person who prepared the dose. It is sound practice never to give an intramuscular injection unless a third person is present. This rule is of especial importance in dental practice, particularly when young female patients are being treated, and the dental chairside assistant should be trained to provide effective assistance to the dentist in such procedures.

Any operator with a past history of allergies should wear clean rubber gloves throughout the procedure in order to minimize the risk of his becoming sensitive to penicillin.

When multiple injections have to be given, care should be taken regularly to change the site of injection in order to reduce discomfort and minimize the risk of muscle necrosis. This precaution is of particular importance when thin persons are being treated.

In obese patients a large amount of fatty subcutaneous tissue overlies the muscles and a needle of adequate length to penetrate the muscle must be selected and employed in such cases. Gently pinching up a fold of subcutaneous tissue permits an estimate of the thickness of the overlying tissues to be made.

An injection should only be given into an immobile site. When children or nervous adults are being treated an assistant should control the part selected for injection throughout the procedure.

Complications

Apprehensive patients may *faint* before, during, or after receiving an intra-muscular injection. The operator can do much to prevent this by acquiring a calm, confident, reassuring, and kindly manner and performing the procedure expeditiously and without an undue display of medical equipment (*see* p. 376).

A simple faint occurring after an injection must be differentiated from a *hypersensitivity reaction*, a much more serious complication. Certain substances called 'allergens' produce reactions of varying degrees of severity when they gain access into the tissues of sensitized individuals by any route. Penicillin and procaine are two such substances. Although patients afflicted with bronchial asthma are especially liable to be hypersensitive to these drugs, otherwise healthy 'normal' people may also react abnormally on occasions. These reactions may vary in degree from local oedema or urticaria at the site of injection to a profound and dangerous *anaphylactic reaction*, which can prove fatal if not treated promptly. In severe cases this comprises a profound degree of shock, with a severe fall in blood pressure, loss of consciousness, respiratory embarrassment, facial and laryngeal oedema, and urticaria. This reaction is due to hypersensitivity to penicillin and unless treatment is instituted immediately it may progress to a fatal termination. Treatment consists of the intramuscular injection of 1 ml of 0·1% (1 in 1000) adrenaline solution, repeated every 5 min until the symptoms begin to subside. Such a heavy dosage of adrenaline is not without its dangers for it can cause acute cardiac failure, but in the presence of severe anaphylactic shock this risk must be accepted if the patient is to survive.

Some vials of 1 in 1000 adrenaline solution should always be conveniently at hand when injections are given, for although they will be required only on very rare occasions, when they are needed, speed is essential if the patient's life is to be saved. Less severe allergic reactions can also be relieved by the slow subcutaneous injection of ½–1 ml of 0·1% adrenaline solution over a period of 2 min or an injection of Hydrocortisone Sodium Succinate Injection BP 100 mg in 2 ml given intravenously, or intramuscularly if a vein cannot be found. These drugs are far better for this purpose than the antihistamines, though to prevent delayed reactions phenindamine tablets BP may be given by mouth, 25 mg three times a day for 1 or 2 days afterwards.

Vials of adrenaline solution should never be placed on the injection tray in case it is confused with the drug which has to be injected (*see Fig*. 9.29). Fatalities have resulted from such errors. Adrenaline should be stored in a cool dark place and only clear colourless solutions should be used. The drug deteriorates rapidly in daylight to form a brown or pink solution.

The serious nature of hypersensitivity reactions to penicillin makes it essential that all patients for whom the drug is prescribed should be carefully and thoroughly questioned about any previous experience of the drug. In the presence of any history of previous reactions to penicillin, however sketchy, another antibiotic should be selected or specialist guidance sought. Although oral administration of penicillin to sensitive persons does not cause so immediate a reaction as parenteral therapy, deaths have followed administration by the oral route.

The dental surgeon must always remember that, in law, an injection is a surgical operation. Thus the consent of the patient, or, in the case of a child, the parent or guardian, must be obtained before an injection is given. Unless this precaution is taken the dentist risks being charged with assault. Should a patient suffer avoidable harm as a consequence of an injection being given in an unskilful or negligent fashion, he is entitled to sue those responsible for damages.

SUGGESTED READING

Adekeye E. O. and Adekeye J. O. (1982) The pathogenesis and microbiology of idiopathic cervicofacial abscesses. *J. Oral Max. Fac. Surg.* **40**, 100–6.

Aderhold L., Knothe H. and Frenkel G. (1981) The bacteriology of dentogenous pyogenic infections. *Oral Surg.* **52**, 583–7.

American Heart Association (1977) Prevention of bacterial endocarditis. Committee Report. *Circulation* **56**, 139A–143A.

Birn H. (1972) Spread of dental infections. *Dent. Pract.* **22**, 347–56.

British Society for Antimicrobial Chemotherapy (1982) The antibiotic prophylaxis of infective endocarditis. Report of a Working Party. *Lancet* **2**, 1323–6.

Cawson R. A. (1981) Infective endocarditis as a complication of dental treatment. *Br. Dent. J.* **151**, 409–14.

Garrod L. P. (1972) Causes of failure in antibiotic treatment. *Br. Med. J.* **4**, 473–6.

Greer Walker D. (1947) Severe infections of the mandible. *Proc. R. Soc. Med.* **40**, 309–16.

Kay L. W. (1960) The management of pericoronitis. *Dent. Pract.* **11**, 80–5.

von Konow L., Nord C. E. and Nordenram A. (1981) Anaerobic bacteria in dento-alveolar infections. *Int. J. Oral Surg.* **10**, 313–22.

Kramer I. R. H. (1956) Antibiotic therapy in dental practice. *Br. Dent. J.* **100**, 69–80.

Moule A. W. (1948) Acute infections arising from teeth. *Dent. Gaz.* **15**, 125–38.

Sims W. (1974) The clinical bacteriology of purulent oral infections. *Br. J. Oral Surg.* **12**, 1–12.

Speirs C. F. and Stephen K. W. (1968) Antibacterial drugs for oral infections. *Br. Dent. J.* **125**, 158–62.

Tonge C. H. and Luke D. A. (1981) Dental anatomy: the spread of infection. *Dent. Update* **8**, 291–301.

Tozer R. A., Boutflower S. and Gillespie W. A. (1966) Antibiotics for prevention of bacterial endocarditis during dental treatment. *Lancet* **1**, 686–8.

Waite D. E. (1960) Infections of dental aetiology in the mandibular and maxillofacial region. *J. Oral Surg.* **18**, 312–18.

Walton J. G. and Thompson J. W. 1970) Pharmacology for the dental practitioner. *Br. Dent. J.* **128**, 32–36, 85–88, 134–42.

Woods R. (1981) The changing nature of dental pyogenic infections. *Austr. Dent. J.* **26**, 209–13.

Woods R. (1981) Diagnosis and antibiotic treatment of alveolar infections in dentistry. *Int. Dent. J.* **31**, 145–51.

Chapter 10
Surgical aids to denture construction

Despite great advances in the dental prosthetist's art, and the advent of many admirable new materials, there remains an appreciable number of patients who never achieve the comfort and efficient service from their dentures which they had hoped for, desired, and confidently expected. These prosthetic failures may be due to a variety of general and local causes, for many factors govern the success or failure of a denture.

Unfortunately some patients cannot, or will not, wear dentures, however well designed, expertly constructed, and aesthetically perfect they may be. Other patients will wear, quite contentedly, ill-fitting, badly designed monstrosities. The psychological make-up of the patient and his attitude to both his environment and his dentures are the critical factors in many cases. The person who lives a full active life usually perseveres with, and masters, his dentures because he realizes their importance to him as he takes his place in society. On the other hand, patients who have little regard for their appearance, the social graces, or intercourse with the society in which they live, do not bother either to obtain dentures or to master any constructed for them. As age advances, a large percentage of patients fall into the latter category, and it is sound practice to avoid the need for dentures by conserving the natural dentition of an elderly patient who is unlikely to succeed in the difficult transition from natural to artificial teeth, though in a younger patient a dental clearance would be indicated. The ageing process is characterized by atrophy and the tissues supporting a denture are affected in the same way as those in other parts of the body, and these changes may make it more difficult to fit and to wear a satisfactory prosthesis.

Whilst most of the general factors are not amenable to alteration, many of the local factors can be either prevented or remedied by surgical treatment.

Many dental prosthetists hold conflicting views about the importance of local factors in the determination of the success or failure of dentures, but all agree that the edentulous denture-bearing area should be devoid of dental remnants and pathological lesions. Most of them desire that the base of the denture be supported by as much of the jaw as is possible. This bony foundation should be covered with a mucoperiosteum of even thickness, which is neither so thin that it ulcerates under denture pressure nor so thick that it undermines the stability of the denture by its excessive movement or uneven compressibility. The denture-bearing area should be free from tender soft-tissue scars and sharp bony prominences which may cause pain when pressed upon by dentures. Positive retention can only be obtained upon a denture base by utilizing the inherent elastic recoil of the

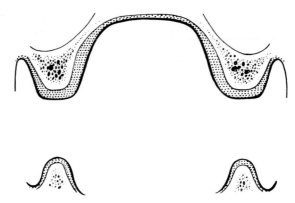

Fig. 10.1. Diagrammatic transverse section of ideal alveolar ridges and sulci for denture construction.

reflected mucous membrane at its periphery. Extensive buccal and labial under-cuts or prominent fibrous bands destroy border seal and thus prejudice retention (*Fig.* 10.1).

Most general surgeons recognize the problems of their colleagues, the limb-fitting surgeons, and plan their operations to assist them whenever possible. This close co-operation contrasts vividly with the lack of forethought and planning which accompanies the straightforward extraction of teeth and their replacement with a denture. Usually the dental surgeon who removes the teeth also provides the dentures for the patient and, by an inexplicable lack of foresight at the time of extraction, creates many of his future prosthetic difficulties.

Every dental surgeon should have a thorough knowledge of the conditions which favour success in denture construction, for carefully planned and executed surgery can prevent the occurrence of many undesirable features and can eliminate others, either at the time teeth are extracted or later.

PREVENTIVE MEASURES DESIGNED TO REDUCE PROSTHETIC DIFFICULTIES

A simple, but most effective way in which the dental profession could facilitate the construction of successful dentures is by raising the standards of tooth extraction. Multiple radiographic surveys of symptom-free clinically edentulous patients conducted in different parts of the world reveal that about a quarter of those examined have retained or buried roots. The intelligent use of pre-extraction radiographs enables the dental surgeon to anticipate and deal with any difficulties or complications encountered during tooth removal (*see* p. 92).

Provided that the patient's total exposure to radiation permits, a complete intra-oral periapical radiographic survey should be peformed whenever a dental clearance is indicated. Careful interpretation of the films and meticulous extraction technique will greatly reduce the incidence of retained root fragments and patho-logical lesions and the need for further radiographs. Radiographic examination of 'edentulous areas' to exclude the presence of buried teeth, retained roots, or intra-bony pathology is of special importance. Whenever a tooth has been extracted with forceps, the socket should be carefully compressed between the finger and thumb so that the expanded alveolar bone is repositioned. Attention to this simple manoeuvre prevents a prominent sharp bony spur being left to make the task of the prosthetist and his patient more difficult. Loose pieces of alveolar bone fractured during tooth removal should be sought for and removed. A loosely tied suture should be inserted to reposition the soft tissues if they show a tendency to gape.

If a root fractures during forceps extraction, the method employed to remove it should ensure that the maximum amount of alveolar bony support for a denture is preserved. The oral surgeon is often requested to remove buried teeth and roots from clinically edentulous patients. It has been shown that retained roots seen in radiographs to be surrounded by a periodontal membrane of normal thickness have vital pulps. They are no danger either locally or to the individual as a whole, but should be removed if liable to be exposed by either resorption or pressure from a denture. Any root which radiographs show to be related to either a granuloma or a cyst must be removed.

The operative technique employed to remove a buried tooth or root should be designed to ensure that the alveolar ridge is left as normal as possible at the completion of the operation. Roots can often be removed via an 'apicectomy' window, thus reducing the amount of bone excised. The alveolar ridge may also

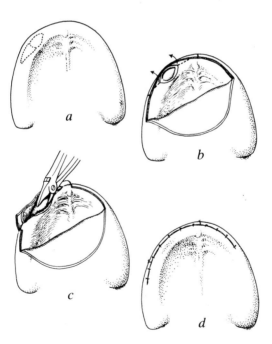

Fig. 10.2. The use of an osteoplastic flap to preserve ridge form (*see* text for explanation).

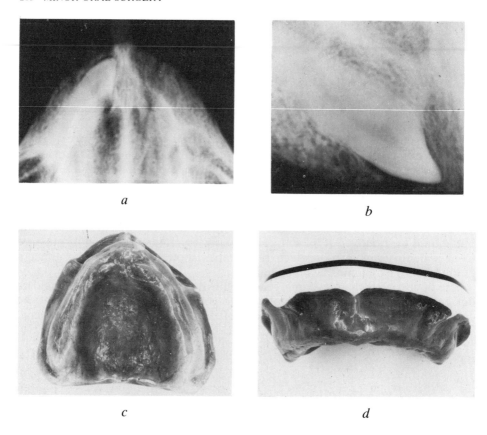

Fig. 10.3. A clinical case in which ridge form was preserved by the use of an osteoplastic flap. *a, b,* Preoperative radiographs showing 3| to be in the alveolar ridge. *c, d,* Postoperative model showing ridge form.

be preserved by sectioning buried teeth and dividing roots, and delivering the separated portions with minimal removal of bone.

It is sometimes possible to conserve bone by the use of an osteoplastic flap during the removal of buried teeth or a cyst. The use of this technique in the removal of a buried right maxillary canine lying in an edentulous alveolar ridge is illustrated in *Fig.* 10.2. After making an incision along the crest of the ridge and raising a palatal mucoperiosteal flap, bone is removed to expose the crown of the buried tooth. Sharp taps upon a chisel, placed as indicated by the dotted line, fracture the buccal plate outwards (*Fig.* 10.2*b*). Vertical incisions are made in the buccal mucoperiosteum about one-quarter of an inch from the bony fracture lines and the osteoplastic flap hinged outwards on its attached soft tissues (*Fig.* 10.2*c*). After extracting the tooth with forceps, removing the follicle, and smoothing the bone edges, the ridge is reconstituted by replacing the flap and closing the wound with sutures (*Fig.* 10.2*d*).

After-pain appears to be slightly more marked when an osteoplastic flap is used, but this disadvantage is outweighed by the preservation of ridge-form obtainable only by this method (*Fig.* 10.3).

Earlier claims that alveolar ridge form and proprioceptive sense could be retained by the use of the so-called root submergence technique have not been substantiated.

Gingival inflammation should be eliminated by pre-extraction scaling of the teeth whenever possible. At least a week should elapse after scaling before extractions are undertaken in order to allow the inflammation to resolve. This simple measure materially speeds healing.

PROSTHETIC DIFFICULTIES AMENABLE TO SURGICAL CORRECTION

The prospective denture wearer should be examined from a prosthetic viewpoint before dental extractions are undertaken for, whenever possible, prosthetic difficulties should be eliminated at the time the teeth are removed. A little

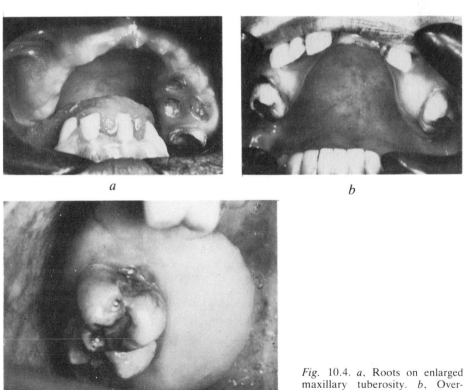

a

b

c

Fig. 10.4. *a*, Roots on enlarged maxillary tuberosity. *b*, Over-erupted maxillary molars. *c*, Fibrous enlargement of tuberosity.

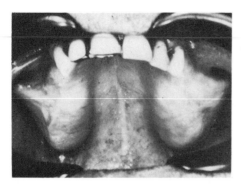

Fig. 10.5. Giant tuberosities.

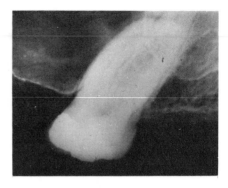

Fig. 10.6. Radiograph of isolated maxillary molar. Note the large antrum.

forethought at this stage may enable the dental surgeon to reduce a socket or a bulbous tuberosity or eliminate a bony prominence or a fibrous band at the time of extraction and thus facilitate the construction of successful dentures. Time spent in pre-extraction prosthetic assessment is always amply repaid. Thus simple forceps extraction of the teeth or roots illustrated in *Fig*. 10.4 would leave maxillary tuberosities of such a size, shape, and consistency as to render denture construction difficult if not impossible. *Fig*. 10.5 shows the maxilla of a patient in whom an extreme degree of enlargement of the tuberosities was present.

In such cases surgical reduction of an enlarged tuberosity at the time the teeth are extracted leaves the mouth in as satisfactory a condition as is possible for denture construction. Pre-extraction radiographs should be taken in these cases as the bony tuberosity is often weakened by an extension into it of the antrum (*Fig*. 10.6).

In other cases examination of an edentulous patient may reveal the presence of one or more unwanted local lesions, causing a prosthetic problem which can be solved by means of surgery. However, it must be recognized that pre-prosthetic surgery is not a panacea, for it can only be used to remedy anatomical obstacles to prosthetic success. Pre-prosthetic surgery is not a substitute for good prosthetics but merely an aid to it.

SPECIAL FEATURES OF PROSTHETIC SURGERY

Prosthetic surgery may demand the full skill of the oral surgeon since the soft tissues may be difficult to work with, due to either the scarring which follows repeated ulceration or friability caused by the atrophic changes of age. In these circumstances it may be extremely difficult to obtain healing by first intention, unless 'tissue craft' of a very high order is displayed. Scar tissue following prosthetic surgery must be minimal in amount and sited in such a position that it is exposed to as little denture pressure as possible. It is essential to keep prosthetic requirements in mind when peforming prosthetic surgery, otherwise the removal

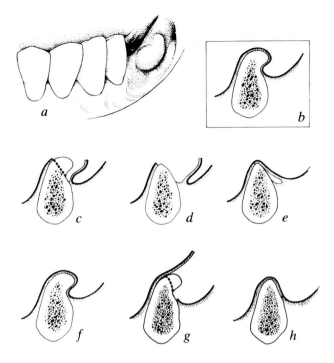

Fig. 10.7. Incorrect and correct techniques employed in the removal of an osteoma from the denture-bearing area. *a*, Clinical appearance of lesion. *b*, Transverse section through the mandibular molar area. *c*, *d*, *e*, Operation performed incorrectly. Note the loss of depth in sulcus. *f*, *g*, *h*, Use of lingually based flap to preserve depth of sulcus. (*see Fig.* 10.17).

of one difficulty may result in the creation of another. *Fig.* 10.7*c, d, e* illustrates a case in which the height of the buccal sulcus has been decreased during the removal of an undercut bony prominence. This complication could have been avoided by the use of a mucoperiosteal flap with its base situated lingually instead of buccally (*Fig.* 10.7*f, g, h*).

Many of these patients possess ill-fitting dentures and, if they attempt to wear them postoperatively, the soft tissues will be damaged and healing delayed. The dental surgeon may either retain the dentures at the time of operation or, by modifying them by the addition of green composition tracing-stick and lining them with either zinc oxide and eugenol impression paste or a tissue conditioner, use them as a protective splint for the healing tissues. If the appliances are utilized in this way, it is essential to ensure that no excess of the lining material enters the suture lines and so delays healing. In some cases, as for example after tuberosity reduction has been performed, resolution of the wound is assisted if the patient wears the upper denture continuously for a week postoperatively, removing it daily, after the first 48 hours, to rinse it free of food detritus.

Although frequently more than one abnormality is present in the same patient, it is more convenient to discuss each lesion separately.

ENLARGED MAXILLARY TUBEROSITIES

The maxillary tuberosities are found to be abnormally large in a considerable number of edentulous patients and in the vast majority of cases this enlargement is due to an excess of white fibrous tissue (*Fig.* 10.8). In some instances this overgrowth is related to periodontal disease around natural maxillary molars, or is derived from overgrowth of the soft tissues distal to an over-erupted unopposed maxillary molar. Enlarged tuberosities are sometimes seen in patients with unopposed mandibular molars who have been wearing an incompletely extended upper denture which has failed to cover the tuberosity area.

An abnormally large maxillary tuberosity may create prosthetic difficulties for a variety of reasons. It may encroach upon the interalveolar space to such an extent that there is insufficient room for upper and lower denture bases, or the convex outer surface of the tuberosity, in addition to producing a buccal undercut, may also render the space between the alveolar bone and the ascending ramus too narrow to accommodate the buccal flange of an upper denture. As previously mentioned, many of these lesions are composed of fibrous tissue which may undermine the stability of the denture by its excessive mobility.

Whilst prosthetic techniques designed to cope with the problem may preserve border seal despite the presence of a buccal undercut, they do so at the expense of the fit between the edge of the flange and its supporting tissues, and they cannot deal with the other difficulties. Surgical reduction of the tuberosity is a simple procedure and by its use all these obstacles to success can be eliminated. The following technique is both simple and quick to perform and is seldom followed by either pain or swelling.

An incision is made forwards along the crest of the ridge from the hamular process to the premolar region (*Fig.* 10.9*a*). The incision is made down to bone and the tip of the scalpel blade is held slightly more buccally than the handle. In most instances the blade will sink into a mass of fibrous tissue but, on those rare occasions when the enlargement is of an entirely bony nature, the knife will strike bone almost immediately upon entering the tissues. In these circumstances no

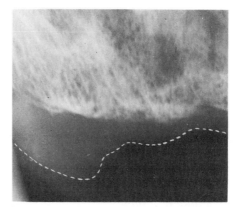

Fig. 10.8. Periapical radiograph of an enlarged maxillary tuberosity showing it to be largely composed of fibrous tissue.

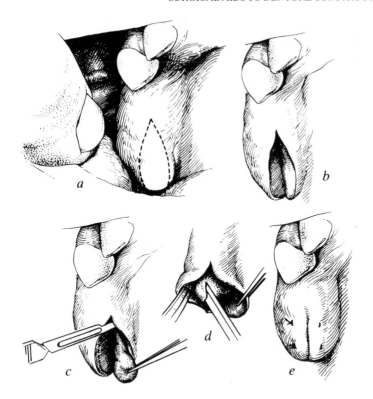

Fig. 10.9. Technique of tuberosity reduction viewed from below (*see* text for explanation).

second incision should be made, but in all other cases a second incision should be made situated buccally to the first, with the tip of the scalpel blade placed slightly more palatally than the handle. This incision should also be down to bone and the ellipse of fibrous tissue outlined by the two incisions can then be lifted from the wound with a pair of curved artery forceps. The angulation of the scalpel blade, when the incisions are made, leaves the cut surfaces of the soft tissue sloping so that the junction between the excess of white fibrous tissue and the mucosa is easily seen (*Figs*. 10.9*b*, 10.10*b*). This facilitates the undercutting of buccal and palatal flaps of mucous membrane and the removal of the underlying fibrous tissue (*Figs*. 10.9*c*, 10.10*c*).

If required, the exposed bone can be trimmed with a chisel and bone file and bone removal is facilitated if the anterior part of the incision is extended in a curve towards the buccal sulcus. The tuberosity often contains an extension of the maxillary air-sinus and bone removal could involve the antrum. If a chisel is used the exposed antral lining often remains intact, whilst perforation usually occurs when a bur is employed (*Figs*. 10.9*d*, 10.10*d*). The mucoperiosteal flaps are approximated and any excess is trimmed off the palatal flap. This preserves the height of the buccal sulcus and sites the scar in a favourable position. The trimmed flaps are then apposed with interrupted mattress sutures (*Figs*. 10.9*e*, 10.10*e*). If

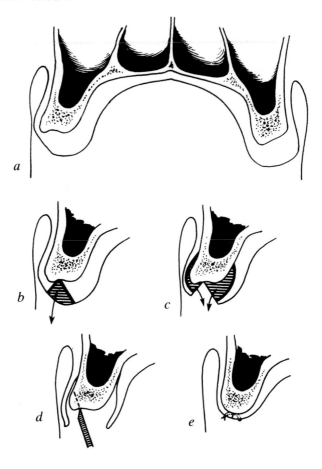

Fig. 10.10. Technique of tuberosity reduction. Transverse section (*see* text for explanation).

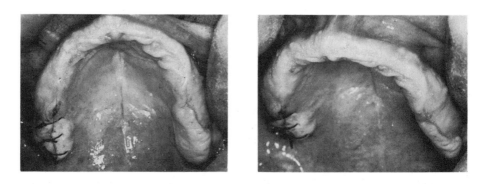

Fig. 10.11. Identical enlarged maxillary tuberosities after surgical reduction of the right one.

the patient has an upper denture, it is lined with either zinc oxide and oil-of-cloves impression paste or a tissue conditioner and worn as a splint for the wound (*Fig.* 10.11).

There is no obvious cause for abnormal enlargement of the maxillary tuberosity or the tendency for the lesion to recur, which is sometimes observed when surgical reduction is not followed by the construction and prompt insertion of dentures.

The treatment of bulbous bony tuberosities is often rendered difficult by the fact that usually such tuberosities are composed of a thin cortical plate, within which are soft putty-like contents, almost fluid in consistency. This material is a poor supporting tissue for a denture, whilst the sharp cut edges of the cortical plate can be readily palpated through the soft tissue.

Despite these difficulties surgical reduction produces much better results than any other form of treatment of the enlaged maxillary tuberosity.

FRENA AND FIBROUS BANDS

Frena or bands of scar tissue resulting from injury or inflammation may have a high attachment on the alveolar ridge. Their presence may necessitate a localized reduction in height of the labial and buccal flanges of a denture. In addition to weakening the denture this adjustment may prejudice its retention by interfering with border seal. In these circumstances surgical elimination of these structures may be indicated.

When a frenum is excised for orthodontic purposes, it is essential to remove all the fibrous tissue present in the median suture and between the central incisors. Postoperative scar-tissue formation is of little consequence. When the operation is performed to remove a prosthetic difficulty, the fibrous band which raises the fold of mucous membrane must be eliminated and the alveolar bone of the deepened sulcus left covered with enough resilient soft tissue to withstand the pressure of a denture base. In order to avoid confusion between the two differing surgical procedures, the term *frenoplasty* is used to describe those operations performed for prosthetic reasons and *frenectomy* for the orthodontic procedure described on p. 174).

Prominent labial frena causing a prosthetic difficulty can be excised in the following manner: An assistant holds the patient's lip at right-angles to the outer surface of the maxilla so that the fibrous band is tensed (*Fig.* 10.12*a*). The mucous membrane is incised on either side of the fibrous band from the alveolar attachment to a point well out into the lip (*Fig.* 10.12*b*). The lower end of the fibrous band is gripped in a pair of fine haemostatic forceps, its alveolar attachment severed, and the whole band excised (*Fig.* 10.12*c*). This exposes the intact periosteum which is still attached to bone. After freeing the edges of the mucous membrane from the underlying tissues and dividing any fibrous adhesions to the periosteum by blunt dissection (*Fig.* 10.12*d*), the mucous membrane is sewn to the periosteum with black silk (*Fig.* 10.12*e*). This suture, which regains the depth of the sulcus, is termed the 'anchor' suture and the use of a Hagedorn needle facilitates its insertion (*see Fig.* 3.37*b*). This needle can be passed easily under the periosteum on its side, and then rotated and brought out of the periosteum with minimal disturbance of the periosteal attachment to bone.

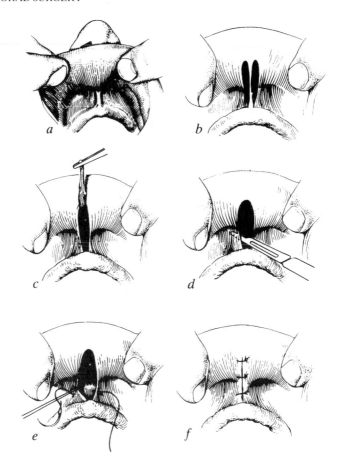

Fig. 10.12. Labial frenoplasty (*see* text for explanation).

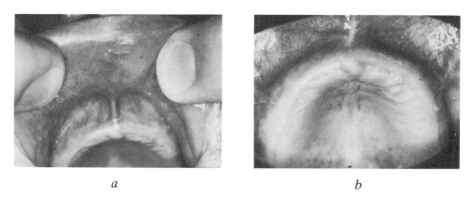

Fig. 10.13. Prominent labial frenum. *a*, Before frenoplasty. *b*, After frenoplasty.

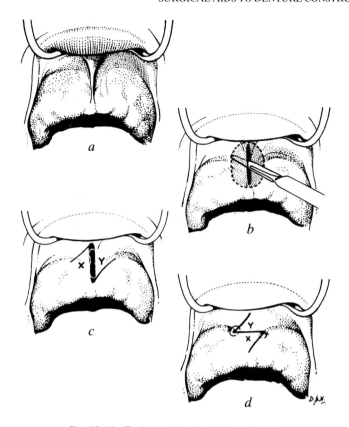

Fig. 10.14. Z-plasty (*see* text for explanation).

The edges of the labial wound are then apposed with interrupted sutures, each knot being carefully placed to one side of the suture line (*Fig.* 10.12*f*).

This technique can be performed in a few minutes under local anaesthesia and *Fig.* 10.13*b* illustrates a typical end-result.

In the mandibular premolar region the presence of the mental nerve makes the insertion of the 'anchor suture' more difficult. The periosteum in the premolar region is more friable and more loosely attached to bone, and the 'anchor suture' does not hold well.

It is good practice to perform a Z-plasty in this situation after excising the fibrous strand and undercutting the mucous membrane widely (*Fig.* 10.14*b*). The resulting flaps should be at least 1 cm long and are transposed and sutured to the cut edges of the attached mucoperiosteum and buccal mucosa (*Fig.* 10.14*c* and *d*). It has been demonstrated that the maximum benefit is obtained by means of Z-plasty when flaps with an angle of 60° at the tip are utilized. It is important to ensure that all fibrous adhesions to the periosteum are divided by means of blunt dissection before the mucosal flaps are repositioned.

When multiple or very wide scar-tissue attachments exist, the insertion of an epithelial inlay is the most satisfactory way of eliminating them and deepening the sulcus, and the patient should be referred to a specialist oral surgeon for opinion and treatment (*see* Chapter 16).

Healing by first intention is essential in frenoplasty if scar formation is to be kept to a minimum and for this reason techniques employing electrosurgery or those which involve crushing tissues are contra-indicated. The unwanted fibrous strand should be excised and the exposed mesodermal tissues covered either with under-cut mucous membrane or by skin. This dissection is facilitated if an assistant holds out the lip and tenses the frenum throughout the operation. The use of a sharp scalpel is imperative if healing is to be satisfactory, and the excision should be carried well out into the lip to prevent the formation of residual tags of soft tissue.

Labial frenoplasty is often followed by postoperative soreness out of all pro-portion to the size and severity of the operation. Labial tenderness may make suture removal difficult and the application of a topical anaesthetic paste to the area facilitates the procedure.

Although histological examination has failed to reveal the presence of muscular tissue in sections of excised frena, it is possible that these folds are raised by the fibrous attachments of muscles. Clinical experience does not support the oft-stated view that excessive removal of the labial frenum permits the upper lip to curl unattractively.

In the anterior lingual region many prosthetists extend the flange of the lower denture to the sublingual folds and utilize the inherent elastic recoil of the soft tissues in this area to develop positive retention upon the anterior part of the denture base. The presence of a short lingual frenum may render impossible this use of the anterior lingual region for prosthetic purposes. In these circumstances

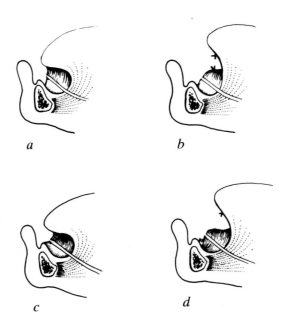

a   *b*

c   *d*

Fig. 10.15. Lingual frenotomy (*see* text for explanation).

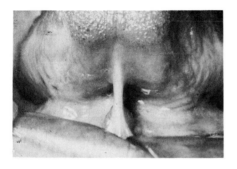 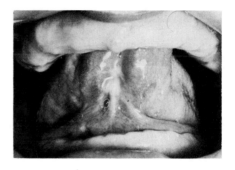

a   *b*

Fig. 10.16. Tight lingual frenum. *a*, Before lingual frenotomy. *b*, Two weeks after operation.
Note the position of the scar.

the elimination of this structure may be indicated by means of the surgical
procedure known as *lingual frenotomy*.

When treating tight lingual frena, the oral surgeon has the problem of eliminating
the tense, short fibrous band without leaving an excess of fibrous tissue in a region
where the prosthetist desires only soft tissues which can be readily distorted. The
problem is best solved in the following manner.

After passing a suture through the tip of the tongue traction is applied to tense
the frenum (*Fig*. 10.15*a*), whilst its attachment to the undersurface is divided
transversely and sewn up vertically (*Fig*. 10.15*b*). The division of the frenum must
be bold and at least one-half of an inch in length, if the tension is to be relieved.
This method has the advantage over all other techniques that the resulting scar is
situated on the undersurface of the tongue, well away from the area which
concerns the prosthetist. If a tight lingual frenum has a high attachment to the
ridge it should be divided vertically and sewn up horizontally as illustrated in
Fig. 10.15*c* and *d*.

Although the patients have slight slurring of speech for a few days postoperatively, this appears to be due to discomfort and disappears after the sutures
are removed (*Fig*. 10.16).

FIBROUS NODULES

Firm nodules are sometimes present in the attached mucoperiosteum and pressure
upon them produces acute pain. Although in rare instances these lesions are
amputation neuromata, the vast majority are composed of fibrous tissue. These
fibrous knots may be either due to the healing of a sinus or secondary to either
irritation by a denture or the presence of an underlying bony spur. They may be
single or multiple and occur more frequently than the failure to mention them in
the literature might imply. Whilst in some cases it is possible to either design or
relieve the denture so that it does not press upon the lesion, it is usually preferable
to deal with the nodule by surgical means.

Before undertaking surgery a radiograph of the area must be taken to exclude the presence of underlying pathology. In the absence of such pathology or a bony spur, the lesion may be readily 'burred out' under local anaesthesia—a procedure which lasts only a minute or two. After pressing a sharp probe into the lesion to confirm that no bony spur is present, a round bur (size 5) running slowly in a straight handpiece is applied to the lesion, which is systematically excised in this fashion down to the level of the periosteum. No sutures are required and the wound is left to granulate.

In those cases in which a pathological area or a bony spicule is present, a soft-tissue flap should be raised and the underlying lesion excised. The wound is closed with sutures after the bone has been smoothed with either a bone file or a 'vulcanite bur'. The area should be re-examined when healing is complete and any remaining tender fibrous knot excised. In most instances no further surgery is required.

BONY PROMINENCES AND TORI

One of the main problems with which the dental prosthetist has to contend is lack of an adequate area of bony support for his denture base. Paradoxically, the presence of local excesses of bone may make his task more difficult. Pain may be caused when the mucoperiosteum is pressed against a sharp bony spur, retention may be impaired if an undercut created by a bony elevation destroys border seal, and the stability of a denture may be upset because the thin mucoperiosteum covering such a lesion lacks the compressibility of the remainder of the soft tissues supporting the denture.

In addition to painful bony spurs caused by faulty extraction technique and failure to compress the socket digitally following tooth removal, osteomata may occur in the denture-bearing area (*Fig.* 10.17).

Bony prominences may be the cause of deep undercuts when present on the buccal and labial plates of the maxilla, and may also occur just lateral to the greater palatine foramen.

Tori are small developmental anomalies that occur in constant sites on the jaw bones. A *torus palatinus* is an exostosis along the suture line of the hard palate

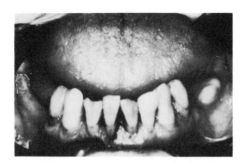

Fig. 10.17. Undercut osteoma in mandibular molar region (*see Fig.* 10.7).

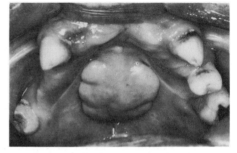

Fig. 10.18. Torus palatinus.

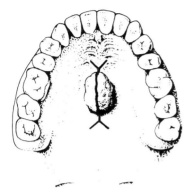

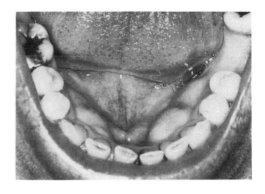

Fig. 10.19. Incision for removal of an enlarged torus palatinus.

Fig. 10.20. Bilateral tori mandibulares.

(*Fig.* 10.18). Although many authorities have stressed the importance of removing palatal tori, the lesion is frequently observed but only occasionally requires surgical correction, and it should not be excised unless it interferes with the retention of a denture. The overlying mucoperiosteum is thin in places and the elevation of the soft tissues from the lesion is often the most difficult part of its surgical removal. Subperiosteal injections of either a local anaesthetic solution or normal saline facilitate dissection.

The incision illustrated in *Fig.* 10.19 provides excellent exposure. The lesion is divided by anteroposterior and transverse bur cuts, and the sections are removed with a mallet and chisel. The cut surface of the bony palate should then be smoothed with either bone files or a 'vulcanite bur', and the mucoperiosteal flaps replaced and loosely sutured together. The soft tissues should not be trimmed but moulded against the vault of the palate. Some surgeons construct a maxillary base-plate on a carved model preoperatively and insert it at the end of the operation to hold the soft tissues in place without the use of sutures. Such plates must be made of clear acrylic resin so that the operator can detect undue pressure by noting blanching of the soft tissues. Unless this precaution is taken sloughing may occur under the appliance.

Torus mandibularis is an exostosis, unilaterally or bilaterally situated on the lingual aspect of the mandible above the mylohyoid line in the region of the premolars (*Fig.* 10.20). Bilateral mandibular tori occur more frequently than unilateral tori and the lesions may be either single or multiple. They may extend backwards to the mandibular third molar region. The aetiology of these painless lesions is unknown, but they are more common in Mongoloid races than in Caucasian or Negroid ethnic groups.

The excision of mandibular tori is only justified if they are either causing difficulty in denture construction or are likely to do so. Prominent tori mandibularis may be excised either at the time a lower clearance is performed or immediately after the teeth have been removed. The technique is as follows.

After making an incision along the crest of the ridge the lingual soft tissues are elevated with a periosteal elevator to expose the bony exostosis, which is excised

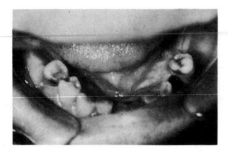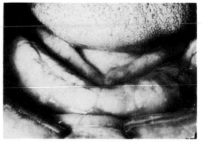

b

Fig. 10.21. Bilateral tori mandibulares excised at time of tooth extraction. *a*, Before surgery. *b*, After surgery: on left side 2 weeks postoperatively; on right side 1 week postoperatively.

with chisels, burs, or rongeurs. The cut surface of the bone is smoothed, excessive soft tissues resected, and the mucoperiosteal flap sutured back into place. When teeth are standing, it is better to use a three-sided flap based on the lingual soft tissues and involving the lingual cervical margins of the gingivae. Whilst bone is being removed, a metal retractor should be placed under the lesion to protect the mucoperiosteal flap and prevent bone fragments from being lost in the soft tissues (*Fig.* 10.21).

DENTURE GRANULOMATA

These lesions are associated with the wearing of an ill-fitting denture (*Fig.* 10.22*a*). It is widely believed that, as resorption occurs, the denture settles and its flanges dig into the adjacent soft tissues, causing the formation of ulcers and granulation tissue. Organization of the granulations into fibrous tissue makes the lesion permanent. In other cases it is possible that denture granulomata are caused by the soft tissues being sucked into the space between the base of an ill-fitting denture and the atrophied ridge which supports it. Whatever the aetiology, there can be no doubt that in the early stages of their formation denture granulomata will shrink and even disappear if the offending denture is either not worn for a period or relieved extensively. New dentures should then be constructed. If fibrosis has occurred within the lesion it will persist and should be excised before new dentures are constructed (*Fig.* 10.23). As these soft-tissue masses are related to the borders of the denture they tend to undermine both the stability and retention of the appliance. The surgical problem is to remove the unwanted lesion without substituting another prosthetic difficulty in its place. Denture granulomata are usually associated with gross alveolar resorption, and great care and skill are required to preserve the little sulcus that remains after their excision.

It is best to remove these hypertrophic masses by a combination of sharp and blunt dissection, leaving the underlying periosteum or muscle intact, using the following technique.

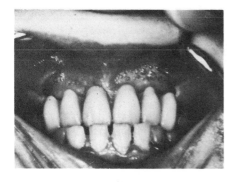 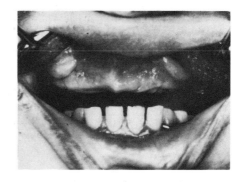

a   b

Fig. 10.22. *a*, Elderly vulcanite gum-fitted denture in situ. *b*, Class 2 denture granulomata related to 'wings' on denture.

A suture is passed through the lesion and then traction is applied to raise it from its bed. In larger granulomata, tissue forceps may be employed (*Fig.* 10.24*b*). The mucosa around the base is incised and the lesion dissected out with a Howarth periosteal elevator, persistent adhesions being divided with a scalpel (*Fig.* 10.24*b*, *c*). The excised specimen is lifted from the wound and sent for section (*see* Chapter 13).

When treating granulomata in the mandibular buccal sulcus, careful blunt dissection facilitates the identification and preservation of the mental nerve, although slight impairment or sensation and/or paraesthesia may persist for a week or two postoperatively in such cases.

The treatment of the resulting defect is determined by the size and precise situation of the base of the lesion, and for this purpose it is convenient to divide them into:

Class 1: Granulomata based entirely upon the attached mucoperiosteum.

Class 2: Granulomata attached entirely to the mucous membrane of the cheeks, lips, or floor of mouth.

Class 3: Granulomata with attachments which straddle and obliterate the reflection of the mucous membrane (*Fig.* 10.25).

Defects resulting from Class 1 lesions (*see Figs.* 10.23, 10.24*a*) heal well with minimal scarring if the exposed periosteum is covered with a base-plate, lined with either black gutta-percha, zinc oxide and oil-of-cloves impression paste, or a tissue conditioner which is worn continuously for the first week postoperatively (*see Fig.* 10.24*d*, *e*). Wounds created by the excision of Class 2 granulomata (*see Fig.* 10.22) usually heal by first intention if the inherent elasticity of the mucous membrane is utilized to cover the exposed muscle after extensive undercutting has been performed. Following the removal of very extensive Class 2 or Class 3 lesions, attempts to obtain coverage of mesodermal tissues by this means either fail completely or are followed by obliteration of the labiobuccal sulcus. In these cases it is best to advance the undercut mucous membrane as far as possible without tensing it unduly, and then maintain it in this new position by suturing it to the underlying muscle. This procedure reduces the area which heals by second

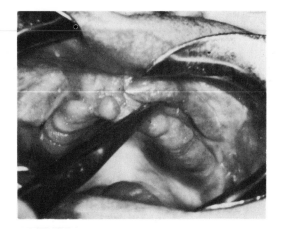

Fig. 10.23.   Class 1 denture granuloma.

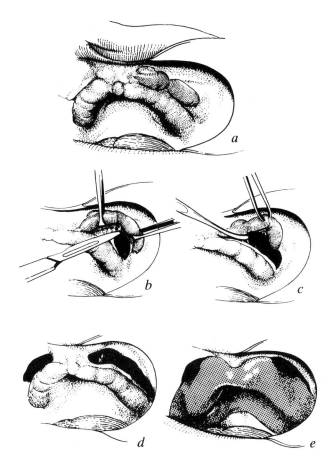

Fig. 10.24.   The removal of a denture granuloma (*see* text for explanation).

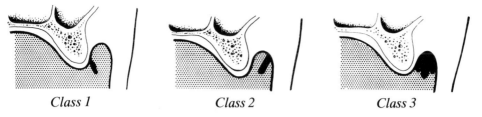

| Class 1 | Class 2 | Class 3 |

Fig. 10.25. The classification of denture granulomata.

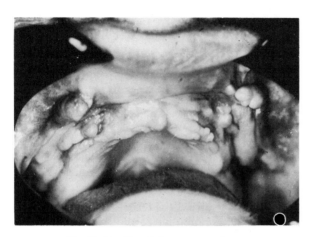

Fig. 10.26. Class 3 denture granuloma.

intention, thus minimizing scar-tissue formation and loss of sulcus depth. This process takes time and the dental surgeon should be neither surprised nor dismayed if the wound looks both swollen and irregular during the first few weeks after operation. Following the excision of very extensive Class 3 granulomata (*Fig.* 10.26), it is sometimes best to cover the resulting defect with an epithelial inlay. In cases of gross resorption of the mandible or maxilla, this latter procedure can be used to regain sulcus depth. Patients requiring this type of surgery should be referred to a specialist oral surgeon (*see* Chapter 16).

Denture hyperplasia occurs in patients who are determined to wear dentures, and therefore appreciate and benefit from relatively slight improvements. For this reason the major procedure of epithelial inlay insertion is seldom required.

LOCALIZED PROBLEMS CAUSED BY GROSS RESORPTION OF THE JAWS

The cause of atrophy of the jaws, unassociated with either infection or metabolic disease, is obscure but, whatever the aetiology, gross resorption of the alveolar bone is a frequent cause of difficulty in denture construction. Any reduction in the denture-bearing area throws a greater load upon the remaining supporting tissues, every part of which has to bear a larger proportion of the total masticatory load. The denture-bearing area may become inflamed, painful, or tender and further resorption of the bone may result. As the height of the ridge decreases, the attachments of the soft tissues to the jaw become comparatively more superficial and the muscles impinge more forcibly upon the denture. It is not uncommon for the mylohyoid ridges and the superior genial tubercles to become the highest points of a grossly resorbed mandible. As the ridge is lost and the denture-bearing surface becomes more flattened, the retention of the denture is prejudiced by the increasing difficulty of obtaining and maintaining 'border seal'. The stability of the prosthesis may also decrease and the contraction of muscles, such as the mentalis, may readily displace a full lower denture.

The increasing frequency and tremendous importance of the prosthetic difficulties caused by gross resorption of the jaws are underlined by the multitude of surgical techniques devised to deal with them. Although in most instances the assessment of, and treatment planning for, such patients is best undertaken by an oral surgeon and a specialist prosthetist working as a team, some of the localized obstacles to prosthetic success can be treated successfully by a dental surgeon.

SHARP TENDER RIDGES

These ridges are often described as 'knife-edge' ridges and are most commonly found in the anterior part of the mandible. The patient is often a postmenopausal woman who complains of localized tenderness over the crest of the ridge when dentures are worn. Clinical examination reveals a very narrow ridge, covered with thin atrophic mucosa which is tender to palpation. Radiographic examination discloses an unevenly resorbed ridge with an irregular margin which is devoid of compact bone (*Fig.* 10.27). If the lesion is localized it may be eliminated by the use of the following technique.

An incision along the crest of the ridge is made across the affected area. It is important to site the incision so that some lingual mucoperiosteum is available to

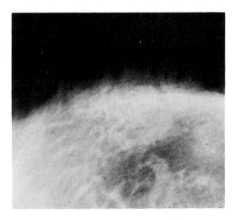

Fig. 10.27. Periapical radiograph of a sharp tender ridge. Note the vertical vascular channels.

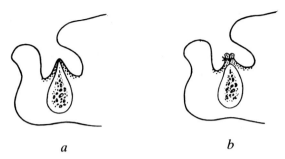

a   *b*

Fig. 10.28. The surgical treatment of a 'knife-edge' ridge. *a*, Preoperative condition. *b*, At end of operation.

hold sutures at the end of the operation (*Fig.* 10.28). The friable soft tissues are carefully elevated from the ridge sufficiently to provide access for the sharp bony ridge to be excised with alveolotomy shears. After smoothing the cut edges of bone with a bone file, the soft tissues are repaired with mattress sutures. The use of horizontal mattress sutures everts the cut edges of the mucoperiosteum and ensures that the treated ridge has an adequate covering of soft tissue. Although the ridge and sulcus height are reduced when this technique is employed, the results on the whole are good, although the lesion may recur unless a really stable and retentive lower denture is provided. In many instances such an appliance cannot be fitted until more major surgery, such as vestibuloplasty has been undertaken by a specialist oral surgeon.

THE FIBROUS RIDGE

Excessive amounts of soft tissue may be present upon, or even replace, the crest of both mandibular and maxillary ridges. They may undermine the stability of a denture, by their uneven compressibility and abnormal mobility, to such a degree that satisfactory dentures can only be constructed and worn following surgical treatment. It is not uncommon to find abnormal flabbiness of the anterior maxillary ridge in patients who have worn a full upper denture opposed by six natural lower front teeth. These patients have either had a partial lower denture which failed to provide the necessary posterior support, or they have never worn a mandibular prosthesis. In these circumstances the full occlusal load is transmitted by the denture to the anterior maxillary ridge and resorption of the supporting bone occurs, leaving only a flabby soft-tissue ridge (*Fig.* 10.29).

Comparatively rarely the retromolar pad is enlarged and interferes with denture construction, either by decreasing the intermaxillary space available for dentures or by undermining the stability of a full lower denture. In other cases the resorbed mandibular alveolar bone is represented only by a fibrous ridge, which may be either mobile or compressible enough to interfere with denture construction. Surgical treatment of flabby ridges should only be undertaken if it is felt that the need for stability outweighs the resulting loss of depth in the sulcus. One surgical technique commonly employed to treat a fibrous anterior maxillary ridge is as follows.

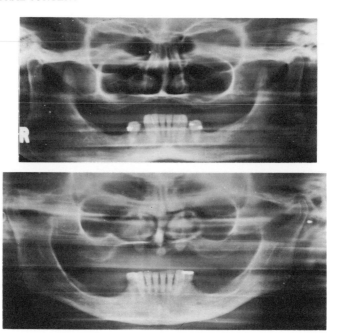

Fig. 10.29. Rotographs showing that the resorption of bone in the anterior part of the maxilla has occurred in areas opposed to standing mandibular teeth.

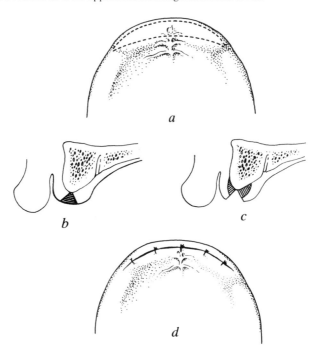

Fig. 10.30. The surgical treatment of a fibrous maxillary ridge (*see* text for explanation).

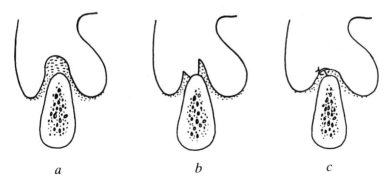

Fig. 10.31. The surgical treatment of a fibrous mandibular ridge (*see* text for explanation).

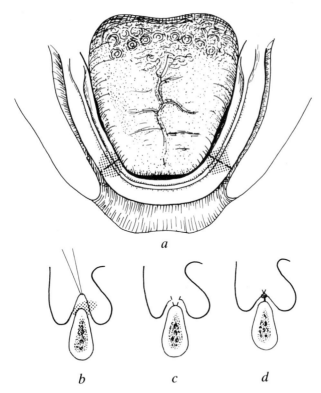

Fig. 10.32. Treatment of a lingually undercut fibrous mandibular ridge (*see* text for explanation).

An incision is made along the crest of the fibrous ridge from the left premolar region to the right premolar region. The scalpel is angled so that its blade is labial to the handle, whilst the incision is carried down to the bone. A second incision is made situated labially to the first and the ellipse of fibrous tissue outlined is removed (*Fig.* 10.30*a*, *b*). The mucosa is separated from the underlying fibrous tissue which is then removed (*Fig.* 10.30*c*). There is often a brisk haemorrhage from the cut tissues despite the presence of a vasoconstrictor in the local anaesthetic solution. This bleeding can be controlled by firm pressure upon the palatal soft tissues. After smoothing the underlying bone, the soft tissues are repaired with interrupted horizontal mattress sutures (*Fig.* 10.30*d*). Any impinging teeth in the opposing jaw should then be extracted.

Often a loss of anterior maxillary ridge height does not create a prosthetic difficulty if the patient has well-preserved posterior ridges and deep buccal sulci; but if the buccal sulci are shallow also, vestibuloplasty with or without the insertion of an epithelial inlay may be required.

A mandibular fibrous ridge can be treated by excising a wedge of fibrous tissue from its crest (*Fig.* 10.31). It is most important to preserve sufficient lingual mucoperiosteum to hold sutures and this can be achieved by making the most lingual of the two incisions as vertical as possible (*Fig.* 10.31*b*, *c*). On occasions a mandibular fibrous ridge may be tilted lingually thus producing an undercut (*Fig.* 10.32*a*, *b*). If such a ridge is present the technique described above must be modified as follows if a postoperative relapse is to be avoided. Bilateral transverse full thickness incisions are made in the canine regions and the soft tissues are elevated from the underlying bone both in front of and behind them thus releasing the tension (*Fig.* 10.32*a*). Each of the resultant three sections of lingually-inclined fibrous ridge is uprighted using a Gillies skin hook (*Fig.* 10.32*b*) and filleted as previously described (*Fig.* 10.32*c*). The small denuded areas of bone exposed in the canine regions are left to granulate, no attempt being made to obtain soft-tissue coverage of them (*Fig.* 10.32*d*).

A technique similar to that employed for tuberosity reduction is used to treat abnormally large retromolar pads (*see Figs.* 10.9, 10.10).

BUCCAL AND LABIAL UNDERCUTS

It has been argued by some that as undercuts provide a valuable means of retention they should be retained. However, it is only possible to utilize an undercut to assist the retention of a full denture, without sacrificing either fit or peripheral seal elsewhere, if each and every undercut in the jaw is parallel to all the others, or very nearly so, in all planes. They never are and so undercuts should be regarded as an obstacle to prosthetic success rather than an aid to it, and eliminated when necessary.

As mere excision of the bony overhang would produce a knife-edge ridge in many cases (*Fig.* 10.33*a*), it is better to rebuild ridge width and obliterate the undercut by subperiosteal packing.

The technique is illustrated in *Fig.* 10.33. A vertical midline incision is made down to bone and the labiobuccal soft tissues are elevated from the bone by subperiosteal dissection. A Mitchell's trimmer or a Cumine's scaler is a useful instrument for this purpose. Care must be taken to free the soft tissues from the

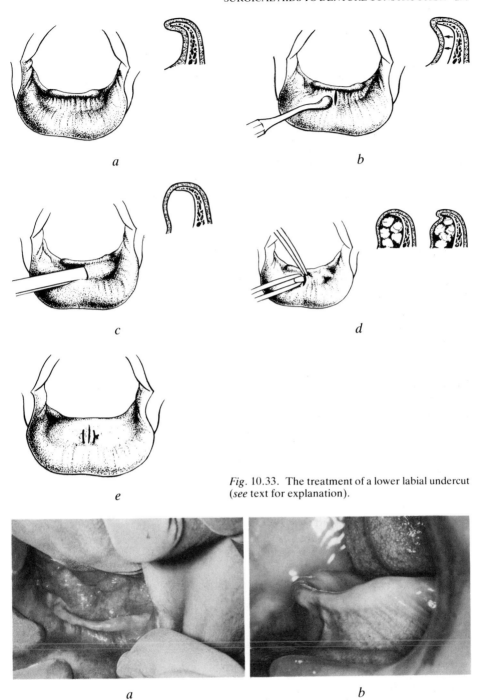

Fig. 10.33. The treatment of a lower labial undercut (*see* text for explanation).

Fig. 10.34. Labial undercut in mandibular ridge (*a*). Three years after a sulphasuxidine pack-out (*b*).

edge of the bony overhang (*Fig*. 10.33*b*, *c*). If this is not done, an undercut persists postoperatively and the patient may experience tenderness when the soft tissues are pressed on to the underlying bone by a denture (*Fig*. 10.33*d*). Broken up sulphasuxidine tablets or fragments of some other packing material are then inserted via the incision to splint the periosteum in its new position. If small pieces are used rather than a block there is less likelihood of the entire pack-out being lost if there is any breakdown of the wound during the postoperative period. The incision is closed with vertical mattress sutures which are left in situ for 2 weeks. Whilst sulphasuxidine has the advantage of being a chemotherapeutic agent which is readily available and cheap, it does seem to delay blood clotting, and it is wise to close the incision with mattress sutures and to warn these patients to expect marked discoloration of the overlying soft tissues due to oozing into the tissue spaces. A number of other substances have been used for the purpose including hydroxyapatite, de-epithelialized fibrous tissue and bone taken from sites elsewhere in the mouth such as enlarged maxillary tuberosities. Clinically the results appear to be similar regardless of the material used. In some cases the raised periosteum appears to lay down new bone, especially in the maxilla, whilst in others the undercut seems to be obliterated with fibrous tissue. Clinically, whichever occurs the prosthetic difficulty is overcome (*Fig*. 10.34).

Whatever the material employed there is always considerable shrinkage during the postoperative period, and so it is advisable to overdo the pack-out.

MYLOHYOID RIDGE RESECTION

The most severe prosthetic problems are those associated with gross atrophy of the jaws.

In the grossly atrophied mandible the genial and mentalis turbercles and the mylohyoid ridges may be the highest points of the jaw and it has been shown that in such cases a full lower denture is displaced from side to side and backwards during chewing. Thus surgery should be designed to eliminate these bony prominences and improve resistance form and stability without impairing retention. In many cases these objectives can be achieved by the technique of mylohyoid ridge resection. By the use of this comparatively minor procedure the prominent sharp mylohyoid ridge and the portion of muscle inserted into it can be removed, thus permitting the use of posterior lingual flanges which provide resistance form to lateral movements of the denture.

This procedure is one of the few oral surgical techniques which is easier to perform under local anaesthesia in the dental chair than with the patient lying anaesthetized on the operating table. It is best performed under local infiltration anaesthesia rather than a mandibular block. When the supraperiosteal injections have had time to work a series of subperiosteal injections are given with the bevel of the needle close to the bone. These injections assist dissection by elevating the rather friable soft tissue from the underlying bone.

The surgical technique is illustrated in *Fig*. 10.35. In most instances a fibrous strand is all that remains of the alveolar bone.

A transverse incision in front of the retromolar pad is joined by an incision in the buccal sulcus just above the reflection of the mucous membrane (*Fig*. 10.35*a*). This incision ensures that the lingual nerve is out of the operative field and

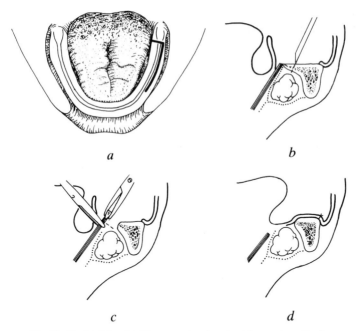

a   *b*

c   *d*

Fig. 10.35. Mylohyoid ridge resection (*see* text for explanation).

guarantees that the sutured incision is supported by bone. This materially assists healing by first intention and minimizes scar tissue formation. The postoperative scar is situated in an area which is acceptable to the prosthetist and the depth of the shallow buccal sulcus is preserved. It is important to ensure that both the incisions are made right down to bone at the point of junction if tearing of the flap is to be avoided. A Mitchell trimmer followed by a periosteal elevator is inserted and the mylohyoid ridge and the attached muscle are exposed by blunt dissection. An assistant supports the mandible whilst a chisel is placed vertically on the mylohyoid ridge and a sharp tap separates the ridge from the mandible (*Fig*. 10.35*b*). It may be necessary to repeat the process until the entire ridge is separated. The assistant then presses upwards with his fingers in the submandibular region enabling each piece of the ridge to be gripped in curved haemostatic forceps and slowly elevated from the wound as it is freed from soft tissue attachments by blunt dissection (*Fig*. 10.35*c*). The muscle is then clamped with a large straight haemostatic forceps which is left in place for at least 1 min. This crushing of muscle fibres materially assists haemostasis in the postoperative period. The muscle is divided as shown in *Fig*. 10.35*d* and the ridge and muscle attachment are removed from the wound. Any sharp bony edge is removed with a bone file pulled in an anteroposterior direction. The lingually-based flap is replaced and the surface of the bone palpated through it to reveal the presence of any sharp prominences. When the ridge is smooth the wound is repaired with interrupted black silk sutures (*Fig*. 10.35*e*).

This procedure has proved to be the most useful pre-prosthetic technique in the treatment of the atrophied mandible and in only a minority of cases is it necessary to supplement it with a labial vestibuloplasty.

ENLARGED SUPERIOR GENIAL TUBERCLES

If the superior genial tubercles are very prominent, they may elevate the fold of mucous membrane between the ridge and the orifices of the submandibular ducts and make the attainment of an anterior lingual seal impossible. They may also be the site of recurrent ulceration when a lower denture is worn (*Fig.* 10.36).

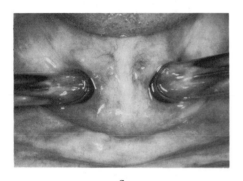
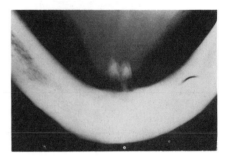

a   *b*

Fig. 10.36. Enlarged superior genial tubercles cause a hard elevation in the midline of the floor of the mouth and are demonstrable clinically (*a*) and radiographically (*b*).

Fig. 10.37 illustrates how they may be resected, leaving a zone of mucous membrane with underlying fibro-elastic soft tissue between the ridge and the orifices of Wharton's ducts. An anteroposterior midline incision should be made and the tubercles exposed by blunt dissection (*Fig.* 10.37*a, b*). If a crest of ridge incision was utilized there would be tension on the suture line every time the patient swallowed in the postoperative period with the resultant risk of breakdown of the wound.

The genioglossus muscle should be transfixed and ligated with catgut prior to the separation of the tubercle using a chisel (*Fig.* 10.37*c, d, e*). Not only does this prevent the separated bony fragment disappearing into the floor of the mouth, but it will help to prevent the brisk postoperative haemorrhage into the floor of the mouth which may otherwise occur in the postoperative period.

After smoothing the cut surface of the bone with a 'vulcanite' bur (*Fig.* 10.37*c*) the wound is closed with interrupted black silk sutures (*Fig.* 10.37*f*).

As previously stated, a brisk haemorrhage into the floor of the mouth may complicate genial tubercle resection. For this reason the procedure should only be undertaken when skilled care is readily available in the postoperative period.

No branch of oral surgery presents more of a challenge to the skill, judgement, and knowledge of the oral surgeon than prosthetic surgery, and the general dental practitioner will be well advised to seek the advice, guidance, and assistance of a colleague who specializes in this type of work whenever his patient requires more than the straightforward surgical elimination of an isolated lesion.

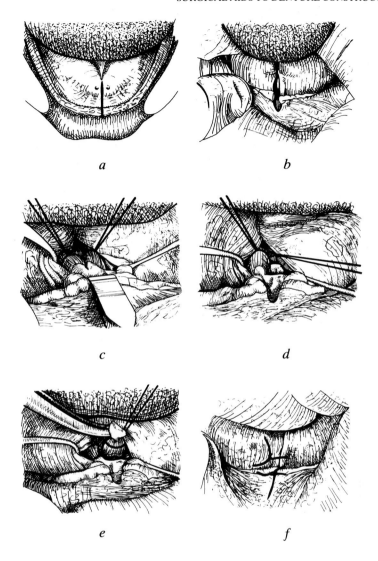

Fig. 10.37. Genial tubercle resection (*see* text for explanation).

SUGGESTED READING

Bear S. E. (1958) Surgical preparation of the mouth for a prosthesis. *J. Oral Surg.* **16**, 3–19.

Behrman S. J. (1961) Surgical preparation of edentulous ridges for complete dentures. *J. Prosthet. Dent.* **11**, 404–13.

Cooper E. H. (1964) Hyperplasia of the oral tissues caused by ill-fitting dentures. *Br. Dent. J.* **116**, 111–14.

Downton D. (1954) Mylohyoid ridge resection. *Dent. Rec.* **74**, 212.

Downton D. (1957) Specialised surgical techniques for the preparation of the jaws for full dentures. *Proc. Br. Soc. Study Prosthet. Dent.* 31–37.

Heartwell C. M. and Peters P. B. (1966) Surgical and prosthodontic management of atrophied edentulous jaws. *J. Prosthet. Dent.* **16**, 613–35.

Howe G. L. (1963) Surgical aids to full denture construction. In: Morrant G. A. (ed.) *Modern Trends in Dental Surgery*. London, Butterworths, pp. 182–95.

Howe G. L. (1964) Surgical preparation of the mandible for prosthesis. *J. Oral Surg.* **22**, 118–22.

Howe G. L. (1965) Preprosthetic surgery in the lower labial sulcus. *Dent. Pract.* **16**, 119–24.

Howe G. L. (1968) Pre-prosthetic surgery. *Int. Dent. J.* **18**, 20–31.

Howe G. L. (1970) Pre-prosthetic operations on the maxilla. *Trans. 3rd Int. Conf. Oral Surgeons, New York* 1968. Edinburgh, Livingstone, pp. 192–7.

Howe G. L. (1973) Oral surgical aids to prosthetic success. *Ann. R. Coll. Surg. Eng.* **52**, 369–79.

Howe G. L. (1976) A less radical approach to the solution of prosthetic problems. *Int. Dent. J.* **26**, 421–6.

Howe G. L. (1982) Recent trends in preprosthetic surgery. *Br. Dent. J.* **153**, 25–6.

Howe G. L. and Leonard M. (1978) Palatal vault osteotomy. *Oral Surg.* **46**, 344–8.

Kent J. N., Quinn J. H., Zide M. F. et al. (1982) Correction of alveolar ridge deficiencies with non resorbable hydroxylapatite. *JADA* **105**, 993–1001.

Lee J. H. and Downton D. (1958) Frenoplasty. *J. Prosthet. Dent.* **8**, 19–21.

Liddelow K. P. (1967) Ideal anatomical conditions for dentures. *Trans. 2nd Congress Int. Assoc. Oral Surgeons* 1965. Copenhagen, Munksgaard, pp. 180–4.

MacEntee M. I., Goldstein B. M. and Price C. (1982) Submucosal root retention. A two-year clinical observation. *J. Prosthet. Dent.* **47**, 483–7.

Obwegeser H. (1964) Surgical preparation of the maxilla for prosthesis. *J. Oral Surg.* **22** 127–34.

Spyropoulos N. D., Patsakas A. J. and Angelopoulos A. P. (1981) Radiographic survey of the edentulous jaws of clinically symptom-free patients. *Oral Surg.* **52**, 455–9.

Urban F. (1966) Pre-prosthetic surgery for the restoration of the masticatory apparatus. *Int. Dent. J.* **16**, 423–8.

Van Wowern N. and Winther S. (1981) Submergence of roots for alveolar ridge preservation. *Int. J. Oral Surg.* **10**, 247–50.

Chapter 11

Surgical aids to the immediate or near-immediate replacement of natural teeth

At the present time, the majority of prosthetists emphasize the desirability of inserting dentures as soon after the extraction of the natural teeth as possible. By this means they hope to prevent the alteration of jaw relationships, the impairment of the patient's appearance, and the development of faulty muscle habits during mastication and speech. When patients know that they will not have to endure the humiliation of being edentulous for a long period, they are less likely

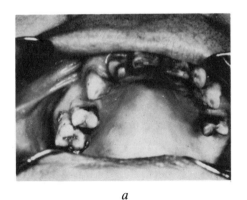

a

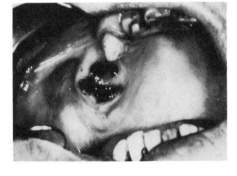

b

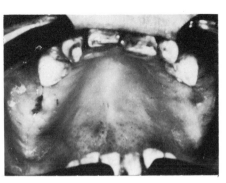

c

Fig. 11.1. The extraction of a right upper premolar and molar (*a*) leaves a buccal undercut, (*b*) which is remedied by judicious socket reduction, (*c*) shows the condition of the ridge one week postoperatively.

to mortgage their general health by retaining septic teeth. Clinically, the denture appears to act as a splint and seems to promote healing. The patient learns to use dentures more rapidly if a prolonged edentulous period is avoided, whilst interference with mastication and speech is minimal.

An *immediate denture* may be defined as a denture constructed before all the remaining teeth are removed and inserted as soon as the extractions are completed. The construction of a *near-immediate denture* is commenced soon after the removal of the teeth and the appliance is inserted within 2 or 3 weeks of the extractions being performed.

Some authorities claim that immediate dentures preserve the integrity of the alveolar bone whilst others believe that immediate dentures speed atrophy of the ridges. Resorption of the ridges is undoubtedly both marked and rapid when the patient wears dentures with poor retention, the occlusion locked, or the vertical height increased at the expense of the 'freeway space'. Conversely, well-designed stable and retentive immediate dentures are worn with comfort and appreciation by many patients for many months before resorption of the alveolar bone renders either relining or replacement of them a necessity. It is therefore imperative that immediate dentures are well designed, properly constructed, and efficient, and there are very few patients in whom it is possible to fit a successful and satisfactory denture soon after forceps extraction of the natural teeth unless some degree of socket reduction is undertaken (*Fig.* 11.1).

TYPES OF IMMEDIATE DENTURE

Before acrylic resins were available for denture construction the appearance of denture-base materials was poor. For this reason it was usual to construct immediate replacement dentures without a labial flange. On these prostheses the fitting surfaces of the anterior teeth are peg-shaped and project below the gingival margins and into the sockets of the extracted teeth. An advantage of this technique is that no surgery, other than clean forceps extraction, is required prior to the insertion of the denture. In most instances the aesthetics of such appliances are good at the time of insertion, although sometimes the lip may have a flaccid appearance. Unfortunately shrinkage of the gingivae soon detracts from the appearance of these dentures and their retention and stability are rapidly undermined. Although it has been shown that permanent irregularities of the alveolar ridge can be prevented by trimming the posts at monthly intervals, few patients are willing, or able, to attend so regularly for these adjustments to be made. Thus the wearing of a denture of this type is frequently complicated by the formation of an irregular resorbed ridge (*Figs.* 11.2, 11.3).

The improved aesthetics of acrylic resins now permit the use of the more retentive and stable type of immediate full denture with a properly extended labial flange. Whilst in some patients it is possible to avoid a slight fullness of the lip by using a very thin labial flange, in most cases some reduction of the labial surface of the alveolar bone is required prior to the insertion of a denture if a good appearance is to be obtained.

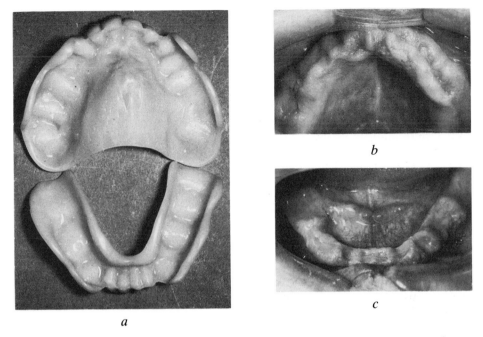

Fig. 11.2. *a*, Unsatisfactory immediate dentures with 'socketing' of the anterior teeth. *b, c*, Ridge form 7 months after the extraction of the teeth.

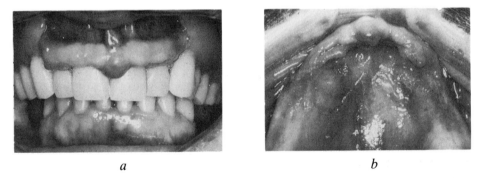

Fig. 11.3. Three-year-old 'socketed' immediate full upper denture which occludes with natural lower teeth. *a*, The necks of the anterior teeth are embedded in the alveolar bone. *b*, Uneven bone resorption behind the labial cortical plate.

CASE SELECTION

Immediate dentures are contra-indicated in patients whose attitudes show them to be unable to appreciate the possibilities and limitations of the service. Intelligent, whole-hearted co-operation on the part of the patient is essential to success. Patients with general medical conditions which contra-indicate surgical procedures

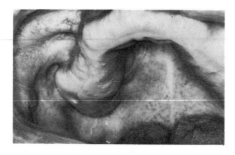

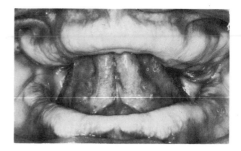

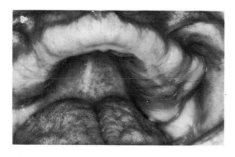

Fig. 11.4. The edentulous ridges of a patient in whom a dental clearance and ridge preparation had been performed three months previously and who had been unable to wear dentures. N.B. The multiple labiobuccal undercuts and enlarged maxillary tuberosities.

incident to removing several teeth and preparing the tissues for dentures at one appointment are not suitable subjects for this technique (*see* Chapter 2). Such local factors as extremely deep overbites, malrelationship of the ridges, or other abnormalities make the successful immediate replacement of teeth difficult, if not impossible.

Immediate replacement of the natural teeth is not usually a satisfactory procedure in patients with a history of difficult extractions, those suffering from severe periodontal disease, or those in whom a marked degree of intrabony pathology is present. A successful near-immediate denture can often be constructed for such patients. There can be no doubt that the immediate replacement of the natural teeth should be undertaken for a larger proportion of patients requiring a dental clearance than is the case at present. Unfortunately some patients and dental surgeons have come to believe that the procedure is neither practicable, satisfactory, nor worth while. It is a matter of regret that in the past this has often been true, for the procedure has not always been carefully planned and well performed (*Fig.* 11.4). Nevertheless, the ease of execution and the success obtained with the techniques now in use render such criticisms unjustified and such opinions obsolete.

SURGICAL PREPARATION OF THE JAWS FOR THE RECEPTION OF DENTURES

The consensus of modern prosthetic opinion stresses the importance of limiting the degree of socket reduction to the minimum amount necessary to facilitate the insertion of a well-designed, stable, and retentive denture. Experience reveals

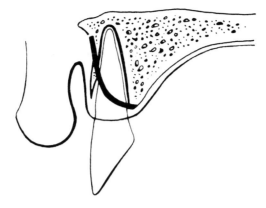

Fig. 11.5. Diagrammatic sagittal section through the maxillary incisor region. The heavy line indicates the outline of the ridge when the teeth are lost.

that, although excessive bone removal is often followed by excessive resorption, conservative surgical reduction of tooth sockets may ultimately preserve more alveolar ridge by facilitating the early insertion of a satisfactory prosthesis, which provides a function for the alveolar bone.

Although it is probable that many prosthetic problems blamed on over-enthusiastic surgery are due really to the pre-extraction neglect of diseased teeth by the patient, the commonest error made during the surgical preparation of the jaws for dentures is the excision of excessive amounts of alveolar bone. Alveolectomy must be performed with both skill and discretion if the natural base for the denture is not to be entirely ruined. It also requires judgement and the dental surgeon must always remember that, however drastically he trims and contours the bone, Nature always remodels and reduces it further. The need for careful extraction with smoothing of bone margins cannot be emphasized too strongly, particularly in those patients in whom the presence of periodontal disease has made the bone margins irregular and uneven.

Bone removal must be minimal and limited to the elimination of sharp points, undercuts which cannot be utilized by altering the path of insertion of a denture, and excessive ridge height, which may reduce the intermaxillary space and so complicate the construction of a satisfactory prosthesis. Whenever possible, bone should be excised from sites from which it would be resorbed by natural means. *Fig*. 11.5 diagrammatically illustrates the typical pattern of resorption in the whole maxilla and the anterior part of the mandible. In the mandibular premolar region, resorption occurs more or less equally in the buccal and lingual cortical plates, whilst in the mandibular molar region more bone is lost on the lingual side.

TECHNIQUES OF SOCKET REDUCTION

Basically, only two methods of socket reduction are available for use by the dental surgeon, namely alveolectomy and intraseptal alveolotomy.

Alveolectomy may be described as the reduction of bony sockets, in which the

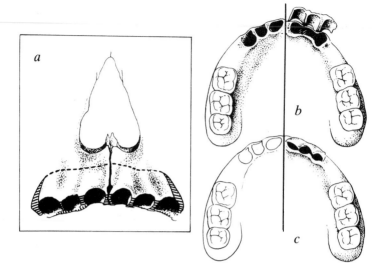

Fig. 11.6. Techniques of socket reduction. *a*, The cross-hatched areas of bone are excised and the labial plate is fractured along the dotted line when intraseptal alveolotomy is performed. *b*, A completed alveolectomy is shown on the patient's right side and the first stage of an alveolotomy on the left. *c*, The intraseptal alveolotomy has been completed.

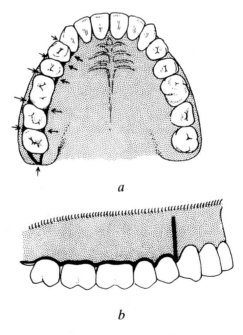

Fig. 11.7. Incisions for alveolectomy in the maxilla (*see* text for explanation).

alveolar trimming is mainly at the expense of the labiobuccal plate and is accompanied by the removal of minimal amounts of the interdental and inter-radicular septa (*Fig.* 11.6*b*).

Intraseptal alveolotomy is the reduction of the bony socket by hinging the fractured labiobuccal cortical plate on its attached mucoperiosteum towards the palatal or lingual wall of the sockets after excising the bony interdental septa (*Fig.* 11.6*b* and *c*).

Both techniques have advantages and disadvantages, advocates and detractors.

Alveolectomy

The use of this technique is indicated in those patients in whom the alveolar bone is dense or intrabony pathology is present, and in those whose teeth resist extraction by forceps. Alveolectomy is the easiest operation in oral surgery to do badly and one of the most difficult to do well. The inexperienced operator always excises too much bone and often loses depth in the labial and buccal sulci by excessive reflection and trimming of the soft tissues.

Gross alveolectomy is rarely indicated and a well-performed alveolectomy is characterized by the amount of alveolar ridge retained and not the amount of bone removed. Only bone which prevents the accurate seating of a denture on its supporting tissues should be excised. The ideal ridge is U-shaped and not V-shaped. The buccal and palatal surfaces of the alveolar bone should be as near parallel as is possible, whilst the top of the ridge should be flat (*see Fig.* 10.1).

The interdental papillae should be trimmed in cases of periodontal disease to eliminate infected granulation tissue but, whenever possible, they should be retained, as they form the basis of a thick tough covering for the crest of the ridge which acts as a cushion for the denture.

The decisions whether to remove or to retain papillae must be made in each individual case according to the clinical picture. In those cases in which it is decided to excise the papillae, buccal and labial incisions should be made along the cervical margins before the teeth are extracted and mucoperiosteal flaps are raised (*Fig.* 11.7*a*). This technique enables the operator to conserve more soft tissue than those which involve the trimming of the margins of a previously raised mucoperiosteal flap. The incised papillae often come away with the extracted teeth (*Fig.* 11.8).

Vertical incisions are then made through the attached buccolabial muco-periosteum and these incisions should not extend to the reflection of the mucous membrane. In the upper jaw the anterior vertical cuts are made in the region of the first premolars (*Fig.* 11.7*b*) whilst posteriorly slightly angled palatal and buccal incisions are made down to the bone and extended backwards across the tuberosity (*Fig.* 11.7*a*). The wedge of soft tissue between these incisions is removed after the extraction of the last standing tooth. Healing is frequently delayed in the mandi-bular canine region if the soft tissues are incised there. This complication can be avoided by making one vertical incision through the labial gingiva in the midline between the two lower central incisors. The mucoperiosteal flap should only be raised sufficiently to reveal the bone enclosing the necks of the teeth, for excessive elevation of flaps causes postoperative discomfort, swelling, and buccal ecchymoses, and may cause loss of depth in the labiobuccal sulcus. The Mitchell trimmer and Cumine scaler (*see Fig.* 3.15) are useful instruments for this purpose.

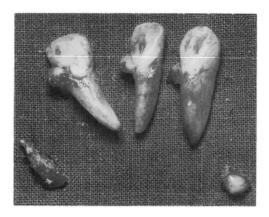

Fig. 11.8. Incised papillae attached to extracted teeth, and triangles of bone and gum cut from the labial plate during alveolotomy.

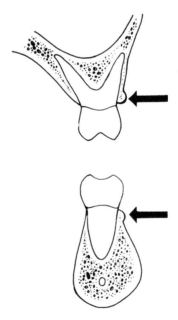

Fig. 11.9. Transverse section through molar region showing beaded rim of bone surrounding the necks of the teeth.

A decision must now be taken whether or not to remove bone before or after the extraction of the teeth. Excision prior to tooth removal enables the amount of bone removed to be controlled more accurately and ensures that teeth, roots, and associated pathological conditions are removed in their entirety. This is particularly so if the teeth are difficult to extract or have a beaded rim of bone around their necks (*Fig.* 11.9). The gingival one-third of the buccal plate should be removed in these cases. Unless the operator ensures that the greatest diameter of the roots is exposed after such bone removal, the septa may be fractured and lost when the teeth are dislocated from their sockets (*Fig.* 11.10). If the bone is brittle or the interdental septa are thin and frail, owing to the teeth being close together, they readily adhere to the teeth and fracture, thus ruining ridge form. In these circumstances, or where severe periodontal disease is present, a better ridge form may be achieved by deferring ridge trimming until several weeks after intra-alveolar extraction.

Once the necessary bone removal has been completed the teeth should be carefully extracted with forceps and elevators. The removal of the canine prior to the extraction of an adjacent lateral incisor and first premolar reduces the risk of the extraction being accompanied by the fracture and loss of a portion of the labial alveolar plate, which is weakened by the empty sockets. When the extractions are

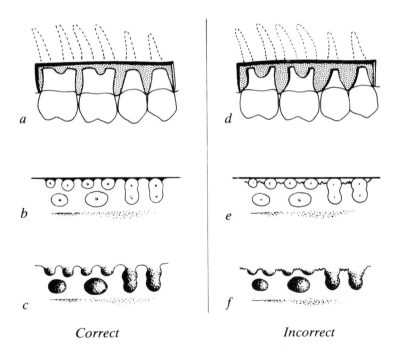

Correct   Incorrect

Fig. 11.10. Correct and incorrect bone removal prior to the extraction of teeth. When viewed from the side the greatest diameter of the roots is visible in *a* but not in *d*. In the transverse section, *b*, it is apparent that the roots can be moved buccally without detaching portions of the interdental septa, as is shown in *e*. The width of the ridge in *c* is greater than that shown in *f*.

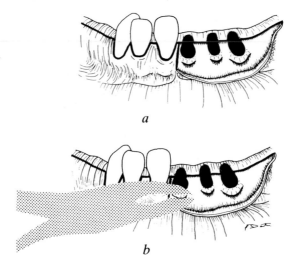

Fig. 11.11. Socket reduction in the mandible should be performed via a midline incision (*a*) using alveolotomy shears (*b*).

completed, all sharp bone edges are lightly trimmed with rongeurs, smoothed with a bone file, and a careful debridement is performed.

In the mandibular incisor and canine regions it is usually preferable to trim the bone after the removal of the teeth rather than before. Vertical incisions in the canine regions heal slowly and so it is wise to avoid using them if possible. Reduction of the beaded alveolar margin is all that is required in most instances. It is convenient to perform this via the midline and crevicular incisions illustrated in *Fig.* 11.11*a* and described above, using a pair of side-cutting rongeurs (alveolotomy shears) for the purpose (*Fig.* 11.15). The instrument is held horizontally with one blade being placed under the beaded rim of bone and the other above it. Closure of the blades removes the desired amount of bone and the process is repeated along the ridge (*Fig.* 11.11*b*). It is sometimes necessary to remove a larger amount of labial plate in the canine sockets in order to eliminate undercuts in that region. Any sharp tips on the interdental septa are removed with the shears, the cut edges of the bone are smoothed with a bone file and the soft tissues apposed with interrupted black silk sutures placed over the interdental septa. It is sometimes necessary to trim away an excess of mucoperiosteum at the midline incision prior to the insertion of a horizontal mattress suture to close the wound.

In those cases in which a more radical alveolectomy is indicated, the ridge should be reduced first in width and then in height, for, if bone reduction is performed in the opposite order, a narrow V-shaped ridge may result. Every effort should be made to preserve the septa, for they form the framework of the ridge. The soft tissues are then held over the alveolar bone whilst its cut surface is palpated through the mucoperiosteal flap. Any sharp edges detected in this manner should be either excised or smoothed. The operator who palpates the bone surface itself often fails to detect the presence of small spicules of bone lying

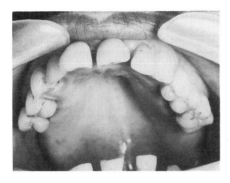
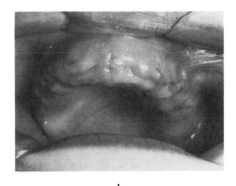

a   *b*

Fig. 11.12. This patient had periodontal disease, hypercementosis of the roots, and sclerosis of bone. *a*, Condition before extractions, alveolectomy, and immediate replacement performed. *b*, Two weeks after surgery.

under the base of the flap. These fragments are readily felt when the bone surface is palpated through the soft tissues. The lingual soft tissues are then raised sufficiently for the bone margins to be smoothed. Although trimming of lingual bone should be minimal it is sometimes required, especially in the mandibular molar region.

The mucoperiosteal flaps are then replaced and loosely sutured. When a whole jaw has been prepared at one sitting the first suture should be placed in the midline, and in the maxilla the incisive papilla and labial frenum are easily identifiable landmarks. Further interrupted sutures are then inserted between the labiobuccal and palatal flaps from the midline backwards on each side. Each suture should pass across and be supported by a septum if the desired ridge form is to be obtained. Sutures should be loosely tied and no attempt should be made to draw the cut edges of the buccal and lingual flaps together (*Fig*. 11.12). Overtight suturing tends to obliterate the buccal sulcus, whilst accurate co-aptation of flaps can often only be obtained at the expense of loss of sulcus depth or by excessive bone removal. However, in severe cases of periodontal disease bone loss may be of such a degree as to permit co-aptation of the soft tissues without tension.

If the tissues have been handled carefully and the procedure performed skilfully, after-pain is seldom marked and is easily controlled by the use of analgesics such as those containing aspirin (*see* p. 84). In many cases there is some local swelling and this is accentuated if the soft tissues have been sutured too tightly. Overtight sutures may 'cut out' of the gingivae when postoperative oedema occurs.

Intraseptal alveolotomy

The advocates of this technique of socket reduction claim that it has the advantage of preserving the compact bone with an unimpaired blood supply and produces a better and broader ridge than alveolectomy. When dentures are worn, the compact bone is less likely to undergo resorption than the cancellous bone which is retained after alveolectomy.

The following technique of intraseptal alveolotomy has been used successfully for many years.

If the papillae are to be excised the method described earlier should be employed (*Fig.* 11.13*a*). The teeth are then extracted cleanly with forceps, the canine being extracted first, followed by the lateral and central incisors, in an attempt to preserve the integrity of the labial cortical plate (*Fig.* 11.13*b*). As the outer plate is to be moved towards the inner plate, which is the arc of a smaller circle, it is necessary to reduce the anteroposterior length of the labial plate. This is performed by excising two triangular pieces of mucoperiosteum and bone at the posterior end of each canine socket (*Figs.* 11.6*a*, 11.13*c, d*).

The alveolotomy shears are then inserted as far into the alveolus as is practicable, with one blade in a canine socket and one in the adjacent lateral socket, and the flat surface of the blades held as close to the inner surface of the labial wall of the socket as possible. As the side-cutting rongeurs are closed, thus severing the labial plate from the septum, the instrument is rotated outwards and this causes a

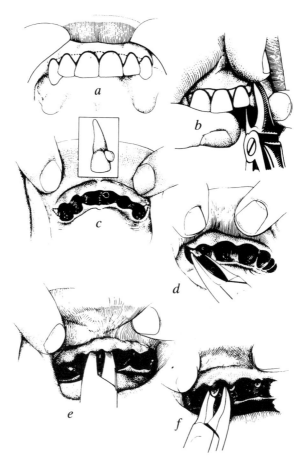

Fig. 11.13. Intraseptal alveolotomy (*see* text for explanation).

horizontal fracture in the labial cortical bone (*Fig*. 11.13*e*). It is essential to insert the shears as deeply into the alveolus and keep the blades as close to the labial wall of the socket as possible in order to obtain a thin, easily fractured, outer cortical plate. The labial ends of each of the septa are divided in turn and the forceps are then reversed and used to cut the palatal attachments of the septa, which drop out of the wound (*Fig*. 11.13*f*).

The palatal cut should be carefully positioned in order to ensure that a sufficient amount of septal bone is excised in the apical area to permit the repositioning of the outer plate to be performed without undue difficulty. This leaves the labial cortical plate of bone hinged outwards upon its attached mucoperiosteum (*Fig*. 11.13*g*). The edge of the palatal mucoperiosteum is then elevated sufficiently to permit any sharp socket margins to be excised with the shears (*Fig*. 11.13*h*). The ridge is then moulded into shape by means of compression between the operator's fingers and thumbs, which is easier to perform if the dentist stands above and behind the patient (*Fig*. 11.13*i*).

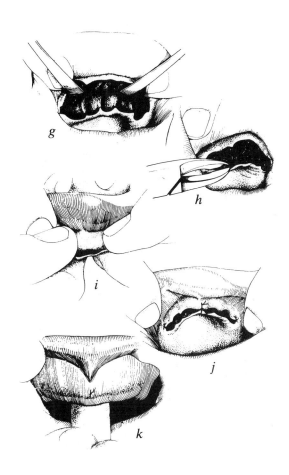

Fig. 11.13. *Continued.*

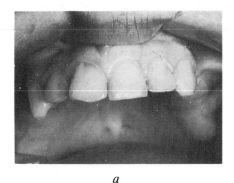 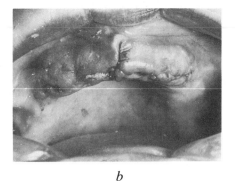

a b

Fig. 11.14. Miss S. P. *a*, Anterior maxillary teeth prior to extractions and intraseptal alveolotomy. *b*, One week after surgery.

If an immediate denture is to be fitted, a clear acrylic surgeon's guide (*see Fig.* 11.17) is then inserted and any blanching of the tissues, indicating a pressure point, is noted. Whenever it is possible, the denture should be eased to relieve the 'high spot'. In those cases in which the bone must be trimmed to relieve a pressure point, bone must be excised from the palatal side of the socket. This is necessary because, if the operation has been performed correctly, the labial plate should be composed almost entirely of thin cortical bone, which is likely to necrose if it is separated from the attached mucoperiosteum from which it derives its blood supply. Loosely tied sutures are used to hold the tissues in place and the denture is then inserted (*Fig.* 11.13*j*).

Intraseptal alveolotomy is a quick simple technique for reducing the sockets of anterior maxillary teeth, which can be performed efficiently by operators who lack the degree of surgical skill and experience to perform well an alveolectomy (*Fig.* 11.14). The method can only be employed if it is possible to execute clean forceps extractions of the teeth with minimal disturbance of the bony socket.

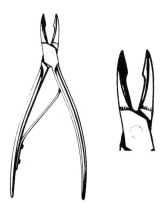

Fig. 11.15.   Ash's No. 5 S side-cutting rongeurs (alveolotomy shears).

Patients whose teeth resist this method of extraction are not suitable candidates for alveolotomy. If the alveolar bone is very dense it makes the creation of the horizontal fracture line (*see Fig.* 11.6*a*), on which the labial plate is hinged, difficult to achieve.

The ease and speed of the technique described are due to the use of the side-cutting rongeurs (alveolotomy shears) (*Fig.* 11.15). The narrow width of the sockets of anterior mandibular teeth and the inaccessibility of the sockets of cheek teeth limit the use of this instrument in these areas, and for this reason the technique is best suited to socket reduction in the anterior part of the maxilla. The method provides only limited access for the removal of roots and intrabony pathology, and in such cases alveolectomy is the technique of choice.

CHOICE OF METHOD

The decision whether or not to fit an immediate replacement denture is not governed by social and economic factors alone. Unless it is decided to leave the patient edentulous and without dentures for some months, some degree of socket reduction will be indicated in practically every case, and the type and amount of surgery which will be required to ensure that the denture is satisfactory should be estimated and the patient carefully assessed to confirm that he or she is fit enough and willing to undergo it. The age and general condition of the patient are of great importance in reaching a decision (*see* Chapter 2).

The immediate replacement of the natural teeth should be performed whenever it is considered to be in the best interests of the patient and is practicable. Both alveolectomy and intraseptal alveolotomy are of value if each method is used only when indicated. The advantages and the disadvantages of the two techniques should be considered before the decision to use one or the other is made. Techniques should always be fitted to patients rather than patients fitted to techniques. In many instances a prosthetic problem in one part of the mouth may be solved by the use of alveolectomy, whilst intraseptal alveolotomy may be used elsewhere in the same mouth to eliminate another difficulty.

Preoperative treatment planning should include the elimination of localized obstacles to prosthetic success. It is sometimes possible to remove mandibular tori or to reduce a tuberosity at the time that surgery for immediate replacement of teeth is undertaken (*see Figs.* 10.4*c*, 10.21). In those cases in which a prominent labial frenum is present frenoplasty (*see Fig.* 10.12) should be performed several weeks before impressions for immediate replacement dentures are taken as postoperative soreness in the operative site may complicate the wearing of complete dentures otherwise.

The technique of immediate replacement following multiple extractions is fraught with many difficulties and it is usually necessary to reline the denture within a period of 3 months from the time the teeth were extracted. It is usually preferable to remove all the posterior teeth and by minimal trimming of the sockets prepare the ridges so that they are ready to withstand denture pressure in 2 or 3 weeks. Then an immediate denture can be fitted after the extraction of the anterior teeth and socket reduction. The 'two-stage' procedure has the disadvantage that undoubtedly some alterations of facial contour and jaw relationships occur between the time that the posterior teeth are extracted and the immediate replacement of the anterior teeth is performed. Some minor degree of change is inevitable with any immediate replacement technique, but there is minimal loss of tissue tone if only 2 or 3 weeks are required for the ridges to heal. Clinically, the 'two-stage' procedure appears to give excellent results.

In patients who exhibit gross bony irregularities, due to either severe periodontal disease or intrabony pathology, or have teeth which resist extraction with forceps, it is sound practice to prepare the ridges at the time the teeth are extracted and then construct and insert near-immediate dentures 2 or 3 weeks postoperatively. The measurement of individual periodontal pockets is subject to many inaccuracies and is not a reliable guide when the models are carved prior to the construction of an immediate denture.

In practice, immediate full upper dentures are found to be more successful than immediate full lower dentures. Whilst some operators relieve the socket area of an immediate full mandibular denture by inlaying a piece of black gutta-percha on the fitting surface, others prefer to use near-immediate dentures in the lower jaw. If used, the black gutta-percha should not extend to the margins of the denture and should be replaced with acrylic resin 2 or 3 weeks after the insertion of the denture.

THE PREPARATION OF MODELS FOR THE CONSTRUCTION OF IMMEDIATE DENTURES

The amount of model carving required is determined by the site and amount of socket reduction which is necessary in each individual case. It is also true that the amount of bone which must be excised to permit the insertion of an immediate denture is determined by the carving of the ridge of the model on which the denture is constructed. For these reasons the carving and preparation of the cast for an immediate replacement denture should be undertaken by the dentist and not by the technician. The study and preparation of the model are of the greatest assistance to the dental surgeon when he is planning his operation.

An immediate replacement full denture must be designed as a full denture and not as a partial denture to which teeth have been added. It is therefore essential to work from a good impression, the correctly supported margins of which extend to the reflection of the mucous membrane and the 'vibration line' of the palate. A mandibular impression must cover both retromolar pads. The jaw relationships are then recorded by the use of a 'squash bite'. The models are cast in a mixture of equal parts of artificial stone and plaster-of-Paris, and duplicated. One set of models is mounted upon an articulator, whilst the other is kept as a record of the size, shape, and arrangement of the natural teeth.

A sharp pencil is used to mark out the gingival crevices of the teeth standing on the disarticulated model (*Fig.* 11.16A). Then a line is drawn on the labial surface of the attached mucoperiosteum, at a distance from the gingival margins which varies with the amounts of bone to be excised and the position of any undesirable undercut. In the upper jaw it is convenient to determine the position of this line clinically in the following manner.

The patient is encouraged to slide his upper lip up over the teeth and supporting structures as high as possible, by the unaided use of its intrinsic musculature. The

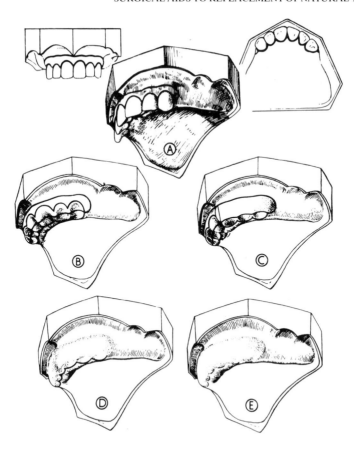

Fig. 11.16. The preparation of models for the construction of immediate dentures (*see* text for explanation).

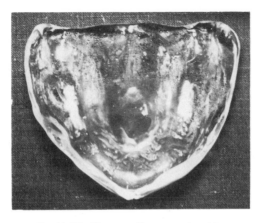

Fig. 11.17. Clear acrylic surgeon's guide.

resulting 'high or retracted lip line' is then recorded and transferred to the model (*Fig.* 11.16A).

The nearer the labial line is drawn to the gingival margin, the less the amount of labial bone which will be sacrificed and, conversely, the farther apart the gingival margins and the 'lip line' are, the greater the amount of bone to be excised. In the average case the distance is between 2 and 3 mm.

Then the teeth are removed from the model and the cast reduced until the areas between the labial and palatal cervical lines are flat. A series of points is drawn half-way between the labial and palatal lines and joined to form a continuous line (*Fig.* 11.16B).

A sharp knife is used to carve the model until a flat surface connects the mid-points of the tooth necks and the 'lip line' (*Fig.* 11.16C). After the path of insertion of the denture has been determined, the cast is scraped to 'round off' any sharp edges and remove any undercuts which cannot be utilized (*Fig.* 11.16D, E). Preparation of the model in this fashion does not involve any carving in the region of the reflection of mucous membrane and thus a 'border seal' can be obtained on the resulting denture.

When the preparation of the model is completed, it should be duplicated to provide a second model on which a clear acrylic 'surgeon's guide' can be constructed. This transparent base-plate must be an exact replica of the fitting surface of the denture, for it is used by the surgeon to check the accuracy of the surgical preparation of the denture-bearing area (*Figs.* 11.13*k*, 11.17).

When either tuberosity reduction or the excision of a torus is to be performed at the time immediate replacement of the teeth is undertaken, the necessary carving of the models must be carried out before dentures are constructed. It is usually preferable either to undertake these procedures prior to commencing the construction of immediate replacement dentures or to perform the surgery and fit near-immediate prostheses.

SUGGESTED READING

Dean O. T. (1941) Intra-septal alveolotomy. *Dent. J. Aust.* **13**, 172–9.

Gazabatt C., Parra N. and Meissuer E. (1965) A comparison of bone resorption following intraseptal alveolotomy and labial alveolectomy. *J. Prosthet. Dent.* **15**, 435–43.

Hayward J. R. and Thompson S. (1958) Principles of alveolectomy. *J. Oral Surg.* **16**, 101–8.

Hedegard B. (1962) Some observations on tissue changes with immediate maxillary dentures. *Dent. Pract.* **13**, 70–8.

Johnson K. (1966) A clinical evaluation of upper immediate denture procedures. *J. Prosthet. Dent.* **16**, 799–810.

Neill D. J. (1959) Immediate full dentures. *Br. Dent. J.* **106**, 105–11.

Pietrovski J. and Massler M. (1967) Alveolar ridge resorption following tooth extraction. *J. Prosthet. Dent.* **17**, 21–7.

Radden H. G. (1959) Local factors in healing of the alveolar tissues. *Ann. R. Coll. Surg.* **24**, 266–87.

Sealey V. T. (1948) Septal alveolectomy. *Aust. J. Dent.* **52**, 25–9.

Van der Ven J. G. (1954) Immediate full dentures. *Int. Dent. J., Lond.* **4**, 354–65.

Watt D. M. (1962) Impression techniques for full dentures. Introduction. *Dent. Pract.* **13**, 155.

Wictorin L. (1964) Bone resorption in cases with upper denture. *Acta Radiol.* Suppl. 228, 84–90.

Chapter 12
Surgical aids to endodontics

Since the introduction of broad-spectrum antibiotics, great advances have been made in root-canal therapy. The use of these drugs, combined with more accurate diagnosis, care in case selection, and the widespread adoption of precise techniques, has made it possible to preserve more natural teeth for further useful life without hazard to the patient. These advances in conservative root-canal therapy have modified both the indications and the need for surgery in many cases.

Apicectomy may be defined as the surgical amputation of the apex of a tooth root, whilst *periapical curettage* is the removal of pathological material present in the periapical region by means of surgical curettage. After it had been demonstrated that in many cases the pulp communicated with the periodontal membrane via multiple channels rather than a single apical foramen, the operation of apicectomy was introduced to eliminate this 'apical delta', which could not be sterilized by the means available at that time. Though freely acknowledging the great value of this operation in the past, most endodontists practising today feel that the 'apical delta' can be sterilized by employing modern techniques of root-canal therapy, including the use of poly-antibiotic pastes.

Other authorities believe that pulpal remnants in the delta retain their vitality after the extirpation of a live pulp, and in view of these opinions less emphasis is being placed upon apicectomy and far more upon periapical curettage. However, the resection of a portion of the apex facilitates the complete removal of pathological material present in the periapical area and enables the operator to check and ensure that the apical end of the pulp canal is effectively sealed. For these reasons apicectomy is still used by most oral surgeons at the present time.

FACTORS GOVERNING THE RETENTION OF A PULPLESS TOOTH

The presence of either congenital or rheumatic valvular heart disease is a positive contra-indication to root-canal therapy, due to the risk of subacute bacterial endocarditis. It is unfortunately true that root-canal therapy of some pulpless teeth, even when performed by very experienced, skilled and competent endodontists, may fail. In such circumstances the tooth may become a source of bacteriaemia without either the patient or the dentist being aware of it. The potential consequences in these patients are so serious that the sacrifice of the tooth is regarded as the lesser of two evils. In these circumstances the pulpless tooth should be extracted under adequate antibiotic cover (*see* p. 256). A severe attack of rheumatic fever or chorea (St Vitus's dance) may cause scarring of the endocardium, which cannot be detected during clinical examination but may still predispose to endocarditis. For this reason a definite history of either rheumatic fever or chorea is usually regarded as a contra-indication to root-canal therapy.

The relationship, if any, which exists between dental sepsis and certain eye diseases (e.g., iritis and iridocyclitis) is still the subject of debate and, whenever a patient has an eye disease, the opinion of an experienced ophthalmologist should be sought before root-canal therapy is undertaken. Once infection has been eliminated, the natural defence mechanisms of the body usually remove any non-cystic pathological tissue remaining in the periapical region and repair the defect. There is even some evidence that small cystic lesions may resolve following successful non-surgical endodontic therapy. As age advances these defensive and repair mechanisms become less efficient, whilst certain debilitating diseases, such as diabetes mellitus and nephritis, may also impair the efficiency of these protective mechanisms to such a degree as to contra-indicate root-canal therapy.

Like all other forms of specialized and time-consuming dental treatment, successful root-canal therapy depends upon the whole-hearted co-operation of the patient, who must appreciate both the value and limitations of such treatment. If the patient is not interested in obtaining this type of dental care or is unable to attend regularly for treatment, due to either his employment, financial situation, or the distance which he has to travel, it is better to advise extraction of the tooth. Other patients who are about to travel to areas where prompt dental aid is not readily available may prefer not to keep pulpless teeth.

The need to avoid extraction in patients afflicted with haemorrhagic diatheses may govern the decision to use root-canal therapy in circumstances when extraction of the tooth would otherwise be the treatment of choice.

Certain local factors may also influence the treatment of a pulpless tooth. Before undertaking root-canal therapy the dental surgeon should ensure that the oral condition of the patient is such as to justify the use of this treatment. When a patient is already wearing a partial denture to replace missing teeth in the same jaw, it is often preferable to extract any pulpless tooth and replace it by adding another tooth to the denture. Root-canal therapy is usually contra-indicated if the patient's oral hygiene and periodontal condition are poor, or when the caries incidence is high. Certain technical considerations may also influence the decision of the dental surgeon.

He should ensure that it is mechanically possible to clean, prepare, and sterilize the root canal of the tooth in question before undertaking to treat it. This process is easiest in straight, single-rooted teeth and becomes more difficult as the number and complexity of the root canals increase. The dental surgeon should also ensure that it will be possible to restore the crown of the tooth when root-canal treatment has been completed.

INDICATIONS AND CONTRA-INDICATIONS TO SURGICAL ENDODONTICS

It is generally agreed that, whilst non-surgical endodontic therapy is the treatment of choice if a live pulp is extirpated and the canal can be adequately prepared, surgery has a place in the treatment of other pulpless teeth. The exact place is a matter of debate, some authorities believing that the periapical granuloma is a protective mechanism and that exotoxins alone enter the periapical tissues. They argue that the bacteria remain in the root canal, so that if the canal is sterilized the natural defences of the body will deal with the periapical lesion. Other authorities state that granulation tissue may be either infected or non-infected and that, on occasions, the natural defence mechanisms fail to eradicate diseased tissues in the periapical region.

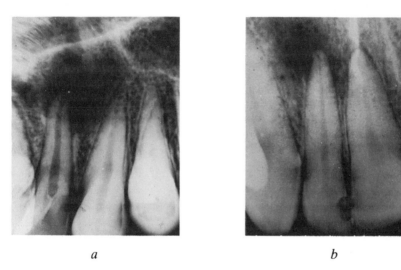

a   *b*

Fig. 12.1. *a*, Chronic abscess. *b*, Periapical granuloma.

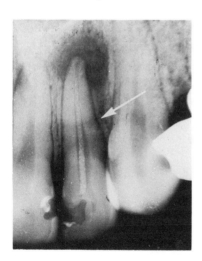

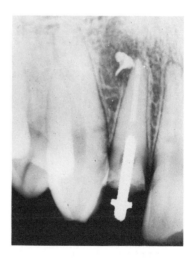

Fig. 12.2. Periapical granuloma. The arrow indicates the lowest point of the lesion.

Fig. 12.3. Excess root filling in the periapical area.

It sometimes proves impossible to cleanse adequately and fill the apical portion of the root canal via the pulp chamber and in such a case periapical surgery is indicated. A substantial majority of dental surgeons believe that surgical treatment is indicated when a pulpless tooth is associated with a chronic abscess. Unfortunately it may be difficult, if not impossible, to distinguish, on clinical grounds,

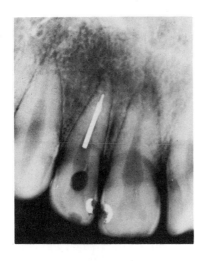

Fig. 12.4. Broken instrument in pulp canal.

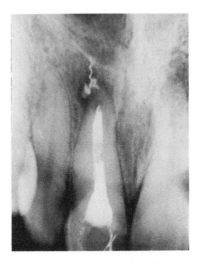

Fig. 12.5. Inadequate root filling with excess root filling and broken instrument in the periapical area.

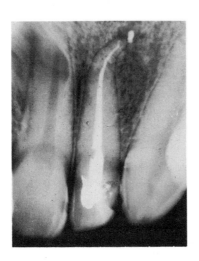

Fig. 12.6. Curved root apex and excess of root filling in periapical area.

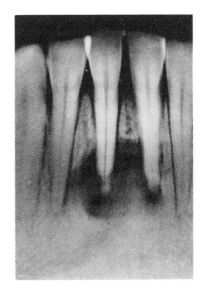

Fig. 12.7. Resorption of apex of lower incisor in abscess cavity.

between a chronic abscess and a periapical granuloma unless a sinus is present (*Figs*. 12.1, 12.2). Surgery eliminates the need for so difficult a differential diagnosis and is an excellent treatment for periapical granulomata, especially in those cases in which diseased tissue extends through the periodontal membrane for a considerable distance from the apical foramen (*Fig*. 12.2). There is some evidence that the success rate in the treatment of pulpless teeth is inversely proportional to the size of the periapical area, and that in the presence of a large periapical area of rarefaction surgical intervention is more likely to be successful than the use of more conservative methods of endodontics.

Surgery may also be required to deal with such foreign bodies as excess root filling present in the periapical area (*Figs*. 12.3, 12.5, 12.6) or cases in which an instrument used in root-canal therapy has been broken in the canal (*Fig*. 12.4). In these circumstances, as in those instances in which it is difficult, if not impossible, to mechanically prepare, sterilize, and fill the root canal, e.g., the presence of a curved apex (*Fig*. 12.6), surgical exposure enables the dental surgeon to effectively treat the tooth and insert a retrograde root filling. This technique is also of value when periapical lesions associated with crowned teeth have to be treated. It is not always possible to decide from radiographs (*see Figs*. 7.6*b*, 12.1*a*) whether a periapical lesion is cystic in nature. If it is, it is best eliminated by surgical means. Although there is debate as to whether erosion of the apex of a tooth (*Figs*. 12.7, 12.8) is an indication for surgery, it is widely held that in those cases in which either conservative endodontic treatment has failed or pulpal death has occurred before formation of the tooth root has been completed, surgery may make it possible to retain an otherwise unsaveable pulpless tooth (*Fig*. 12.1).

Perforation of the tooth root may sometimes complicate the mechanical preparation of the root canal. Some of these mishaps can be remedied by treatment via the pulp chamber, but surgery may be required to deal with others. Perforations situated in the apical third of the root may be treated by apicectomy, whilst in others the site of perforation may be exposed by surgical means and filled. However, the repair of perforations is the least satisfactory of the surgical

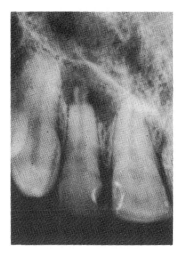

Fig. 12.8. Surgical treatment of this chronic abscess is contra-indicated, for there would be insufficient bony support for the incisor postoperatively.

techniques employed in endodontics and in general the prognosis for a tooth with a perforated root is poor especially if the perforation is of long standing or on the palatal surface of the root.

In some instances, circumstances may dictate that root-canal therapy be completed as promptly as possible, with the minimum number of attendances. Surgical treatment is the quickest technique of conserving a pulpless tooth and in many cases the active phase of treatment can be completed during a single visit.

Apicectomy and periapical curettage should only be used to treat cysts and chronic inflammatory lesions, and both procedures are contra-indicated if acute inflammation is present. In these cases the condition should be rendered chronic by the use of conservative measures and the institution of effective drainage (*see* p. 234). Root resection reduces the bony support of the tooth and should not be undertaken if, due to periodontal disease, there will be insufficient bony support postoperatively (*Fig.* 12.8). When required, temporary support may be given by the use of a fenestrated cast-silver cap splint constructed and cemented to the tooth and its neighbours preoperatively and left in situ for at least 6 weeks following apicectomy. If a fracture is present in the apical third of the root the lesser fragment may be removed surgically, but apicectomy is contra-indicated by the presence of a fracture elsewhere in the root.

The proximity of such important structures as the nasal cavity, maxillary antrum, or the inferior dental and mental nerves always renders successful operative interference more difficult and may contra-indicate the surgical treatment of a pulpless tooth in some cases. Occasionally the nerve and blood supply of the pulp of an adjacent vital tooth is in such a position that it could be damaged if a periapical lesion were removed by means of curettage. It is sometimes possible to deal with such a problem by draining the periapical lesion via either the pulp canal or alveolar bone, or both, and deferring the excision of the diseased tissue until some bone regeneration has taken place.

The aims of endodontic surgery are to eliminate diseased tissue in the periapical area and to ensure that the apical end of the cleansed pulp canal is effectively sealed. Inadequacy of an apical seal is a common cause of failure in root-canal therapy and surgery has the advantage of facilitating inspection of the apical end of the root filling. Any deficiencies which are noted during such an inspection can be remedied by means of retrograde root filling.

There would now appear to be widespread agreement amongst dentists that surgical endodontics should be undertaken only when conventional orthograde root-filling techniques are either impracticable or have failed. The results of utilizing a retrograde approach to obturate a root canal are less satisfactory than those obtained when an orthograde approach is employed. Thus the retrograde approach should be reserved for use when the coronal parts of the root canal are either impassable or inaccessible and can neither be instrumented nor filled.

PREOPERATIVE ASSESSMENT

Success in surgical endodontics is dependent upon thorough preoperative assessment of the difficulties in each individual case. A careful history should be supplemented by both clinical and radiographic examination. In addition to the important factors already mentioned some further points merit attention. The age of the patient may be reflected in the degree of apical development and the rate of healing which can be anticipated and, when considered in conjunction with the patient's temperament and general health, may influence the choice of the form of anaesthesia to be employed (p. 27).

Clinical examination may reveal that the arch is crowded whilst the inclination of the crowns of the pulpless tooth and its neighbours may indicate that the roots of adjacent teeth may be close to one another, and that apices of some teeth may be more easily exposed than others. Particular attention should be paid to the presence of periodontal pocketing around, or an excessive occlusal load upon, the pulpless tooth. A deep overbite may result in a tooth with a shortened root loosening in response to occlusal interference during the postoperative period. Any such occlusal trauma should be remedied and a splint constructed if its use is indicated. Gingival recession may make it more difficult to obtain a good aesthetic restoration and reduce sulcus depth, whilst the presence of a chronic sinus indicates that perforation of the cortical plate has occurred. This usually facilitates both the location and the surgical exposure of the apex.

The pulpal status of the teeth adjacent to the pulpless tooth should be determined prior to endodontic surgery being undertaken, for should a neighbouring tooth fail to respond preoperatively, any necessary adjustment to the treatment plan can be made in consultation with the patient.

Meticulous examination of a good periapical radiograph should reveal the degree of root development and apical closure and disclose any external resorption of the apex which may be present. The use of a hand lens for this purpose is of great value. Although thinning and perforation of the cortical bone is more clearly shown in radiographs than defects in cancellous bone, some idea of the size and shape of the periapical lesion and the involvement of adjacent teeth may also be deduced from such a film (*Figs.* 12.2–12.8).

TECHNIQUE OF APICECTOMY AND PERIAPICAL CURETTAGE

These operations can be conveniently performed under local anaesthesia provided that acute inflammation has been adequately treated. In the maxillary incisor region the supraperiosteal injections used to secure infiltration anaesthesia are sometimes exceedingly painful, even when carefully given. If a piece of cotton-wool, wound upon the end of an orange stick, is soaked in a 10% solution of cocaine and placed on the floor of the nose, via the nostril, the degree of anaesthesia which is produced within a few minutes permits these injections to be given almost painlessly.

The design of the mucoperiosteal flap is governed by the need for good exposure of the periapical lesion and the necessity to leave the flap margins supported by bone at the end of the operation. The semilunar incision illustrated in *Fig.* 12.9 is often used and passes through the frenum where necessary. A band of attached mucoperiosteum, 5 mm wide in its narrowest part, must be left between the incision and the cervical margin, if the vitality of these soft tissues is not to be prejudiced. Such an incision should extend for the width of the affected tooth and the width of the two teeth immediately adjacent to it. Whilst the resultant semilunar mucoperiosteal flap fulfils all the criteria detailed on p. 64 when the periapical lesion is sited around and above the root apex, it fails to do so

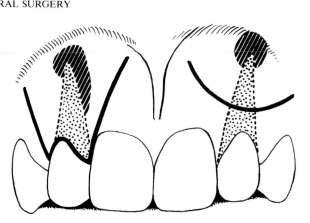

Fig. 12.9. Incisions for apicectomy.

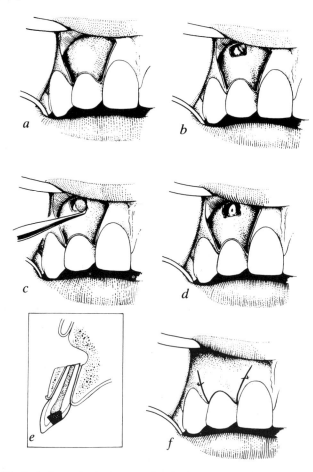

Fig. 12.10. Technique of apicectomy and periapical curettage (*see* text for explanation).

when the diseased tissues spread through the periodontal membrane and along the surface of the root. In these circumstances, which are present in most cases, the 'classic' three-sided flap illustrated in *Fig.* 12.9 should be employed even though its use occasionally produces a slight recession of the gingiva related to the pulpless tooth which may disclose the margin of a post crown and thus detract from its appearance. This problem may be avoided by making the horizontal incision about 2 mm apical to the gingival crest and dividing the soft tissues obliquely until the bone surface approximately 2 mm below the margin of the bone is reached. This incision should be carried apically to any periodontal lesion. Full thickness diverging vertical incisions are then made at each end of the horizontal incision and the mucoperiosteal flap raised from the bone.

With this sole exception all incisions should be made firmly through both layers of the mucoperiosteum. After reflection of the flap, the bone should be examined for the presence of a sinus communicating with the periapical lesion. If such a bony defect is present it can be enlarged, by the use of either chisels, hand gouges, or burs, to form a bony window of such a size as to afford good exposure of the periapical lesion. In those cases in which no sinus is present a small rose-head bur should be used to create a bony window of reasonable size in the labial plate, after the position of the root apex has been determined by a careful clinical examination supplemented by a detailed study of the radiograph (*Fig.* 12.10*b*). These positional checks are of particular importance when the apex of the maxillary lateral incisor is to be exposed, for due to the developmental position of this tooth the bony labial plate in relationship to its apex is often rather thick, a factor which can make accurate localization more difficult.

An endeavour to visualize the position of the apex should be made by estimating the root length and noting the angulation of the crown and the inclination of the root in all planes. If the tooth is either very proclined or its root is very curved it is often wise to make the initial exposure of the surface of the root at a level which is closer to the crown than would otherwise be the case in order to facilitate identification of it. Once the root has been identified positively the apex can be exposed by judicious bone removal. In most cases it is only necessary to expose slightly more of the length of the root apex than the amount it is planned to resect. However, judicious removal of some of the bone overlying a periapical lesion which extends along the lateral surface of the root towards the crown of the tooth may facilitate greatly the removal of the diseased soft tissues.

Once the granulomatous sac has been exposed it should be separated from the bony wall of the cavity by careful dissection. The round end of a Mitchell trimmer, an angled Warwick James elevator (*Fig.* 12.10*c*), or a dental excavator is useful for this purpose. The apex of the root should then be exposed and removed with a small round bur. Only that amount of apex necessary to facilitate the removal of all pathological soft tissue from the periapical region need be resected and this is usually about 3 or 4 mm long. If the cut surface of the retained root is made to slope towards the opening in the labial plate (*Fig.* 12.10*d, e*), it facilitates checking of the apical seal and the insertion of a retrograde root filling if required. When the periapical lesion extends farther down one side of the root than the other, an oblique cut in the lateral dimension ensures that the maximum amount of bony support for the tooth is retained.

After careful curettage and debridement of the bony cavity have ensured the elimination of *all* diseased tissue, the area is irrigated with sterile saline and any sharp bony edges are smoothed. The cut surface of the root end is smoothed, with either a large round surgical bur or a so-called 'vulcanite bur', and is then inspected using a sharp probe in order to ensure the adequacy of the apical seal. Any deficiency which is detected may be remedied by means of the technique of retrograde root filling (*see* p. 325).

Some authorities seal the open dentinal tubules on the cut end of the root by painting the surface with ammoniacal silver nitrate solution and then applying oil of cloves to produce a black precipitate of silver. If this technique is employed care must be taken to ensure that the medicaments are applied to the cut end of the root alone. The mucoperiosteal flap is then replaced and loosely tied sutures inserted to hold it in place (*Fig.* 12.10*f*). Whenever it is practicable, the apicectomized tooth should be taken out of occlusion during all excursions of the mandible by means of judicious grinding of the opposing teeth preoperatively. If desired, temporary splintage may be applied, either by the use of an acrylic or cast-silver cap splint or by ligaturing the tooth to its neighbours. Suture removal is undertaken on the seventh postoperative day.

PREPARATION AND FILLING OF THE ROOT CANAL

It is generally agreed that careful reaming, adequate preparation, cleansing, and disinfection of the root canal are essential to success in endodontics, and that the most important portion of the root filling is that part which occludes the apical third of the root canal and seals the apical foramen. Only by means of inspection following surgical exposure is the dental surgeon able to confirm with certainty that the apical end of the root canal is sealed adequately, for root canals which appear upon radiographic examination to be filled perfectly are often found at operation to be either overfilled or underfilled.

Although the majority of dentists would agree that the pulp chamber should be opened and the canal cleansed and reamed prior to surgery, there is considerable debate concerning the optimum time for filling the root canal of a tooth which is to be apicected. Many endodontists believe that they can ensure that the canal is cleaner and the root filling more closely adapted to the walls of the canal if the root filling is inserted prior to surgery. If this technique is used there should be no delay in apicecting the tooth if the risk of precipitating a flare-up of acute inflammation is to be avoided. When a pulpless tooth is to be restored by means of a post crown, both the canal and post must be prepared prior to surgery and the post crown should be cemented into place at operation. This ensures that the maximum length of root canal is utilized for purposes of retention and facilitates condensation of the amalgam, if retrograde filling of the apical portion of the canal is required. The apical seal must be inspected in every case and any excess filling material eliminated via the operation wound. Following apicectomy it may be difficult to prepare a root for the reception of a crown without displacing the apical seal, unless the 'fractured silver point' technique has been employed.

Some dental surgeons prefer to fill the root canal after resecting the root apex, and it is very easy to ensure that the root filling is adequate and to remove any excess of filling material when this procedure is employed. However, should any difficulty be experienced in securing haemostasis, contamination of the root canal by blood may cause discoloration of the tooth, in addition to interfering with the seal of the root filling.

RETROGRADE FILLING OF THE ROOT CANAL

Regardless of whether the root canal is filled before or after apicectomy, the canal should be prepared and sterilized prior to surgery whenever this is feasible. It is not always possible to do this, for cases occur in which the apical part of the canal cannot be adequately cleansed and filled via the pulp chamber, due to the presence of either an abnormal root pattern or obliteration of the canal by either calcific degeneration of the pulp or a previously inserted silver point. It is usually possible, by histological means, to demonstrate the presence of a very narrow strand of pulpal tissue in those teeth in which calcification of the pulp appears to be complete on clinical and radiographic examination. Some of these teeth can be salvaged either by eliminating the untreated apical portion of the root by means of apicectomy or by the insertion of a retrograde root filling at operation. The latter technique may also be used to provide an effective apical seal in pulpless teeth with incompletely formed roots and 'immature' root-canal patterns, in addition to those in which inspection at operation reveals the canal to be underfilled.

It cannot be overemphasized that the adequacy of the apical seal can never be accurately assessed by radiography alone, for, even if errors in technique, angulation, and interpretation are ignored, a radiograph cannot detect deficiencies on the labial or palatal aspects of a root filling. Retrograde root filling may also be employed in the treatment of apically infected pulpless teeth, bearing either a post or porcelain jacket crown or a bridge abutment of the three-quarter crown variety.

The technique is not without its disadvantages. Thus, in order to provide sufficient access to treat the apical end of the canal, more bone and root have to be cut away than are normally removed during either apicectomy or periapical curettage. As the apical part of the root canal is opened up, cleansed, prepared, and filled at one operation, there is no opportunity to employ antibiotics in an attempt to sterilize the canal. It is often difficult to keep the apical cavity dry when inserting the filling and it is impossible to condense the amalgam unless the cervical portion of the canal is obtunded by a previously inserted root filling or crown post.

Retrograde filling of the root canal is performed in the following manner. The apex and the pathological tissues related to it are exposed and removed in the manner illustrated in *Fig.* 12.10*a–d*. The labial orifice of the resultant bony cavity is enlarged, mainly at the expense of the bone forming the roof of its anterior part, to permit instrumentation (*see Fig.* 12.10*e*). After all the sharp edges of bone have been smoothed the cavity is irrigated with sterile saline, dried with pledgets of cotton-wool, and packed with either sterile gauze soaked in a local anaesthetic solution containing adrenaline or a haemostatic sponge, e.g. absorbable gelatin sponge with dequalinium chloride 0·1% (Dequaspon), so that the dried cut surface of the root end is isolated from the remainder of the bony operation wound. As has been stated previously, the angulation of this cut surface should be such as to facilitate inspection. This point is of particular importance when retrograde root filling is envisaged, for the apical end of the pulp canal must be

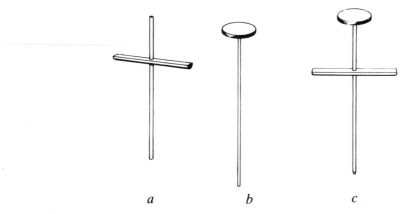

Fig. 12.11. Amalgam carrier (*c*) made out of 1-mm diameter stainless-steel orthodontic wire (*b*) and 1-mm internal diameter tubing (*a*) and used for retrograde root filling.

identified and its location confirmed with the tip of a sharp probe. This aperture is first enlarged, using sterile small round burs held in the miniature head of a right-angled handpiece, and then an undercut cavity is prepared of such a size as to permit filling with the special amalgam carrier illustrated in *Fig.* 12.11. This apical cavity should be 2 mm in depth and in cases in which the presence of more than one apical foramen is detected the intervening dentine should be removed to create a single cavity. If the root canal has been filled with gutta percha care should be taken to remove any tags left after cavity preparation using either a small excavator or a sharp Briault probe for the purpose.

After irrigating the cavity with either sterile saline or local anaesthetic solution to remove all the debris present, it is dried with either paper points or pledgets of cotton-wool and absolute alcohol applied to its walls. A small amount of either silver–tin or copper amalgam is mixed and conveyed to the cavity in the special amalgam carrier. A small spoon-ended excavator is used to condense the amalgam into the undercuts, and further amalgam is added and condensed with suitable plastic instruments until the cavity is filled completely. Care should be taken to ensure that a bulk of amalgam does not build up on the cut surface of the root tip. Any excess should be removed before a new increment is placed. The cavity should be slightly overfilled and as soon as the amalgam has partially set it should be carved flush with the root surface using an inverted large round excavator with a chisel-like action. All excess filling material is carefully removed from the root surface and the haemostatic sponge or gauze is then removed from the wound. The bony wound is then irrigated with sterile saline, dried, and carefully inspected for the presence of any pieces of excess amalgam, which should be removed with either excavators or a fine sucker end. Particular attention should be paid to the undersurface of the mucoperiosteal flap and the upper surface of the bony cavity when searching for retained debris. The wound is then insufflated with a mixture of polymyxin, neomycin, and bacitracin (Polybactrin spray) and closed with interrupted black silk sutures, which are left in situ for 1 week. A postoperative radiograph should be taken either immediately after the placement of sutures or at the first postoperative visit. The patient should be advised to keep the wound clean using hot saline mouth baths and not to raise the lip repeatedly to examine the wound.

POSTOPERATIVE PROGRESS

The patient should be seen at regular intervals following root-canal therapy, regardless of which method of therapy has been employed to conserve the pulpless tooth. The condition of the tooth should be checked by both clinical and radiographic means at each visit. The patient is usually seen 1 week after operation and on this occasion the clinical condition is checked, the pulpal responses of neighbouring teeth are determined, especial care is taken to ensure that the treated tooth is still out of occlusion, and the sutures are removed. A periapical radiograph is taken in order to reveal the periapical condition of the tooth in the immediate postoperative period, and similar films taken at periods of 3, 6, 12, and 24 months following surgery are used to determine the amount and speed of bone regeneration which occurs. Treatment of a pulpless tooth is usually considered to be successful if the tooth remains clinically symptomless and functional for 2 or more years and the radiographic appearances return to normality as the bony cavity fills up with new bone. Unfortunately some periapical radiolucency may persist following the surgical treatment of large periapical areas, and in such cases biopsy often reveals that the cavity has been partially obliterated by healthy scar tissue. In these circumstances the periodontal membrane shadow can usually be traced around most of the apicected root and the radiolucent area often appears to be isolated from the root-tip. In the absence of symptoms and signs, active intervention is not indicated but serial radiographs should be utilized to ensure that the radiolucent area is either static or is decreasing in size. Should breakdown of the wound occur the cause should be sought and remedied. Inadequate sealing of the root canal, incomplete removal of infected periapical granulation tissue, occlusal interference, and death of the pulp of an adjacent tooth must all be excluded as possible aetiological factors for breakdown. If indicated, periapical curettage may be repeated.

In theory the prognosis of all teeth, regardless of their location, should be similar once a satisfactory apical seal has been placed. However, anatomical factors make the endodontic treatment of cheek teeth more difficult than that of single-rooted anterior teeth. Multiplicity and complexity of root canals combine with the problems of access to make successful surgical endodontics on cheek teeth difficult to achieve consistently.

THE TREATMENT OF LOWER ANTERIOR AND CHEEK TEETH

In the maxilla it is virtually impossible to use a palatal flap for access due to the high position of the apices of the palatal roots. In the mandible it is difficult to reflect the soft tissues sufficiently to provide good vision of and access to the operative site. Furthermore, both the position of the mental nerve and bleeding during surgery frequently cause problems. Nevertheless, some teeth can be treated and each individual case must be judged on its merits and endodontic treatment should not be undertaken unless a successful outcome can be reasonably expected. The presence of a large apical lesion is not a contra-indication for it may actually provide working space. Competently performed endodontic surgery may fail on occasions for no apparent reason and so success can and should never be guaranteed.

It is difficult to treat *two-rooted upper premolars* because the depth at which the palatal root is placed makes both surgery and vision difficult. Access to both roots should be obtained via a buccal approach. It is necessary to sacrifice a greater length of buccal root to provide access to the palatal root. Inter-radicular bone is then drilled away until part of the palatal root is located. The apex is then sculpted out with a small bur, resected obliquely, and treated. Small perforations of the antrum may be ignored.

If possible, it is preferable to root-fill the palatal root of either *a first premolar* or *a first maxillary molar* by conventional means and confine surgical endodontics to the buccal root or roots. It is fortunate that the palatal root canals of first molars tend to be both wide and straight, thus facilitating the conservative approach to be employed as the surgical treatment of such roots is extremely difficult. The cut root face of upper cheek teeth should slope downwards and forwards to facilitate the search for and treatment of the root canals. The position of the zygomatic process of the maxilla makes access to the buccal apices of the *maxillary second molar* especially difficult and it may be necessary to identify the root at a relatively coronal level.

The apices of *lower incisors* are slender and are usually sited deeply in the bone. Both vision and access can be extremely limited and oblique resection of the apex is essential to success. The apices of *lower premolars* are relatively deeply placed in dense bone and the presence of the mental nerve limits access.

In molar surgical endodontics the application of methylene blue on a cotton-wool pellet to the cut surface of the root outlines for 2 min enables the root canals and isthmus to be seen more readily and stains the periodontal ligament thus clearly outlining the root.

Lower first molars are notoriously difficult to treat surgically principally because of difficulties with access. The apices should be resected obliquely with a fissure bur and elevated upwards and outwards. This procedure may be extremely difficult due to the buccolingual breadth of the roots and the width of the buccal plate of the alveolus.

INTENTIONAL REPLANTATION

Intentional replantation has been described as the purposeful extraction of a posterior tooth to perform extra-oral endodontic treatment of it, curettement of the apical soft tissues when required and the replacement of the tooth in its socket. It is essentially a technique of last resort and should only be used when more conventional endodontic therapy cannot be undertaken or has failed, and conventional surgical intervention would be either impracticable or unlikely to succeed, and the extraction of the tooth is the only alternative. The technique should not be employed if the patient is either medically compromised or insufficiently motivated to appreciate both the value and the limitations of the service. If the periodontal condition of the tooth is poor or its roots are extremely divergent or curved and so liable to fracture reimplantation is also contra-indicated.

The technique requires two operators, one of whom acts as the surgeon whilst the other acts as the endodontist and is performed as follows:

The tooth is restored and the pulp chamber filled with restorative material in an endeavour to strengthen the crown of the tooth. Meticulous aseptic technique is required throughout the procedure. The tooth to be extracted is isolated and it and the tissues around it are swabbed with an antiseptic solution. Both operators should wear sterile rubber gloves and the 'dental surgeon' carefully and gently removes the tooth, preferably without using either an elevator or rotatory movements in an attempt to avoid crushing the periodontal ligament. The socket is curetted and covered with gauze to prevent contamination whilst the 'endodontist' holds the tooth in gauze soaked in a solution of tetracycline in saline and either simply amputates the root apices or inserts retrograde root fillings. Any blood clot is carefully removed from the socket which is then irrigated with either sterile saline or local anaesthetic solution before the tooth is gently replaced, generally being inserted from the lingual aspect towards the buccal. The buccal and lingual walls of the socket are compressed and the tooth is splinted with either wire or liquid cement (enamel adhesive) and covered with a periodontal pack which is left in situ for 2–4 weeks. Care should be taken to ensure that the replanted tooth is free of occlusal contacts during all excursions of the mandible. Proximal contacts should be maintained as they prevent drifting.

The procedure must be completed as expeditiously as possible for if the tooth is out of the mouth for more than 30 min the chances of long-term success are markedly diminished.

Follow-up radiographs are taken at 6-monthly intervals for at least 3 years which is regarded as the critical period for resorption or resolution to occur. If required the replanted tooth can be brought into occlusion with its opponents by means of either an onlay or a crown. Continued long-term monitoring is advisable. A case can only be regarded as completely successful when the tooth is asymptomatic, the adjacent gingival tissues are healthy and the radiographic appearances of both the periodontium and the periapical tissues are normal. Using these criteria various workers have claimed success rates of between 55 and 65%.

FOCAL SEPSIS

The day has passed when dental sepsis was thought to be the prime cause of many diseases of unknown aetiology. The obvious consequences of gross visible 'open' sepsis are likely to be of more importance than any part it may play in the causation of such chronic conditions as arthritis. It is convenient for purposes of discussion to apply the term 'closed' oral sepsis to those clinical conditions, such as a periapical lesion not accompanied by sinus formation, in which the products of infection do not drain directly into the mouth. Periodontal and other lesions which drain directly into the mouth are described as being 'open' foci of oral sepsis. Although it was originally believed that the infected contents of 'closed' foci of sepsis drained into the blood and lymphatic system, and that drainage of the so-called 'open' lesions was into the gastro-intestinal tract, it is now realized that no such clear distinction exists and that one lesion may exhibit both characteristics.

There is no doubt that subacute bacterial endocarditis can be considered to be one of the direct results of either form of dental sepsis (*see* p. 40).

Whether heart valves are damaged or not, all dental sepsis must be eliminated for the general well-being of the patient. In the case of valvular heart disease or iritis and iridocyclitis, where either life or sight may be at stake, all pulpless teeth should be removed under antibiotic cover (*see* p. 256). In all other cases, if there is an indication for retaining a tooth on aesthetic or other dental grounds, root-canal therapy is justified and, provided that a normal radiographic appearance is restored and maintained and the tooth is clinically sound, there is no danger to the health of the average fit dental patient.

The exclusion and elimination of a dental focus of sepsis

Most medical practitioners, when considering the problem of focal sepsis, tend to think in terms of a dental focus of sepsis in general and of pulpless teeth in particular. Infected gingival pockets are probably more important and frequent sources of dental sepsis than well-treated pulpless teeth, whilst organs elsewhere in the body, such as infected tonsils, air sinuses, or gall bladders, may also constitute septic foci. These factors must be borne in mind when a patient is referred for an opinion regarding the possibility of a dental focus of sepsis being present.

When dealing with such a request the dentist should take a careful history and perform a painstaking examination of the teeth and their supporting structures. This examination should include probing of the gingival crevice and pulp testing where indicated, and a full-mouth intra-oral radiographic survey should be undertaken as a routine. It has been demonstrated that retained roots seen in radiographs to be surrounded by a periodontal membrane of normal thickness have vital pulps and are no danger to the individual as a whole. Any tooth or root which is either affected by untreatable periodontal disease or is seen in radiographs to be related to either a granuloma or a cyst must be removed before an oral focus of sepsis can be excluded. Before undertaking active treatment it is usual to send a report of the dental findings to the doctor concerned, accompanied by an offer to eradicate any dental sepsis present and emphasizing that no guarantee can be given that any improvement or cure of the underlying disease will result from the proposed dental treatment.

Antibiotic cover (*see* p. 256) must be provided when either scaling is performed or teeth are removed from such a patient.

SUGGESTED READING

Allen F. J. (1961) Incisor fragments in the lip. *Dent. Pract.* **11**, 390–1.
Barnes I. A. (1981) Surgical endodontics—introduction, principles and indications. *Dent. Update* **8**, 89–92, 95–97, 99.
Barnes I. A. (1981) Surgical Procedures—Part 1. *Dent. Update* **8**, 159–60, 162–3, 165–8.
Barnes I. A. (1981) Surgical Procedures—Part 2. *Dent. Update* **8**, 227–31, 233, 235–6.
Barnes I. A. (1981) Surgical Procedures—Part 3. *Dent. Update* **8**, 303–5, 307–10, 312–13.
Barnes I. A. (1981) Surgical Procedures—Part 4. *Dent. Update* **8**, 423, 425–7, 429–31, 433, 435—6.
Barnes I. A. (1981) Prognosis, follow-up, correction and preoperative assessment. *Dent. Update* **8**, 497, 499–500.
Barnes I. A. (1981) The repair of perforations. *Dent. Update* **8**, 503–5, 508–9, 511, 513.

Fish E. W. (1952) Focal infection. *Med. Press.* 82–6.

Grossman L. I. (1982) Intentional replantation of teeth—a clinical evaluation. *JADA* **104**, 633–9.

Harty F. J., Parkins B. J. and Wengraf A. M. (1970) Success rate in root canal therapy. *Br. Dent. J.* **128**, 65–70.

Helsham R. W. (1960) Some observations on the subject of roots of teeth retained in the jaws as a result of incomplete exodontia. *Aust. Dent. J.* **5**, 70–7.

Lubin H. (1982) Intentional replantation: report of a case. *JADA* **104**, 858–9.

Malmström M., Perkki K. and Lindquist K. (1982) Apicectomy—a retrospective study. *Proc. Finn. Dent. Soc.* **78**, 26–31.

Mitchell R. and Maclennan W. D. (1983) A modified flap for apicectomy. *Br. J. Oral Surg.* **21**, 21–6.

Nicholls E. (1962) Retrograde filling of the root canal. *Oral Surg.* **15**, 463–73.

Nicholls E. (1963) Assessment of the periapical status of pulpless teeth. *Br. Dent. J.* **114**, 453–9.

Nicholls E. (1965) The role of surgery in endodontics. *Br. Dent. J.* **118**, 59–67.

Nicholls E. (1965) Research and clinical practice in endodontics. *Dent. Pract.* **16**, 81–90.

Nosonowitz D. M. and Stanley H. R. (1984) Intentional replantation to prevent predictable endodontic failures. *Oral Surg.* **57**, 423–32.

Rushton M. A. (1953) Rise and fall of focal sepsis. *Dent. Rec.* **72**, 374–9.

Slack G. L. and Pogrel H. (1955) Root and canal therapy. A carrier device. *Br. Dent. J.* **98**, 447–8.

Storms J. L. (1969) Success in endodontic treatment. *J. Can. Dent. Assoc.* **35**, 83–97.

Chapter 13

Oral surgery in relationship to pathology

The dental surgeon should not undertake the surgical treatment of intra-oral lesions unless he has a sound knowledge of pathology and can arrange for a histopathological examination of the excised tissues to be performed by a pathologist with experience in the diagnosis of oral lesions. In many cases it is necessary to supplement a clinical diagnosis with a histological diagnosis before a definitive diagnosis can be made. In the vast majority of instances the histological examination merely serves to confirm the clinical diagnosis, but even experienced clinicians are occasionally surprised by the findings of the pathologist. The omission of this essential procedure may result in the future health of the patient being jeopardized.

All excised surgical specimens should be sent for pathological examination, even when the operator is certain that his clinical diagnosis is correct and that the lesion is benign. A histological diagnosis forms a permanent record and is invaluable on those occasions when it becomes necessary to confirm that an excised lesion was benign. Thus a patient who is found to have a malignant lesion may give a history of having had a tumour removed from the tongue some years previously. It will then become important to determine whether the malignant lesion is either a primary growth or a secondary deposit related to the lingual tumour, before the prognosis of the patient can be assessed or a treatment plan prepared. If a histological report on the intra-oral lesion, or better still a microscope slide, is available for examination the problem is readily resolved.

As a general rule it is better for a general dental practitioner to refer any patient with a lesion which appears to be malignant to a specialist, who has all the facilities required to investigate and treat the patient. In all other cases the surgical specimen should be sent to a pathologist for examination.

Most pathologists will send a slide of the lesion in addition to a written report if asked to do so, and advantage should be taken of such a service, for it enables the clinician to extend his knowledge of disease processes.

THE VALUE OF BIOPSY

A *biopsy* may be defined as a histopathological examination of tissue removed surgically and it may assist the surgeon in a variety of ways. Diagnosis is the responsibility of the clinician and not the pathologist, but, although it must always be remembered that histological diagnosis is only a link, albeit an important one, in the process of forming a definitive diagnosis, biopsy may confirm a clinical

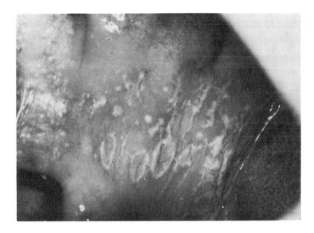

Fig. 13.1. Lichen planus affecting the mucosal lining of the right cheek.

diagnosis (*Fig.* 13.1). In other cases it may exclude the presence of malignancy and save the patient from either mutilating surgery or needless radiotherapy. A positive biopsy report is the only acceptable diagnosis of malignant disease and this is important when the surgeon has to tell either the patient or his relatives the nature of the condition. It is also essential for the purposes of treatment, records, and research. In malignant disease the histological appearances of the lesion may be of great assistance in determining the prognosis of the patient and may provide some indication of the likely response of the tumour to radiotherapy (*Fig.* 13.2).

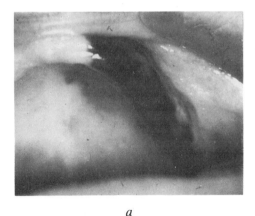

a

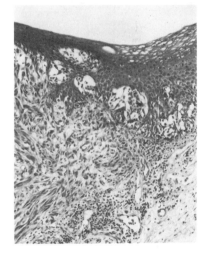

Fig. 13.2. Malignant melanoma of maxilla. This type of lesion is relatively radioresistant. *a*, Clinical appearance. *b*, Histological section. (× 72.)

b

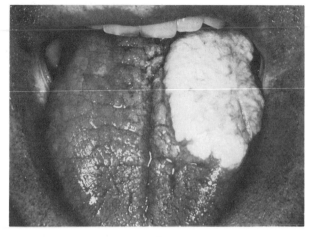

a

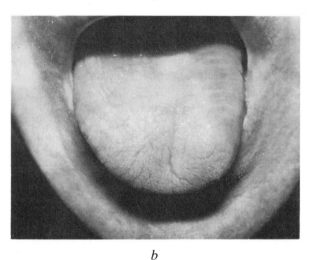

b

Fig. 13.3. Leucoplakia of the tongue. The Wassermann reaction was positive. *a*, Lesion at patient's first attendance. *b*, Tongue after excision biopsy and repair of the resulting defect utilizing local tissues.

Serial biopsies, that is biopsies taken at regular intervals, are sometimes employed to determine the progress and response to treatment of such chronic conditions as white lesions of the oral mucosa (*Fig.* 13.3*a*).

Although biopsy may be of great value in both diagnosis and treatment planning, it must always be remembered that in many tumours the histological pattern may vary in different parts of the same lesion, and so other methods of diagnosis must not be neglected. Both histological diagnosis and clinical acumen are required if the patient is to receive the best possible treatment.

Some authorities criticize surgery for biopsy purposes in cases of suspected malignant disease and believe that the practice increases the likelihood of metastases occurring. Although clinical experience does not lend support to these beliefs, and it is widely agreed that the proven value of biopsy in clinical practice far outweighs this theoretical objection, care should be taken to minimize the risk. Thus the tissues should be handled very gently at all times and local anaesthetic solution should be injected well away from the tumour site. The microscopical appearances of the specimen may be distorted by 'artificial waterlogging' unless the injections are made at least 2 cm away from the lesion. If the suspected cancer is related to a bone, care should be taken not to penetrate the periosteum when a biopsy specimen is removed.

AIDING THE PATHOLOGIST

The accuracy of histological diagnosis varies as widely as that of clinical diagnosis and the surgeon can assist the pathologist to eliminate errors in several ways. If possible, the pathologist should see the patient with the surgeon so that both the site and extent of the biopsy can be mutually determined. This is not possible in the majority of cases and so when the specimen is sent to the laboratory it must be accompanied by such details as the patient's age, sex, the site of the lesion and its clinical features such as its size, colour, texture and consistency. It should also be noted whether the lesion is painful or tender, mobile or fixed, or has caused any functional difficulty such as limitation of tongue movements and whether the regional lymph nodes are enlarged. Other details of importance include the duration of the illness, the clinical diagnosis and the treatment given, particularly if it is likely to affect microscopical appearances. In some instances radiographic appearances and the results of other tests (e.g., serum calcium, phosphorus and alkaline phosphatase levels) may help the pathologist in his task.

An adequate amount of tissue must be removed for purposes of biopsy. It must always be remembered that excised tissue shrinks and the excised specimen should be at least 1 cm × ½ cm in size. Any small and accessible lesion should be excised completely and sent for histological examination. No good purpose is served by submitting a patient to two operations if one will suffice. The specimen should not be crushed, torn, or burned. Some surgeons use electrosurgery to remove biopsy specimens because they believe that it may lessen the risk of metastases occurring. Clinical experience does not support this view and there is good evidence that burning tissue makes histological examination more difficult.

Quite obviously the tissue must be taken from the right area if an accurate histological diagnosis is to be made. An attempt should be made to determine the macroscopic junction of the lesion and the normal tissue adjoining it. The specimen removed for biopsy purposes should include tissue on either side of this macroscopic junction and necrotic areas should always be avoided. When intra-oral biopsy specimens are being taken from the cheeks in cases of suspected lichen planus, sites other than the occlusal line must be used because frictional hyperkeratosis is often found in this area. The specimen should be sent to the pathologist accompanied by a drawing outlining the lesion and clearly indicating the exact spot from which the biopsy specimen was taken.

The sooner the specimen is fixed, the better the section will be, for inadequate fixation allows autolysis to proceed unchecked and may make the subsequent interpretation of microscopical appearances either difficult or even impossible. The dental surgeon should have suitable containers, of varying size and containing 10% formol saline, readily available. For ideal fixation a piece of tissue should be immersed in at least ten times its own volume of fixative. Immediately the specimen is removed from the wound it should be dropped into an already labelled container and promptly sent to the pathology department. When the specimen has to be sent to the laboratory through the post either an unbreakable container or a carefully packed glass bottle can be used. If for any reason a jar of fixative is not available, the specimen should not be put into either water or normal saline which will hasten autolysis, but should be taken whilst still fresh to the laboratory. If this is not possible for several hours, the specimen should be wrapped in moist cotton-wool and kept in a refrigerator.

INDICATIONS FOR BIOPSY

The surgeon should take a biopsy specimen without delay whenever difficulty is experienced in diagnosing the true nature of a lesion, except when the possibility exists of a blood dyscrasia being present. In these circumstances surgery is contra-indicated and a detailed examination of the blood must be performed. On the rare occasions upon which the histological diagnosis and the clinical diagnosis do not agree, a full discussion between the surgeon and the pathologist will usually either resolve the difficulty or suggest further investigations which may clarify the picture.

When the lesion appears to be malignant on clinical grounds but the biopsies fail to confirm the suspicions of the surgeon, further specimens should be obtained and examined, for in many cases the first biopsies will have been taken in the wrong place or at the wrong depth. Most pathologists like to make a diagnosis of malignant disease on a paraffin section and regard cytological examination (*see* p. 340) as an adjunct only and frozen sections as being of limited value in this respect.

The management of a patient with a chronic lesion, such as a hyperkeratotic area, may require repeated biopsy examinations to be performed at varying intervals of time. By means of this technique, which is known as serial biopsy, the progress of the lesion or its response to treatment may be determined. Specimens are usually obtained by using the incisional method, although cytological examination is sometimes used for the purpose.

Three different techniques are used in clinical practice to obtain a specimen of tissue for biopsy purposes and they may be described as excision biopsy, incisional biopsy, and drill biopsy respectively.

EXCISION BIOPSY

When dealing with lesions which, upon clinical examination, appear to be benign this technique should be employed whenever it is possible to do so, for not only is

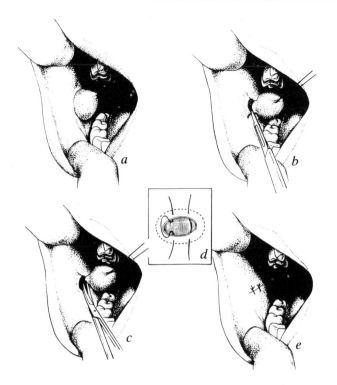

Fig. 13.4. Excision biopsy of 'fibroma' of cheek (*see* text for explanation).

the whole of the lesion made available for examination, but complete excision of the lesion is usually the only form of treatment available for most of the conditions liable to be the subject of histological examination. In these circumstances, complete excision of the lesion for biopsy purposes also constitutes the required treatment and so no further operation is required. All too often specimens obtained in this manner are ruined by being crushed by the use of either toothed forceps or haemostats. This complication can be avoided by transfixing the lesion with one or more sutures, which can then be used to move and control the specimen and to tense the soft tissues during its removal. In vascular areas, such as the tongue and lips, excessive haemorrhage may be controlled either by the application of pressure by an assistant (*see Fig.* 3.46) or by the insertion of stay sutures, which enclose a large amount of soft tissue and render it ischaemic when tension is applied. Traction is applied to the lesion, thus raising it from its bed and stretching the mucosa around its attachment (*Fig.* 13.4*a, b*).

After the mucosa surrounding the base of the lesion has been incised, the specimen is separated from the underlying tissues by a combination of sharp and blunt dissection (*Fig.* 13.4*b, c*). The detached specimen is placed immediately into an already labelled specimen bottle or jar containing fixing solution. If the resulting wound is on a surface covered with attached mucoperiosteum, it is usual to cover the defect with either a base-plate or denture lined with zinc-oxide impression paste or tissue conditioner, or with a ribbon-gauze pack soaked in Whitehead's varnish. In all other sites the mucosa surrounding the wound should be undercut and advanced (*Fig*. 13.4*d, e*). When dealing with pedunculated and small lesions with a sessile base, it is often possible by this means to close the mucosal defect without tension and so obtain healing by first intention. In other cases it may only be possible to reduce the size of the area left to heal by granulation, by advancing the undercut mucosa and sewing it to the underlying mesodermal tissues.

INCISIONAL BIOPSY

When this technique is employed, only part of a lesion is removed for biopsy purposes and it is usually used to obtain specimens of lesions which might prove difficult to excise completely, owing to either their extent or situation. In the mouth the commonest lesions of this type are the white hyperkeratotic lesions which affect the oral mucosa. In such cases bleeding, ulcerated, painful, or indurated areas should always be removed for biopsy. The most thickly keratinized areas should not be chosen for examination, as the areas covered with thin atrophic mucosa or granulation tissue are potentially more dangerous. Antiseptics should not be applied to the lesion prior to surgery and care must be taken

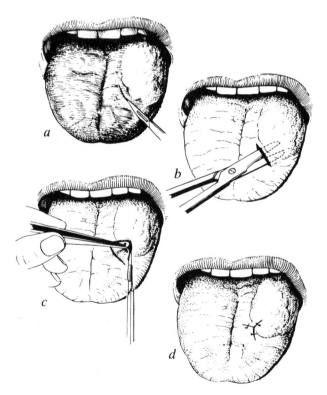

Fig. 13.5.   Technique of incisional biopsy (*see* text for explanation).

to ensure that local anaesthetic solution is deposited well away from the site from which the tissue is to be removed. An incision made in front of the lesion permits the area selected for examination to be first undermined and then excised (*Fig.* 13.5*a, b, c*). The surrounding tissues are then undercut and repaired with sutures (*Fig.* 13.5*d*). If the removed tissue tends to curl, it should be laid on a piece of blotting paper before it is put into the fixing solution.

Incisional biopsy should not be performed on either pigmented or vascular lesions. Melanomas are highly metastatic and so pigmented lesions should be excised with a generous margin of macroscopically normal tissue around and beneath them. A clinical diagnosis of haemangioma can often be confirmed by the aspiration of blood from the lesion into a glass syringe via a wide-bore needle.

DRILL BIOPSY

Specimens for biopsy can be obtained from the mouth by the use of a suitably modified Ellis biopsy drill, which fits into a straight dental handpiece (*Fig.* 13.6).

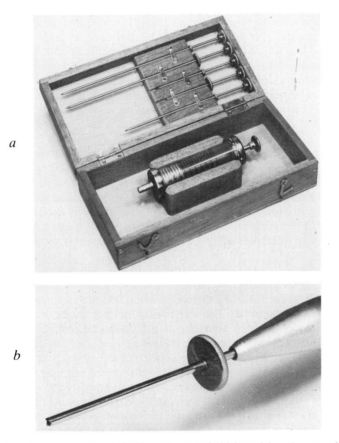

a

b

Fig. 13.6. *a*, Ellis biopsy drill. *b*, Drill, on the end of which teeth have been cut, in straight handpiece.

This instrument can be used to obtain specimens 1·2 cm long and 1·4 mm in diameter. It is particularly useful for obtaining biopsy material from central fibro-osseous lesions in the jaws, being easy, safe and suitable for use under local anaesthesia on out-patients. The technique provides a specimen in depth which is ideal for the examination of bony dystrophies, but the specimen is so small that it may not be truly representative, whilst the heat which may be generated during the procedure, unless great care is exercised, may cause distortion. A negative drill biopsy must never be accepted, for it is very easy to miss the lesion when inserting the drill. In such cases further biopsies should be taken.

CYTOLOGY

Great developments in the techniques of cytological examination, that is the microscopic examination of the characteristics of individual cells, have been made in recent years. Despite the undoubted value of the technique it must only be regarded as an adjunct to biopsy rather than a substitute for it. Any lesion which appears on clinical grounds to be malignant should be biopsied. The use of oral cytology is indicated when the surgical removal of specimens for biopsy purposes either is not feasible, or is refused by the patient, or does not seem to be warranted. The technique is of especial value when diffuse or multicentric lesions have to be examined, or when repeated examinations have to be performed over long periods as in the follow-up of patients who have previously been treated for oral cancer. Oral cytology should be employed when it is decided to keep a lesion under observation in preference to performing a biopsy. As many early oral cancers appear innocuous the trivial appearance of an abnormal area should not be regarded as obviating the need to perform a cytological examination. The technique may be used in conjunction with biopsy examination, for it is always possible that the tissue sample removed for biopsy examination may not be truly representative of the lesion. A positive cytology result in such circumstances would then emphasize the need for a repeat biopsy. A planned series of cytological smears taken from a lesion with a large surface area may be used to select the most suitable sites for the surgical removal of specimens for biopsy. Whenever doubt arises during the interpretation of cytological material a biopsy should be performed.

As the accuracy of cytological examination is dependent upon the smear consisting of cells representative of the lesion with the minimum of extraneous material and saliva, care must be exercised when taking the smear if false-negative results are to be minimized. The method is simple, quick, causes little or no discomfort, and can be repeated as frequently as desired even after radiotherapy without prejudicing the welfare of the patient.

Material is obtained by scraping the surface of the suspect area with either the straight edge of a dental flat plastic instrument, or the edge of a wooden tongue depressor moistened in tap water, several times in one direction. A moist surface bathed in saliva is desirable and the mucosa should be moistened if it is abnormally dry. Whilst a little haemorrhage will not interfere with microscopic examination it should be avoided if this is possible. The lesion should not be wiped or dried prior to being scraped, unless it is covered with a slough. Sloughs should be removed either with gauze moistened with normal saline solution, or by gentle scraping before specimens for examination are taken. Keratinized lesions present special problems, for scraping the surface of a thickly keratinized lesion will produce keratin rather than cells of diagnostic value. Scrapings taken from the deeper levels of any fissures present in such a lesion will yield representative cells, but it is often better to perform a biopsy in these circumstances. Difficulty may be experienced in obtaining satisfactory cytology specimens from labial lesions due to either crust formation or keratinization. These obstacles to success must be removed prior to scraping if a specimen containing representative cells from the deeper layers of the epithelium is to be obtained. Lesions on the vermilion border of the lip can be softened by soaking with wet gauze for at least 15 min prior to scraping. Cytology is a painless procedure except when ulceration is present. Satisfactory scrapings can be obtained without pain from an ulcerated surface after the application of a topical anaesthetic.

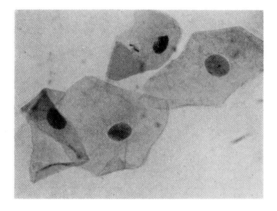

a

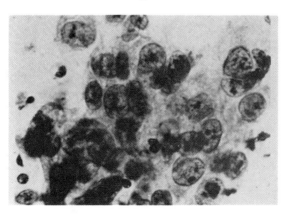

b

Fig. 13.7. Cytology specimens. *a*, Inner layer squamous cells. (× 455.) *b*, Smear from malignant tumour showing variation in cytoplasm/nucleus ratio. (× 455.)

The material obtained is carefully spread on a clean previously labelled slide by using the edge of another slide. After any excess of saliva has been allowed to evaporate the slide is put into a jar containing a mixture of equal parts of ether and 95% ethyl alcohol for at least 15 min. Immediate fixation of the smear is essential if distortion of the cells due to drying is to be avoided. It is usually advisable to prepare at least two slides and place them back to back in the jar. Paper clips or elastic bands may be put on the ends of the slides to keep them apart whilst they are in the container. The slides are removed from the jar when convenient and allowed to dry in the air without heating. When slides for cytological examination have to be sent to the pathology laboratory through the post, it is often more convenient to fix the cells immediately after spreading them on the slides by using a proprietary spray (e.g., Cytospray or Spraycyte). Care should be taken to pack the slides in such a way as to ensure that they are kept apart during their journey to the laboratory. The interpretation of cytological smears can present problems and so the laboratory chosen should be one in which there are personnel who have especial competence and experience in this work (*Fig.* 13.7).

VENEPUNCTURE

Every dental surgeon should familiarize himself with the technique of vene-puncture, for not only does it enable him to obtain blood samples for either haematological or biochemical examinations (*Table* 13.1), but in a case of emergency, e.g., adrenal crisis (*see* p. 41), he must be able to give an intravenous injection if the patient's life is to be saved.

Before taking blood for either haematological or biochemical examination, the dental surgeon should ascertain the amount required for the purpose and ensure that the appropriate container is available, labelled, and ready for use. When small quantities of blood are required a 2-ml disposable syringe fitted with a No. 1 needle may be used (*see Fig.* 9.30). When larger amounts are required a 10- or 20-ml syringe fitted with an eccentric nozzle and a No. 1 needle should be employed (*Fig.* 13.8).

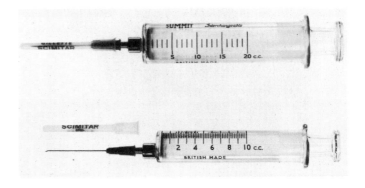

Fig. 13.8. Glass syringes with eccentric nozzles.

Table 13.1. Some Physiological Normal Values

	Erythrocytes (millions/c mm)	Haemoglobin (g/100 ml)	Packed cell volume (per cent)	Leucocytes (per c mm)	Differential leucocyte count (per cent)	Platelets (per c mm)
Men	4·5–6·5	13·5–18·0	40–54	4000–10000	Neutrophils: 40–75 Eosinophils: 1–6 Basophils: Up to 1 Lymphocytes: 20–50 Monocytes: 2–10	Range varies considerably with the method used: 150000–400000
Women	3·9–5·6	11·5–16·4	36–47			
Children (1 year)	4·5 (average)	11·2 (average)	35 (average)	6000–18000	Blood counts in children show a wide range of variability, which tends to decrease as the child grows older At 4 years the percentage of lymphocytes is roughly equal to the percentage of neutrophils At puberty the count reaches adult proportions	
Children (10 years)	4·7 (average)	12·9 (average)	37·5 (average)	4500–13500		

Colour Index: 0·85–1·15
Proteins (g/100 ml plasma or serum):
  Total   6·0–8·0
  Albumin   3·5–5·5
  Globulin   1·5–3·0
  Fibrinogen 0·2–0·4
Sugar (venous) (mg/100 ml whole blood):
  Fasting 65–105
  After meal 85–140

Reticulocyte Count: 0·2–2 per cent
Calcium: 9–11 mg/100 ml plasma or serum
Phosphate: 3–4·5 mg/100 ml plasma or serum
Alkaline Phosphatase (King-Armstrong units/100 ml plasma or serum):
  At age 1 year   10–25
           10 years 15–30
           Adult   3–13
Urea: 15–35 mg/100 ml whole blood

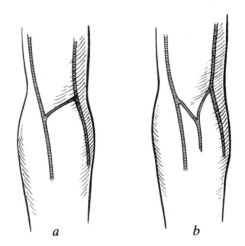

Fig. 13.9. Arrangement of veins at the elbow (*see* text for explanation).

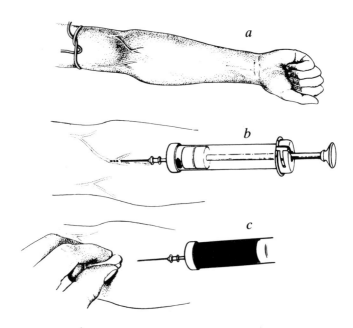

Fig. 13.10. Venepuncture (*see* text for explanation).

The vein chosen for the purpose of venepuncture should be large and strong, near the surface, not too freely movable, and should be capable of being rendered turgid by compression. Unless these criteria are fulfilled the operator may fail to locate the vein, tear its wall, or transfix it without realizing that the vein has been entered. These mishaps cause unnecessary pain and bruising.

The favourite site for venepuncture is within the bend of the elbow, where veins are usually visible and often conform to one of the simple patterns illustrated in *Fig.* 13.9. The veins are arranged in the form of the letter H, the one on the inner side of the arm being called the 'basilic', and that on the outer the 'cephalic' (*Fig.* 13.9*a*). These veins are joined by the 'median cubital' vein, which may be V-shaped, in which case the two arms of the V are known as the 'median basilic' and 'median cephalic' respectively (*Fig.* 13.9*b*). Although the median basilic vein is the most frequent site of venepuncture, the operator should choose the most suitable vein for his purpose.

The patient's elbow is extended and supported either by an assistant or by a pillow placed upon the arm of the dental chair. The veins are rendered turgid by compressing them proximally to the chosen site. This is best done by the hand of the patient or an assistant grasping the upper arm tightly enough to prevent the return of venous blood, but not so tightly that the flow of arterial blood into the limb is impeded. It is sometimes more convenient to use a tourniquet, which can take the form of either a piece of rubber tubing tied with a 'quick-release' tie (*Fig.* 13.10*a*) or a sphygmomanometer cuff inflated to a pressure of 80 mm of mercury. Distension of the veins is speeded by the patient clenching his fist a few times and by the operator lightly tapping the skin overlying the vein. The skin covering the site of puncture is then cleansed with a swab, soaked in ½–1% cetrimide in surgical spirit, and is stretched to steady the position of the vein. The skin is punctured with the long axis of the needle lying parallel to the vein with its bevel uppermost. The point of the needle should be inserted through the skin at a site about 1 cm distal to the place at which the vein is to be punctured and advanced alongside the vein before being introduced into its lumen (*Fig.* 13.10*b*).

With practice the operator can feel when the needle has entered the vein and this fact is confirmed if blood enters the barrel of the syringe when the plunger is withdrawn. After the amount of blood required for examination has been withdrawn the pressure on the upper arm is released, an antiseptic swab is held over the site of puncture, and the needle is withdrawn (*Fig.* 13.10*c*). Pressure over the site of puncture reduces the risk of haematoma formation, but should not be exerted until the moment that the needle is withdrawn, or it will cause pain. Pressure must be maintained for a few minutes if bleeding and bruising are to be prevented and the patient can often hold the swab firmly in position by flexing his forearm.

INTRAVENOUS INJECTIONS

When an intravenous injection is to be given, certain small but important modifications in the technique of venepuncture described above must be made. All air-bubbles must be expelled from the barrel of the syringe before the needle is inserted into the tissues. This is best achieved by holding the syringe vertically, with the needle pointing upwards, and lightly tapping the side of the barrel. This procedure causes any contained bubbles to rise to the top of the barrel of the syringe adjacent to the hub, through which the air can be expelled by depressing the plunger. Once the tip of the needle is in the vein it should be advanced in line with the vessel for 1 or 2 cm and the aspiration test repeated to make sure that it is still in the lumen. After the pressure on the veins has been released the intravenous injection should be given slowly.

Scrupulous care must be taken to ensure that intravenous injections are both prepared and given under aseptic conditions. Every precaution must be taken to ensure that the correct dose of the correct strength of the right drug is given in the correct form to the right patient. After the identity of the patient has been confirmed, the label on the container of the drug and the dosage drawn up for injection should be checked by someone other than the person who prepared the dose. It is sound practice never to give an intravenous injection unless a third person is present and the injection should only be given into an immobile site. When children or nervous adults are being treated, an assistant should control the part selected for injection throughout the procedure.

SUGGESTED READING

Baillie L. W. (1968) Exfoliative cytology in dental practice. *Aust. Dent. J.* **13**, 410–14.
Cannell H. (1975) Excision and biopsy in soft tissue. *Dent. Update* **2**, 129–31.
Cannell H. (1975) The incision and biopsy in soft tissue. *Dent. Update* **2**, 235–7.
Cooke B. E. D. (1958) Biopsy procedures. *Oral Surg.* **11**, 750–61.
'Joint Position Statement on Oral Cytology' (1968) *JAMA* **205**, 523.
Jolly M. (1968) Soft tissue surgery in general dental practice. *Aust. Dent. J.* **13**, 1–16.
Lemmer J. and Shear M. (1968) The biopsy in cancerous and pre-cancerous lesions of the mouth. *J. Dent. Assoc. S. Afr.* **23**, 274–85.
McMillan D. R. (1964) Diagnostic cytology. *Dent. Pract.* **14**, 198–201.
Whitehead R. (1954) Biopsies. *Br. Med. J.* **1**, 1254–6.

Chapter 14

The surgical treatment of periodontal disease

by Ross J. Bastiaan

Gingival and periodontal disease is endemic in our society and comprises a major public health problem. Loss of periodontal support is the major cause of tooth loss in the adult population.

It is now widely agreed that the sole identifiable aetiological agent in destructive periodontal disease is dental plaque and so treatment is designed to eliminate plaque retention. This is of particular importance in the presence of such systemic conditions as pregnancy, diabetes mellitus and leukaemia which modify the response of the periodontal tissues to plaque. Local factors such as the over-hanging margins of restorations, the wearing of partial prostheses and the presence of periodontal pocketing may lead to plaque retention and make it difficult for the patient to maintain an effective level of oral hygiene.

Periodontal surgery is used less frequently than in the past but still has a place in the treatment of periodontal disease. It may be used either to treat damage to the periodontium and alveolar bone in order to capitalize upon the innate potential for healing and repair of these tissues and/or to facilitate the effective removal of plaque. Surgery must be employed judiciously by an operator who has a real understanding not only of the disease process but also of both the values and limitations of non-surgical therapy.

THE STAGES OF PERIODONTAL DISEASE

In health the coral pink, scalloped, knife-edged gingival margin adheres tightly to the tooth surface and conforms closely to the contours of the underlying alveolar bone (*Fig.* 14.1A). The shape of the crowns of the teeth, together with the presence of marginal ridges and intact interdental contact points control the direction of food-shedding during chewing and so protect the gingivae, and prevent food packing. When plaque is allowed to accumulate and mature on the teeth, marginal inflammation of the gingivae occurs and clinically this condition is known as gingivitis. The accumulation of plaque is increased in the presence of dental calculus.

In gingivitis, the gingivae appear on clinical examination to be red and oedematous and to have lost their adhesion to the necks of the teeth. However, histological studies reveal that at this stage neither the attachment of junctional epithelium to the tooth is broken nor has the epithelium proliferated towards the apex on the root surface. At this stage the disease is reversible for if correct treatment is instituted which combines improved oral hygiene techniques with

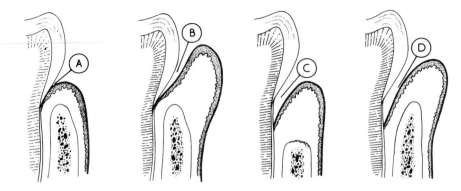

Fig. 14.1. Diagrams showing: A, Normal relationship of a tooth and its supporting tissues;
B, Gingival or false pocket; C, True or periodontal pocket, D, Infra-bony pocket.

scaling and cleaning, the tissues will return to a healthy state. Occasionally, superficial hyperplastic gingival deformities develop and these may require surgical correction either in order to improve access for plaque removal or to improve appearance (*Fig.* 14.1B). If gingivitis is not treated, the disease process may progress to a more advanced stage which is known as periodontitis.

In periodontitis the junctional epithelium proliferates apically to form a perio-dontal pocket in which an inflammatory process with the capacity to destroy both the connective tissue and bony support for the tooth may occur and persist.

The loss of a functional gingival seal around the neck of the tooth allows the apical proliferation of dental plaque and potentiation of the disease process. The tissues may respond by further epithelial migration, connective-tissue proliferation and destruction of the adjacent alveolar bone (*Fig.* 14.1C and D). A proliferative hyperplastic tissue response and a deepening periodontal pocket may combine to retain more plaque and render its removal more difficult for the patient to achieve.

Treatment of the disease at this stage can arrest further tissue breakdown but inevitably some gingival deformity will persist which modifies the natural anatomical protective relationships and makes the maintenance of an effective regime of oral hygiene obligatory if the tissues are to remain in a healthy state.

THE MANAGEMENT OF CHRONIC PERIODONTAL DISEASE

A careful detailed *history* must be taken from each patient following the pattern described in Chapter 1. Special note should be taken of any history of previous periodontal disease, bleeding which occurs on toothbrushing and its frequency, the presence of mobile teeth, recession of the gums, halitosis, or an unpleasant taste in the mouth. Such general factors as pregnancy, diabetes mellitus or the ingestion of either the contraceptive pill or Dilantin Sodium are of especial importance in this context. The patient should be asked whether he or she is aware of either tooth-grinding or tooth-clenching habits or of chewing the lips, cheeks or foreign objects. Details of tobacco smoking habits should also be recorded.

Information should be obtained concerning the frequency and method of toothbrushing, and the use of interdental cleaning aids. The patient's attitude to dental health can also be assessed if enquiries are made into the frequency and reasons for previous dental attention.

Extra-oral *examination* should include palpation of the submental, submandibular and cervical lymph nodes. When either mouth breathing or an incompetent lip seal is present the patency of the nasal passages should be tested.

All the intra-oral soft tissues are then carefully and systematically examined so that if any malignant lesion is present, diagnosis is rapid and treatment quickly undertaken. It is also important to recognize other mucosal lesions, such as lichen planus, which may also affect the gingiva. The colour, consistency and contour of the gingival tissues should be assessed. Pocket depths should be measured on the buccal, lingual, mesial and distal surfaces of the teeth. Furcation involvement should be detected by probing carefully and recorded if present.

Occlusal changes or abnormalities, progressing diastemata and the number of missing teeth together with the reason for any extractions should be noted.

The existence of a pocket does not necessarily imply active disease for it is known that many pockets undergo a quiescent phase and so may not require surgical treatment. It is, therefore, important to note the existence of bleeding or the exudation of pus from the depths of a pocket for the presence of either of these signs indicates the likelihood of active disease. However, measurement by probing can lead to an overestimation of the pocket depth, because the junctional epithelium of an inflamed pocket is readily penetrated by the examining probe. Thus care must be taken to ensure the accuracy of the measurements of pocket depth obtained in this way if they are to be used to assess the progress of periodontal disease. Modern periodontists believe that tissue reaction rather than the depth of pocketing is the critical factor in determining prognosis. Consequently, the earlier concept that the elimination of periodontal pocketing by means of surgery is always indicated, is no longer valid.

The position of the line of attachment of the reflected alveolar mucosa to the attached gingiva, the so-called mucogingival junction, and its relationship to both the gingival margin and the base of the pockets should be recorded. Pockets, the bases of which are above the mucogingival junction, can be eliminated readily by surgical means. Those with bases located beneath the junction are more difficult to treat. The width of the attached gingiva must also be assessed, particularly if it is suspected that a frenum pulls upon it. Until recently, at least 2 mm of functionally adequate attached gingiva was considered to be necessary for good marginal gingival health but the current view is that even this width may not be required if plaque control is good.

Tooth mobility should be recorded on an arbitrary scale of 0–III by the use of two metal instruments applied alternately to the buccal and lingual surfces of the tooth in question. A reading of 0 indicates physiological mobility, I—less than 1 mm horizontal movement, II—more than 1 mm horizontal movement, and III—vertical movement in the socket in addition to over 1 mm horizontal movement.

The occlusion should be assessed with the mandible in the centric relation position, in the centric occlusal position, in lateral excursions and in protrusion. The articulation of the teeth in these various positions and any occlusal interferences must be noted and recorded. The presence of any tilting, spacing or migration of teeth should be charted. Changes in the temporomandibular joint and tenderness in the muscles of mastication should also be sought for, especially if any occlusal disharmonies are present. Tooth mobility will neither initiate nor potentiate periodontal breakdown, but correction of it can enhance patient comfort and function.

Radiographic examination should involve the use of the long cone intra-oral technique, using either RINN X-C-P or Snap-a-Ray film-holding devices to parallel the film with the long axis of the tooth. These radiographs provide an undistorted picture of the relationship between the alveolar crest and the amelo-cemental junction which is of particular importance around the molars when diagnosing the presence of bony defects and their relationship to the furcation areas.

The *response of the pulps* of the teeth should be checked using a thermal pulp tester (*see* p. 8). Endodontically treated and pulpless teeth frequently present with periodontal symptoms and their presence may complicate periodontal assessment and management.

If either excessive gingival inflammation or marked alveolar bone loss is present, *special tests* may be indicated to ascertain whether they are due to a systemic cause, such as agranulocytosis, leukaemia, diabetes mellitus or vitamin deficiencies.

THE PROGNOSIS OF PERIODONTAL DISEASE

Provided that patients treated for gingivitis and periodontitis are able to attain and maintain a high level of oral hygiene the prognosis is good. However, the surgical correction of periodontal damage and defects may be required to eliminate areas in which plaque is retained and so make it easier for the patient to subsequently remove plaque effectively.

The main factors affecting the prognosis of a tooth affected by periodontal disease are as follows:

1. The degree and type of bone loss and, in the posterior teeth, the presence of involvement of furcation areas.

2. Root anatomy and the crown:root ratio.

3. The relationship of infra-bony pockets to surrounding anatomical structures, such as the external oblique ridge or the maxillary sinus.

4. The presence of restorations in the teeth and the condition of their pulps.

5. The mobility of the involved tooth.

6. The standard of oral hygiene maintained by the patient.

7. The patient's general health and attitude to dental care.

TREATMENT PLANNING

Every periodontal treatment plan must be designed to establish and preserve the dentition as a functioning unit. Treatment should not be made up of a series of individual procedures each of which is independent of those performed elsewhere in the mouth. Rather it should comprise a carefully planned and co-ordinated sequence of events designed to meet both the needs and the expectations of the patient concerned.

Once an overall diagnosis has been made a treatment plan is formulated and implemented along the following lines:

1. Emergency treatment, such as the relief of pain, swelling, bleeding, etc. is given.

2. The nature of the problem is explained to the patient and oral hygiene procedures are instituted.

3. Urgent restorations, endodontics or extractions are undertaken.

4. Root planing is performed.

5. The occlusion is adjusted as necessary.

6. Plaque control is reassessed and reinforced.

7. Surgery to treat persistent active lesions or to correct gingival contours is undertaken only if indicated.

8. Conservative and prosthetic treatment is completed.

9. Minor orthodontic movement of teeth may be performed.

10. Regular recall visits are arranged at which the efficacy of the patient's home care is assessed and professional removal of plaque is provided if required.

Other than in exceptional circumstances extensive restorative or prosthetic procedures are best delayed until the periodontal health of involved teeth is established as subsequent periodontal treatment may affect the prognosis of a tooth and make it necessary to alter the overall treatment plan.

Unlike oral surgery which is normally designed to eliminate the disease, the usual aim of periodontal surgery is to combat the progressively destructive effects of a disease which is likely to either persist or to recur if local irritation persists.

In gingivitis and early periodontitis, the sequence of treatment may not be essential to success, but as the complexity of the case increases and other kinds of dental treatment are required, the sequence becomes increasingly important if the desired results of treatment are to be achieved.

THE APPROACH TO TREATMENT

As plaque is the only recognized causative agent in periodontal disease all treatment, whether surgical or non-surgical, should be directed towards assisting the patient to remove it effectively. For many years the culmination of almost every periodontal treatment plan was the surgical elimination of residual pocketing. Today periodontal treatment is directed towards gaining a re-attachment of the gingival tissues to the tooth usually via a long junctional epithelium. The tooth surface adjacent to an infected pocket contains endotoxins and lipopolysaccharides which prevent re-attachment of gingival epithelial cells. The removal of the infected root surface tissue by scaling and root planing procedures is designed to enable the epithelium to reattach and reduce the pocket depth (*Fig.* 14.2).

Thus it is the operator's ability to scale and root plane the affected root surface that will dictate whether a surgical or a non-surgical approach to treatment will be necessary. Different areas of the mouth will require either one or both approaches and accessibility to the affected root surface areas is the factor which determines which approach should be employed. Surgery, although more complicated than the non-surgical approach, provides direct vision and ready accessibility to affected areas. The non-surgical approach requires a higher degree of clinical precision and dexterity than the surgical approach, for by its very nature the root

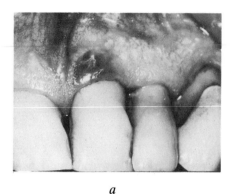

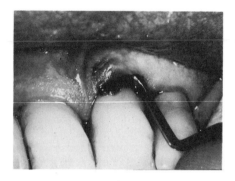

a

b

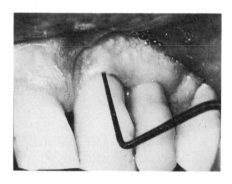

Fig. 14.2. *a*, Large deposit of subgingival calculus, associated with a 5-mm pocket on the labial aspect of the central incisor. *b*, Root planing with a curette removed the calculus and smoothed the surface of the root. *c*, With a clean root surface, the gingiva reattached to the tooth, thus reducing the pocket depth to 2 mm. The pocket did not bleed on probing after root planing.

c

planing is performed without the benefit of direct vision of the affected root surfaces. Nevertheless, every effort should be made to scale and root plane all affected areas before any surgery is undertaken.

NON-SURGICAL MANAGEMENT OF PERIODONTAL DISEASE

Plaque control should be instituted with personalized instruction in the use of the toothbrush and such interdental cleaning aids as dental floss or wood points. An 0·2% aqueous solution of chlorhexidine digluconate is a most effective anti-plaque mouth rinse and when used twice a day for periods of 10 days will improve marginal tissue colour and contour. Occasionally prolonged use of such a mouth rinse can produce staining of the teeth, a partial loss of taste and a brown discoloration of the dorsum of the tongue.

Scaling and root planing are the clinical procedures in which calculus, plaque and infected cementum are removed from the clinical crowns and subgingival root surfaces of teeth, leaving a smooth, hard tooth surface. In root planing, the aim is to produce a root surface free of any pathological changes consequent upon periodontal disease. These procedures are designed to alter the number and types of the bacterial flora in the pocket in addition to removing the potentially toxic material associated with affected root surfaces. Subgingival curettage, a procedure in which the inner surface of the gingival wall of the periodontal pocket is scraped in order to clean out, separate and remove diseased soft tissue and granulation tissue, is no longer widely advocated, for inflamed gingival tissue will heal satisfactorily without being removed if the adjacent infected root surfaces are planed.

Scalers are used to remove large deposits of calculus and bacteria on the tooth surface. It is important to remove overhangs on restorations, thereby both reducing plaque accumulation and facilitating plaque removal by the patient. This is particularly important in the interdental areas where cleaning is more difficult than on the buccal or lingual surfaces of the teeth.

Curettes have finer ends than scalers so making it possible to insert them more readily to the bottom of the pockets. When used skilfully they are the most effective instruments used for periodontal purposes for although ultrasonic scalers are of great value they do not produce as smooth a treated root surface as do curettes.

All hand instruments used must be both sharp and sterile. Good finger rests are essential if laceration of the soft tissues is to be avoided and the working edge of the instrument guided along the root surfaces.

Using minimal force the instrument is inserted into the pocket to enable the position of the calculus to be determined. The working edge of the scaler is then engaged against the calculus and pulled out against the root surface. Then root planing is continued until a hard smooth root surface is obtained. The use of local anaesthesia is desirable as the procedure can cause the patient discomfort when performed thoroughly.

The clinician needs to be patient, persistent and above all systematic when root planing. However, even when this is the case over half the teeth treated will have some small amounts of residual calculus remaining after root planing and a review appointment should be arranged so that this residuum can be removed.

As a rough guide, approximately 10 min will be needed to properly root plane each tooth being treated.

RE-EVALUATION

After scaling and root planing, the patient's standard of oral hygiene and periodontal health should be assessed at intervals of 3 months. Such an assessment must include a thorough clinical examination during which attention should be paid to the following points:

1. The depths of the periodontal pockets and the presence within them of either bleeding or suppuration.

2. The relationship of the base of the pocket to the mucogingival junction.

3. The presence of either trifurcation or bifurcation involvement.

4. The width of the attached gingiva in all areas. This should be of a sufficient width to ensure that the gingival margins are not retracted by any attached frenum.

5. Changes in mobility of teeth (temporary stabilization of loose teeth and gross occlusal reshaping, although not discussed in this book, may also form part of initial periodontal treatment).

6. The relationship of clinical pocket depth to infra-bony depth assessed by means of radiographic examination.

If the breakdown of the periodontal tissues is found to be continuing after root planing has been performed a periodontal surgical approach may be necessary. For example, bleeding or suppuration from a previously root planed pocket may indicate the need for further planing of the affected root surface. Poor access may limit the value of indirect visual instrumentation and so surgery to expose the root surface and permit instrumentation under direct vision may be required.

Time spent in treatment before surgery is undertaken provides the dentist with an opportunity to assess the healing potential of the patient. If, despite the removal of all local irritants and the maintenance of good patient oral hygiene by the patient, the results are still poor, the presence of an underlying systemic disease should be suspected, investigated and excluded.

PERIODONTAL SURGERY

General considerations

A large variety of instruments are available for use in periodontal surgery, and individual preference and experience will determine their selection (*see* Appendix B).

The majority of patients undergoing periodontal surgery do not require pre-medication for the relief of apprehension and anxiety. When indicated, diazepam (Valium) 10 mg by mouth the night before surgery and 10 mg 1½ hours before operation is particularly valuable. The patient should be accompanied to and from the surgery and advised against drinking alcohol or driving for 24 hours following ingestion of the drug (*see* p. 55).

In the maxilla local anaesthesia is obtained by infiltration into the base of the labiobuccal vestibule and into the palatal mucoperiosteum. In the lower jaw a mandibular block is used. Once regional anaesthesia has been obtained localized papillary (interdental) infiltrations are given to tense the tissues. The adrenaline contained in the local anaesthetic solution also aids in haemostasis. A general anaesthetic should neither be employed nor prolonged any more than is necessary. Hurry compromises surgical technique and is to be avoided. Thus, even for patients in whom flap procedures in all parts of the mouth are planned general anaesthesia is seldom indicated. However, there are occasional patients who cannot tolerate surgery under local anaesthesia and in such cases general anaesthesia should be employed.

Periodontal dressings are no longer used routinely after surgery. Whilst such a dressing may reduce the postoperative discomfort and improve healing this is not always necessary if a chlorhexidine digluconate mouthwash is used conscientiously during the postoperative period. Dressings may be used to help stabilize a flap and maintain the close adaptation of the soft tissues to bone thus reducing the risk of haematoma formation. Thus, following a gingival grafting procedure a dressing may be used to immobilize and protect the grafted tissue on the recipient site. However, dressings should never be employed as a substitute for proper suturing.

The dressing is retained by extensions of it being locked into the interproximal embrasures and is left in situ for 1 week. In most instances the insertion of a further dressing is not required.

The two types of periodontal dressing in most frequent use are:

1. Coe-Pak, a proprietary, pink, non-eugenol dressing which is easily mixed and is supplied in preparations with various setting times. It is readily mixed to a tacky paste and, when it achieves a consistency similar to that of plasticine, is applied first interdentally and then buccally and lingually as desired. The operator should coat his fingers with petroleum jelly before applying the dressing which when set presents a smooth surface to both the healing wound and the tissues adjacent to it.

2. An asbestos–rosin dressing, a typical formula for which is:

Powder	g	Liquid	cc
Zinc oxide	63	Eugenol	80
Rosin	30	Olive oil	20
Asbestos fibre	5		
Zinc acetate	2		

The patient should always be warned that there is bound to be some discomfort following periodontal surgery. There may also be some postoperative swelling when flap procedures are employed. Postoperative pain can usually be controlled by analgesics (*see* p. 84). As severe pain may be an indication that either postoperative infection or pulpitis has occurred the patient should be instructed to contact the dentist if severe pain is experienced and told precisely where and how he or she can do this.

To minimize the risk of bleeding the patient should be warned against any activities that may increase the blood pressure, especially during the first 48 hours postoperatively. Alcohol and tobacco smoking should be avoided for a similar period. Nevertheless, postoperative bleeding may occur and if it does the patient should be instructed to sit upright and to apply local pressure directly over the site of bleeding for 20 min.

Eating may become difficult especially when several areas of the mouth are treated at one time. The patient should be encouraged to take soft yet nourishing foods which require minimal mastication and are not served excessively hot.

The most rapid and satisfactory healing occurs if plaque levels immediately adjacent to the surgical sites are low and so a high standard of oral hygiene must be maintained in the rest of the mouth. This may be assisted greatly by the use of chlorhexidine digluconate mouthwashes twice daily for 10 days postoperatively. If dressings are used hot salt water mouthbaths will help keep both the dressings and the mouth clean.

Antibiotics are not used routinely in any type of periodontal surgery except where there are medical indications (e.g. rheumatic valvular heart disease). If an extensive flap procedure and bone removal have been performed the use of antibiotics may be prudent but there is little scientific evidence to support strongly their efficacy in this context.

Contra-indications

Systemic disease may be a contra-indication to periodontal surgery. Terminal illnesses are an obvious contra-indication to surgery whilst patients under psychiatric care and alcoholics are best treated by non-surgical means. The periodontal treatment of patients afflicted with controllable systemic diseases should be planned in co-operation with the physician concerned. In each case a decision whether to treat the patient on either an out-patient or an in-patient basis must be made.

In pregnancy it is wise to delay surgery until after parturition and to rely upon scaling and oral hygiene instruction to control gingival bleeding and inflammation.

When the periodontal tissues are acutely inflamed, as for example in the presence of either acute necrotizing ulcerative gingivitis or an acute periodontal abscess, they are very friable and therefore ill suited to surgery, other than the institution of drainage. Surgery should not be undertaken until the acute condition has been controlled by conservative therapy.

Periodontal surgery is contra-indicated in any patient in whom, despite repeated oral hygiene instruction, plaque is retained around the teeth, for invariably surgery will fail unless effective oral hygiene is maintained.

Extent of surgery

The efficacy of root planing techniques in reducing both the depth of pockets and bleeding from them has resulted in full mouth periodontal surgery being required only rarely. Surgery is now limited to isolated areas of the mouth in which persistent bleeding from pockets exists and may involve only a few teeth in each quadrant. In such cases two quadrants on one side of the mouth may be treated at a single visit. Usually a gap of 2 weeks between surgical visits is advisable. If the periodontal involvement is generalized surgery should be undertaken in each of the four quadrants on separate occasions. The operative procedure should not stop in the midline but continue around to the opposite canine area, thus minimizing the duration of the associated poor aesthetics due to the presence of either exposed dressing or sutures.

Techniques employed in periodontal surgery

Various periodontal surgical flap procedures are available for use. The differences between them are not always well defined and procedures are often combined or overlap.

Periodontal pockets may be eliminated surgically by:
1. Resecting the detached gingival tissue, or
2. Apically repositioning the detached gingival tissue, or
3. Obtaining a reattachment of the soft tissues to the tooth surface at approximately the pre-surgical gingival height.

Resection involves the removal of the tissue forming the pocket wall (*Fig.* 14.3*a*).

Apical repositioning eliminates the pocket by the displacement of the detached gingival tissues on the attached mucoperiosteum in an apical direction along the root surface and alveolar bone by an amount equal to that of the pocket depth (*Fig.* 14.3*b*).

Reattachment aims to produce a new connective-tissue fibre attachment to newly formed cementum on the root surface. Clinically this is rarely achieved and usually a long junctional epithelium forms attaching the gingiva to the root surface. This approach is particularly useful where there are aesthetic consider-ations or root sensitivity problems in an isolated pocket. Such surgical techniques as the modified Widman flap, excisional new attachment procedure and open flap curettage are based on this principle (*Fig.* 14.3*c*).

Choice of method

As the choice of the procedure to be utilized is governed by the needs of the patient being treated the dentist must carefully consider the situation in each portion of the mouth before deciding which of the three methods, or what combination of them, should be employed. Resection techniques waste tissue whereas reattachment and apical repositioning conserve most of the tissues. Both resection and apical repositioning can expose large amounts of root surface

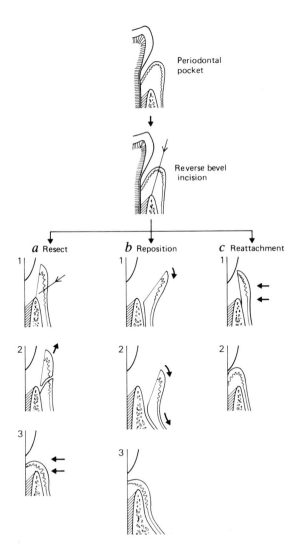

Fig. 14.3. Methods of pocket elimination. *a. Resection.* (1) A further reverse bevel outline incision is made at the appropriate level. (2) The excess tissue is resected and removed. (3) The new gingival margin of the flap just covers the crestal bone. *b. Repositioning apically.* (1) The mucogingival complex is reflected. (2) Flap displaced over alveolar bone in an apical direction. (3) Repositioned flap margin just covering the crestal bone. *c. Reattachment.* (1) The flap is replaced in toto and is firmly adapted to tooth. Any discrepancies between the flap and tooth become filled with blood clot. (2) A long epithelial attachment and not a connective tissue attachment occurs on the root.

whereas reattachment is designed to minimize the extent of such exposure (*Fig.* 14.3).

Reattachment provides the best postsurgical aesthetic results combined with minimal risk of postoperative root sensitivity but places the highest reliance on gaining a complete attachment over a much greater surface of the affected root than either resection or apical repositioning. With these latter two methods the gingiva is placed almost directly over the crestal alveolar bone, thus reducing the area on which postsurgical reattachment must occur.

The decision whether to either resect or reposition the detached gingiva is dependent upon the relationship of the depth of the pocket to the dimensions of the attached gingiva in the affected area. Because of a relatively narrow attachment of the gingiva on the buccal aspects of both jaws a functionally inadequate width of attached gingiva is likely to be the best result of resection of all but the shallowest of pockets in these areas. If the existing attached gingiva needs to be conserved and the reattachment method is not indicated then the repositioning technique should be employed. However, in the palate where a functionally adequate width of gingiva is always present, and in those mouths where an unusually wide band of gingiva exists, as for example in the lingual lower premolar and molar and the buccal upper molar areas, resection of the pocket wall may be utilized. In all cases of doubt, apical repositioning should be performed.

Reverse bevel incision

It has become a routine practice in periodontology to utilize a reverse bevel incision when outlining gingival flaps. Such a flap must provide both visual and mechanical access to the root surface and alveolar bone thus facilitating the direct examination and assessment of the treatment requirements. It can also be modified to cope with various periodontal defects, thus conserving rather than sacrificing the periodontal tissues and so ensuring optimal postoperative mucosal coverage of bone (*Fig.* 14.4).

The reverse bevel incision has three separate components:

1. The positional component which is determined by the decisions as to whether the detached gingiva is to be reattached, apically repositioned or resected. In the first two instances the outline incision is commenced about 1 mm from the gingival margin thus conserving the gingiva (*Fig.* 14.3*b, c*). When the gingiva is being resected the incision is made at a point related to the crestal bone (*see Fig.* 14.3*a*). Failure to site this incision correctly will lead either to the exposure of alveolar bone or to an excess of gingival tissue over the bone.

In order to improve accessibility the incision may be either extended along the gingival crevices of the teeth adjacent to the surgical field or, less frequently, vertical relieving incisions may be made.

2. An outline component consists of a shallow outline or marking cut (no more than a couple of millimetres deep) with the blade directed apically (*Fig.* 14.4*a*). This cut follows the scalloped contour of the gingival margin thus conserving interdental gingival tissue and creating a surgical flap margin that will ensure optimal postoperative coverage of crestal bone interdentally.

3. A thinning component represents the deeper extension of the shallow outline cut directed apically towards the crestal alveolar bone (*Fig.* 14.4*b*). This excision should completely excise the epithelial lining of the pocket wall and thin

the pocket wall to ensure a gingival contour conducive to optimal plaque control. The angle of the thinning incision therefore should be adjusted according to the particular features of the case (*Fig.* 14.5).

The incision thus splits the detached gingiva into two layers, an outer layer of keratinized gingiva and an inner pocket lining referred to as the cervical wedge (*Fig.*14.4*d*).

The thinned flap is then reflected sufficiently to facilitate removal of the now separated cervical wedge (*Fig.* 14.4*d*). This is repeated on the opposite aspect of the tooth following the appropriate reverse bevel incision. Removal of this tissue may be facilitated by a vertical incision down the periodontal pocket prior to removing the cervical wedge tissue with a curette.

Management of the root surfaces and bone

The raising of the flap makes it possible to examine the affected root surfaces. Residual calculus and plaque deposits should be removed and the parts of the root surfaces that have been exposed within periodontal pockets, root planed. Although some clinicians have applied demineralizing agents such as citric acid to planed root surfaces the results of this practice have been equivocal and it is not recommended. Whenever residual soft tissues are attached to the roots of the

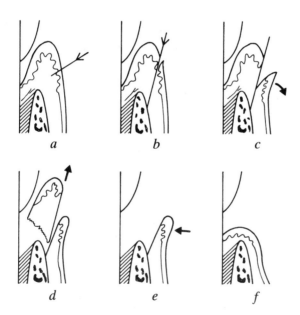

Fig. 14.4. The reverse bevel incision. The stages of the incision when the attached gingiva is being resected. *a*, The positional and outline component. *b*, The thinning component— a deeper and apically directed extension of the shallow outline component towards the crestal bone. Note the thinning of the detached gingiva and the excision of the epithelialized pocket lining. *c* and *d*, The isolation and removal of the cervical wedge. *e*, Gingival tissue pulled towards root surface. *f*, Gingival margin placed so as to cover the crestal bone by approximately an amount equal to the thickness of the flap itself.

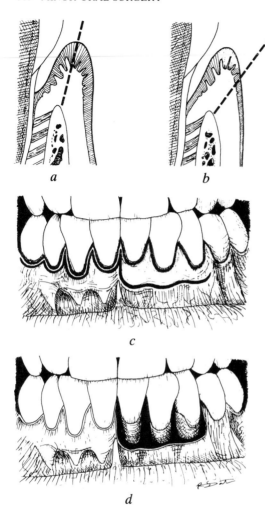

Fig. 14.5 The reverse bevel incision. *a*, Angulation of the incision employed when conserving gingiva. *b*, Angulation of the incision used when gingiva is resected. *c*, Labial view of the lower anterior region in which the dark lines indicate the incisions shown in (*a*) and (*b*). *d*, End result of incisions shown in (*c*). The gingiva has been conserved on the right side and resected on the left.

teeth close to the alveolar crest curettage should be performed. All soft tissues should be removed from the bony surfaces of infrabony lesions but it is not essential to restore the normal bony architecture by means of osseous surgery in such areas. If it proves difficult to adapt the soft-tissue flap to the teeth because of the presence of excessive bony contours some minor bone reshaping with burs or chisels may be necessary. However, this should be kept to a minimum and preferably performed on non-tooth-supporting outer alveolar bone (*Fig.* 14.6).

The results of attempts to restore lost alveolar bone utilizing various osseous graft materials are such that their routine use cannot be recommended at the present time.

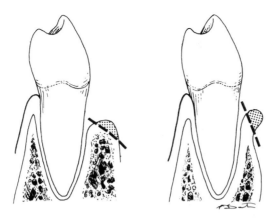

Fig. 14.6. Osteoplasty to reshape thickened buccal alveolar margins. Only the stippled areas of bone are excised.

Management of the flap

Where resection of the soft tissues has been planned the cut margin should be placed so as to cover the crestal bone by about an amount equal to the thickness of the mucoperiosteum itself (*see Fig.* 14.4*f*). The soft tissues are merely adapted to both the crestal bone and the necks of the teeth and sutures inserted and a dressing applied.

Where the incision has been made 1 mm from the gingival margin there will, depending on the preoperative depth of the pocket, be varying degrees of flap tissue coronal to the crestal bone.

When reattachment is attempted the flap must be closely adapted to the root surfaces for close, firm adaptation of the freshly cut flap margin to the tooth will minimize the volume of blood clot and speed the attachment process (*see Fig.* 14.3*c*2). A dressing may inadvertently displace tissue apically and therefore, if used, should be placed carefully, apical pressure being avoided.

When apical repositioning is the objective, the flap complex of gingiva, alveolar mucoperiosteum, submucosa and mucogingival junction is reflected sufficiently with periosteal elevators, to allow it to be displaced over the alveolar bone in an apical direction so that the flap margin just covers crestal bone (*see Fig.* 14.3*b*2 and 3). When the pattern of crestal bone resorption is irregular it is frequently found that the evenly scalloped margin of the flap cannot be readily adapted to the crestal bone as advocated above. Frequently this problem can be solved by positioning the flap margin over the crestal bone of the least involved teeth and then adapting it to the roots of the most involved teeth. In other cases the inherent tissue elasticity of the flap may allow it to be displaced in such a way as to accommodate minor discrepancies between the margin of the flap and the contour of the crestal bone. All alveolar bone must be covered by soft tissue and none should be left exposed above the flap margins. A combination of reattachment and apical repositioning techniques can be used and the flap margins sutured in the new position to prevent further apical displacement when and if the dressings are applied. The sutures will prevent the flaps sliding coronally (*Fig.* 14.7).

Determining the level of resection is fairly simple when the pocket wall is thin

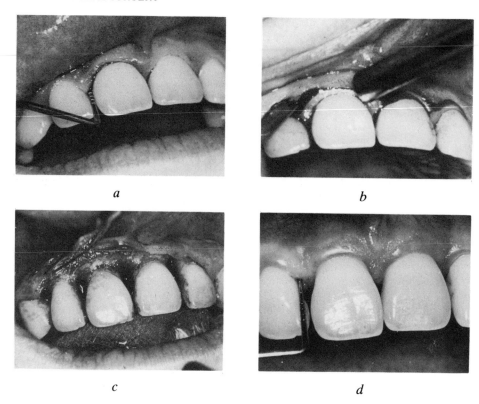

a b

c d

Fig. 14.7. a, A persistently bleeding 7 mm periodontal pocket between an upper right central and lateral incisor. b, After the outlining incision the thinning component of the incision was extended onto the crestal alveolar bone. Note minimal loss of gingival margin, as the incision was kept close to sulcus. c, Reflection of the flap and removal of interdental soft tissue. Root planing has been completed and there was no indication to alter the bone morphology. Flaps replaced and sutured interdentally. d, Three months postoperatively, the interdental areas exhibit healthy gingivae, with 2 mm pocket depths.

and the outer surface of the related alveolar plate is nearly parallel to the long axis of the clinical crown. In such situations the topography of the pocket is readily determined and the surgical margin of the flap can be related easily to the edge of the crestal bone. However, in such areas as the palate where the gingiva is usually thickened, especially around the molar teeth and where, except in patients with a high palatal vault, the surface of the alveolar bone is at an obtuse angle to the clinical crown the appropriate position and angulation of the resecting (thinning) reverse bevel incision is more difficult to establish. Furthermore, the convex shape of the palatal tooth surface may make difficult the effective use of instruments especially when the palatal vault is shallow. Also the cervical wedge so created cannot be removed readily because of its broad base and tough fibrous attachment to the palatal bone.

These difficulties can be minimized by initially reflecting the flap with a periosteal elevator immediately after making an incision along the gingival crevice thus enabling the clinician to assess, in situ, any requirement for osseous surgery and the degree of pocket wall resection and thinning necessary (*Fig.* 14.8*b*).

Root planing and osseous reshaping are performed, the flap replaced, and supported digitally whilst a shallow outline incision conforming to the contour of the related crestal bone and root surfaces is made (*Fig.* 14.8*c*).

The flap is then reduced in thickness, as required, by incising more deeply into this shallow outline incision down to alveolar bone (*Fig.* 14.8*d*). Any obstruction to the use of the scalpel by the related palatal tooth surfaces and cusps can be avoided by deflecting the already mobile palatal mucosa away from the teeth. The cervical wedge usually comes away from bone readily as its attachment to palatal bone has already been severed by the periosteal elevator during the initial reflection of the flap. The soft tissues can now be positioned over crestal bone and sutured in place (*Fig.* 14.8*e, f*).

Surgical management of pockets related to teeth adjacent to edentulous areas
Reverse bevel incisions are continued from the buccal and lingual aspects of affected teeth to meet within the gingival crevice adjacent to the edentulous ridge.

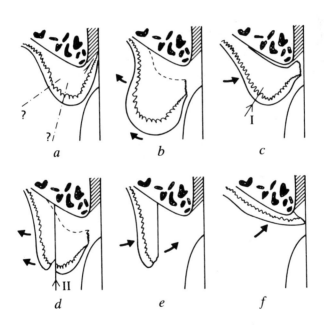

Fig. 14.8. Reverse bevel pocket resection. The method of circumventing the problems associated with the resection of 'thick' pocket walls on the palate. *a*, The correct position of incision (I) is difficult to determine because of the bulk of tissue. *b*, A vertical incision along the sulcus is made and a mucoperiosteal flap reflected. *c*, The flap is then replaced and the outline incision made (I). *d*, The flap is reflected again sufficiently to avoid the crown of the tooth deflecting the scalpel; thereby facilitating the completion of the thinning incision (II). The outline incision (I) is used as a guide when the thinning incision is made. The cervical wedge comes away readily as its attachment to bone has already been severed. *e, f*, The flap is adapted to crestal bone.

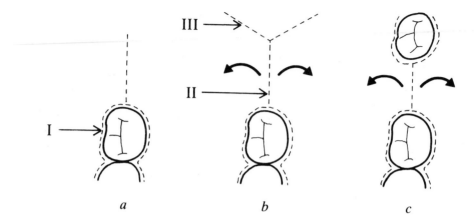

Fig. 14.9. Pocket management about teeth related to edentulous areas *a, b*. Appropriate buccal and lingual reverse level incisions are made about the teeth. (I) These incisions should be made down the gingival crevice if no pocketing is on the buccal or lingual aspects of these teeth. A linear incision is then made (II) from the gingival crevice passing along the crest of the ridge to facilitate adequate reflection of the flaps. Note the relieving incision (III) in (*b*) (if required) and the linear incision linking the crevicular incision on a short edentulous area in (*c*).

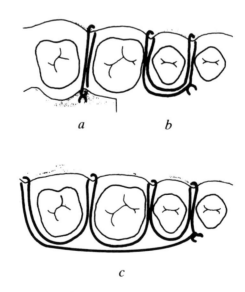

Fig. 14.10. *a*, Interrupted suture securing buccal and lingual papillae with equal tension. *b*, Sling suture securing adjacent papillae without involving papillae on the opposite aspect. *c*, Continuous suture securing a row of adjacent papillae, allowing the papillae on the opposite aspect to be sutured at a different tension.

If neither buccal nor lingual pockets are present crevicular incisions are used (*Fig.* 14.9*a*). A linear incision commencing at the gingival crevice should be extended along the crest of the ridge sufficiently to allow for elevation and reflection of buccal and lingual mucoperiosteal flaps. Vertical relieving incisions may occasionally be required to provide the access for a thinning incision to be performed but the buccal and lingual mucoperiosteal attachments of the alveolar ridge should not be disturbed (*Fig.* 14.9*b*). The flap is supported digitally, thinned using a No. 15 blade, and then bone contouring is performed as required. The flaps are replaced and it will be found that one margin tends to overlap the other dependent upon the size of the connective-tissue wedge removed. This excess tissue can be resected so that the edges of the flaps approximate accurately or a buccal or a lingual flap may be reflected further and apically repositioned.

Suturing

It is best to use interrupted sutures when suturing flaps when either reattachment or resection procedures have been performed. However, if there is a need to vary tension in the flap during apical repositioning on the buccal aspect but on neither the palatal surface nor around isolated teeth in a quadrant, the continuous suture technique allows more variation in suture tension than the use of interrupted sutures (*Fig.* 14.10).

Recall

After surgery, regular 4–6-monthly recall visits for professional cleaning and supervision are essential if the health of the periodontium is to be maintained.

Gingivectomy/gingivoplasty

Gingivectomy is the surgical excision of the soft-tissue wall of a periodontal pocket. *Gingivoplasty* is the shaping of the gingiva when a pocket no longer exists so as to obtain improved contour to facilitate plaque removal by the patient.

The indications for gingivectomy are few compared with those for techniques employing the reverse bevel incision but they include the presence of:
1. Hyperplastic gingival tissues (i.e. Dilantin hyperplasia) (*see Fig.* 2.1).
2. Shallow suprabony pockets without underlying bony deformities.
3. Altered passive eruption in which the gingival margins appear not to recede normally but to remain at the height of the maximum contour of the crowns of the teeth.

The *contra-indications* to gingivectomy are the presence of:
1. Severely inflamed friable tissues which are better treated by root planing the involved teeth.
2. Areas in which surgery would eliminate most of the attached gingiva such as areas buccal to the premolars, sites of mucogingival periodontal involvement or close proximity to frena which may cause retraction of the attached gingiva.
3. Underlying bone deformities, such as interdental craters and thickened buccal ledges.

In the technique of gingivectomy, pocket depths are marked on the outside of the gingivae either with a periodontal probe or a pair of pocket marking forceps (*Fig.* 14.11*a*, *b*). Either a Blake gingivectomy knife with a No. 15 blade or a Goldman Fox No. 7 knife is then used to make a linear incision commencing at a

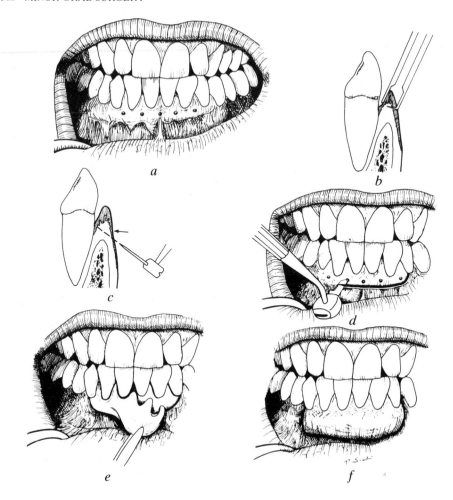

Fig. 14.11. Diagrams showing: *a*, Pocket-marking forceps in position, labial mandibular incisor teeth. *b*, Buccolingual view. *c*, Incision at 45° to the long axis of the tooth. *d*, Labial view: note incision begins at the midline of the tooth and not interproximally. *e*, Removal of excised gingiva. *f*, Periodontal pack in situ.

papilla. The incision is started about 2 mm apical to the bleeding points that mark the base of the pockets and its internal level should end just apical to the base of the epithelial attachment. Its angulation will be dictated by the width of attached gingiva but ideally should be at an angle 45° to the long axis of the tooth (*Fig.* 14.11*c*, *d*). When adequate attached gingiva exists the bevel can be long, but when the gingiva is narrow the bevel should be kept shallow rather than involving the attached mucoperiosteum in the incision. A No. 11 blade is used to sever the papilla interdentally and join the initial incision between the teeth. Curettes are then used to remove the detached tissues (*Fig.* 14.11*e*). Correction of the gingival contour may be carried out by gingivoplasty to the cut surface left by the initial gingivectomy incision utilizing either the No. 15 blade, soft-tissue nippers or high-speed rough diamond stones rotating under a water spray. All tissue tags must be removed so as to leave a smooth wound surface which is then covered with a periodontal pack.

Soft-tissue grafts

Soft-tissue grafts may be utilized to remedy alterations to the normal morphological arrangement between the attached gingiva and the alveolar mucosa at the level of the mucogingival line. The use of soft-tissue grafts may be indicated when areas of gingival recession have resulted in root hypersensitivity, a lack of marginal epithelial seal associated with the presence of a frenum or muscle pull or an unfavourable appearance. Use of them simply to increase the width of the attached gingivae in the absence of any of the above mentioned indications is ill advised. Attached gingivae of a width of less than 2 mm can remain just as clinically healthy as broad widths of attached gingiva if good plaque control is maintained.

Free gingival grafts obtained from normally keratinized mucosa have been used successfully to increase the width of the keratinized gingiva and to cover localized gingival recessions (*Fig.* 14.12).

After obtaining anaesthesia by means of local infiltration an incision along the mucogingival junction is made and the graft bed prepared by sharp dissection. Any existing band of keratinized gingival tissue around the tooth can be retained, thus creating a recipient site with a circumferential blood supply. The alveolar mucosa, muscle attachments and periosteum are displaced apically, thus exposing the surface of the underlying bone.

All extraneous soft tissue on the graft site should be removed and any area of tooth root that is to be covered by the graft vigorously root planed.

The mucosal flap must be mobilized sufficiently to permit apical displacement of it in order to ensure that it will not encroach upon the grafted area during healing. A tin-foil template of the prepared site may be used to aid the correct assessment of the size and shape of the graft to be removed from the donor site.

The keratinized gingiva of the palate is the preferred donor site. The incisions outlining the graft are made at least 2 mm clear of any palatal gingival margins and kept well away from the greater palatine artery. A partial thickness graft about 2·0 mm thick is carefully dissected away from the palate, a procedure which is facilitated if fine tissue forceps are used to elevate carefully the graft and improve visibility.

Once the graft has been detached from the donor site any loose tags of soft tissue on its undersurface are removed and its edges are thinned in an endeavour to avoid bulbous margins.

The graft is then positioned carefully and adapted firmly to the recipient site. Sutures are inserted at its lateral borders making certain that no tension is put on the graft which is then covered with a periodontal dressing which is left in situ for 1 week. If indicated, a suture may be placed at the donor site in addition to the dressing in order to aid haemostasis.

The graft is morphologically distinguishable from adjacent gingiva for many months and may always be slightly bulbous (*Fig.* 14.12e).

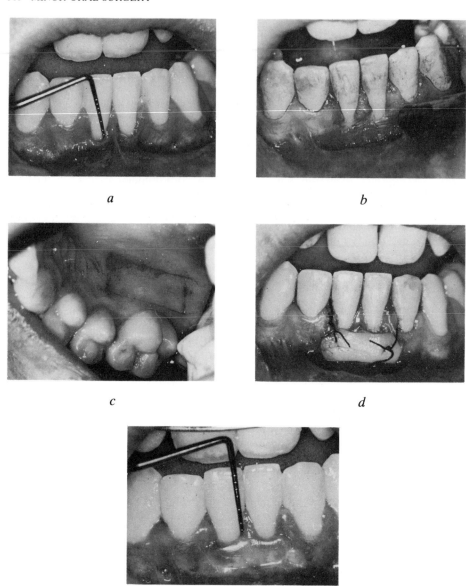

a

b

c

d

e

Fig. 14.12. *a*, Localized gingival recession and an inadequate width of attached gingivae labial to the mandibular central incisors. The gingiva, although not pocketed, bled on probing. *b*, Preparation for the graft bed with a linear incision along the mucogingival junction. *c*, Outline incision around the palatal donor tissue. The incision margins are clear of the greater palatine artery, the gingival margins and fatty glandular tissue of the palate. *d*, Graft secured into position, with two interrupted silk sutures. *e*, Three months postoperatively, the graft is firmly adherent to the underlying tissues. The graft has resulted in a 5-mm band of keratinized gingiva, which has reduced the gingival recession on the incisors by 2 mm.

Laterally repositioned flaps

A laterally repositioned flap may be used to treat a localized area of gingival recession as an alternative to the free gingival graft (*Fig.* 14.13). The laterally repositioned flap retains its direct vascularization, tissue characteristics and vitality. The procedure usually results in a 65% reduction in the amount of recession and the results are more predictable than the insertion of a free gingival graft if a deep, wide, localized area of recession is to be covered. There must be neither dehiscences nor fenestrations of the alveolar plate in the donor area and it is preferable to use a donor site on which the gingiva is relatively thick.

The tissue bordering the defect is thinned and the root surface thoroughly root planed. Ideally, sufficient radicular tissue should be removed to bring the root into alignment with the neighbouring bone margins.

A flap at least one and a half times as wide as the defect is prepared at the donor site. The flap is resected by sharp dissection leaving the periosteum over the donor site intact.

The flaps should be rotated to cover the exposed root surface and sutured into place with 5 × 0 silk without tension. Finger pressure should be applied in order to

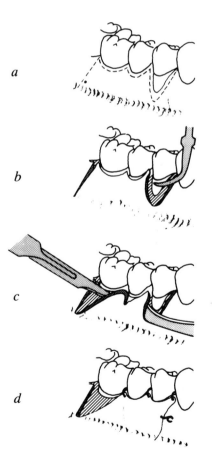

a

b

c

d

Fig. 14.13. *a*, Localized recession on the first premolar. Broken line marks line of incision for preparation of flap. *b*, Incision provides access to root plane exposed root surface with curettes and prepare graft bed. *c*, Flap separated from periosteum by scalpel and periosteal elevator. Flap relieved apically sufficiently to allow lateral displacement without compromising flap vascularity. *d*, Flap laterally displaced and sutured securely over previously exposed root surface.

minimize the size of the blood clot beneath it before a soft periodontal dressing is applied.

The exposed area at the donor site often heals without forming a defect whilst the flap becomes attached to the tooth by both connective tissue and a long epithelial attachment.

Root amputation and hemisection

The loss of both the hard and soft supporting structures of multirooted teeth is often so severe that the only way in which adequate access for plaque control by the patient can be provided is by removal of either a root (root resection) or half the crown and a root (hemisection). Frequently the only alternative to such a procedure is the extraction of the involved tooth.

The indications for root amputation or hemisection are:

1. Severe vertical bone loss involving either one root of a mandibular molar or a combination of either one or two roots of a three-rooted maxillary molar.

2. Close proximity of other roots associated with interdental bone loss.

3. Multirooted teeth with fractures of individual roots complicating endodontic treatment.

4. Single roots of multirooted pulpless teeth which are not accessible to normal endodontic procedures.

5. Teeth serving as abutments for fixed bridges with an otherwise hopeless prognosis due to periodontal disease.

These procedures are contra-indicated by inadequate bony support around the root or roots to be retained, fusion of the roots apically to the area of bone destruction or the impracticability of treating the roots to be retained by endodontic means.

Whenever possible, endodontic therapy should be undertaken before such periodontal surgery is performed. If the involved tooth is pulpless all its root canals should be treated endodontically and amalgam should be inserted into the root canal just apical to the planned level of root section.

At operation a full-thickness mucoperiosteal flap should be raised just apical to the site of the most extensive bone loss. The exposed soft tissues investing the root are then removed by curettage to allow the direct visual assessment of the bone contour, the root morphology and the mechanical access to the site of amputation (*Fig.* 14.14).

Sufficient bone is then removed with bone burs under saline irrigation to expose the most coronal aspect of the furca. The root is separated from the rest of the tooth with either a long fissure bur or a tapered diamond bur run under saline irrigation. Root division should begin in the furcation and proceed outwards, care being taken to ensure that the level of section is as close to the furcation as is practicable in order to avoid the creation of areas in which plaque may accumulate later. The best test to determine whether separation is complete is to apply pressure to the root in order to establish that it moves independently from the remainder of the tooth.

The root is then delivered with elevators and forceps, a process which can often be facilitated by dividing the amputated roots into smaller segments. After this either a bur or a diamond stone is used to contour and smooth the bone in order to

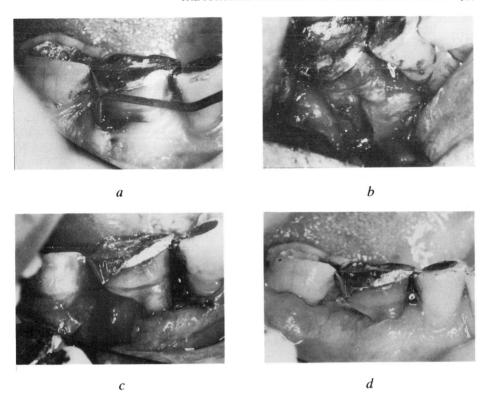

Fig. 14.14. *a*, Lower first molar with a 12-mm pocket associated with the distal root. The mesial root is well supported by bone and surrounded by a healthy periodontium. *b*, Full-thickness periodontal flap raised. A longitudinal root fracture was evident on the distal root and good bony suport around the mesial root and furcation area was noted. *c*, Amputation of split root was achieved by using a high-speed diamond bur. *d*, One year postoperatively, the gingival tissues have healed with no residual pocketing. In order to facilitate effective plaque control the overhanging distal section of the crown should be resected and the single root either restored as a premolar or utilized as an abutment for a bridge with a sanitary pontic.

ensure that the overlying gingival tissues are both smooth and readily cleansed once healing is complete. If a vital tooth is sectioned the exposed pulpal tissue should be capped directly with a sedative dressing such as zinc oxide and eugenol.

The mucoperiosteal flap is repositioned and quite often conforms to the depression created by the loss of the root. It may be retained with a pack inserted into the defect for a week.

Occlusal adjustment of the tooth must then be undertaken to ensure that it is neither subject to excessive lateral forces nor extreme mobility. Once healing is complete restoration of the retained tooth may be restored.

Orthodontic perincision

A tendency to relapse characterizes orthodontic treatment during which teeth are rotated around their vertical axes. This is believed to be due to the stretching of supracrestal fibres of the periodontal membrane. *Perincision* is the division of these stretched fibres during the retention phase of orthodontic treatment and is best performed 8 weeks prior to debanding.

Although various techniques of perincision have been described a simple, practicable and effective method is to insert a No. 11 scalpel blade (*see Fig.* 3.11*b*) through the anaesthetized gingival sulcus against the root in a vertical and an apical direction. The blade is then passed through the periodontal membrane all round the root in order to sever all its fibrous attachments down to a depth of approximately 2 mm below the crest of the alveolar bone. No excision of either the attached or marginal gingiva is undertaken. A dressing is normally not required and postoperative discomfort is minimal.

ACUTE PERIODONTAL ABSCESS

Periodontal abscess formation is due to an acute inflammatory reaction occurring in an existing periodontal pocket. The pathway along which pus and exudate normally drain from the pocket is blocked and swelling and sinus formation may occur if the lesion is left untreated. Acute periodontal abscesses commonly occur in furcation areas.

The lesion usually occurs suddenly and is associated with swelling and pain in the related area of gingiva. The pain is typically less severe than that associated with an acute periapical abscess whilst the involved tooth may be tender to percussion and responds to pulp testing. In some cases the patient will be pyrexic and complaining of malaise.

Certain features aid differential diagnosis between an acute periodontal abscess and an acute alveolar abscess. Thus, in the presence of the former, both the involved tooth and its neighbour and adjacent teeth respond to pulp testing; the pain is less intense than that associated with an acute pulpitis and the gingival swelling is usually more marginally placed than that of an apical abscess. A probe can always be inserted into a pocket if the lesion is periodontal but usually cannot if it is a periapical abscess.

Treatment is in two phases, the first being designed to remedy the immediate acute inflammation and the second, which is given at a later date, is aimed at eliminating the chronic infection within the residual pocket.

Drainage can usually be obtained by gently inserting a periodontal curette or ultrasonic scaler tip to the base of the pocket. The use of local anaesthesia may be necessary. Pus and exudate then drains from the abscess thus relieving tension within the lesion. If the abscess has pointed, drainage may be instituted by means of direct incision using a No. 15 scalpel blade. The incision should not involve the gingival margin and the abscess cavity should be carefully curetted via the incision in order to facilitate the release of more infected material.

Especially in the presence of furcation involvement, the tooth may be over-erupted and a selective minor occlusal adjustment may be required. Minimal

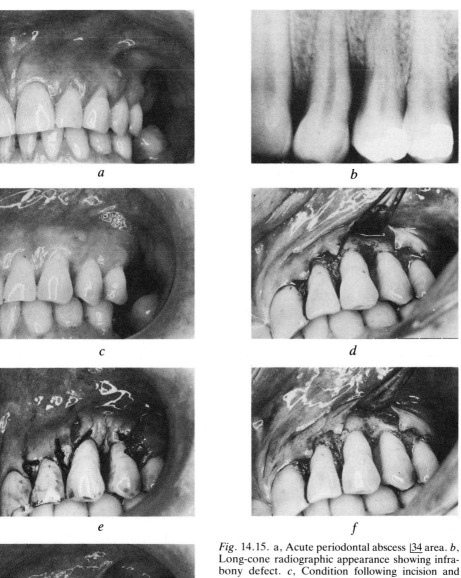

Fig. 14.15. a, Acute periodontal abscess |34 area. *b*, Long-cone radiographic appearance showing infrabony defect. *c*, Condition following incision and drainage. *d*, Reflection of full-thickness mucoperiosteal flap with exposure of osseous deformity. *e*, Osteoplasty to the bone between |34 is performed to assist the final gingival contour. *f*, The flap is apically repositioned and collapsed into the defect and sutured. It is important that any exposed bone should lie interdentally rather than over the thin cortical bone covering the convexity of root surfaces. *g*, Postoperative appearance: elimination of pocket depth has been achieved, together with the most satisfactory tissue contour that the patient can maintain. (*Courtesy of Mr J. S. Zamet.*)

cuspal removal and gentle finger pressure on the tooth during grinding will ease the discomfort of the patient.

Antibiotic therapy is indicated if the patient is pyrexic and unwell. Hot salt-water mouth baths, used three times a day for 3 days postoperatively, will further assist drainage of pus and resolution of the lesion.

Once the acute phase has been controlled subsequent treatment may involve root planing the involved tooth or even flap surgery (*Fig.* 14.15). The occurrence of acute periodontal abscesses may indicate the terminal stages of periodontal disease and if so the teeth affected are best extracted.

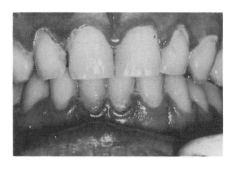 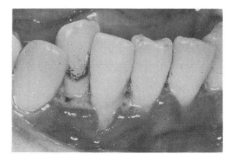

a   b

Fig. 14.16. Acute necrotizing ulcerative gingivitis. The gingiva is swollen and haemorrhagic. Necrosis of the gingival margins, especially in the interdental papillary region is characteristic of the condition.

ACUTE NECROTIZING ULCERATIVE GINGIVITIS

The acute symptoms of pain and bleeding need immediate treatment which involves the removal of plaque and calculus deposits around the teeth with curettes or the ultrasonic cleaner. Careful manipulation of hand instruments is important as the affected tissues are very tender. Ultrasonic cleaners are of particular value in this context as the pain experienced by the patient during their use is less than that associated with the use of curettes and the water spray removes soft-tissue debris.

Oral hygiene instruction should be instituted immediately and directed towards the removal of plaque from the teeth without damaging the infected gingiva. Chlorhexidine digluconate mouthwashes should be used twice daily for 10 days. The routine use of antibiotics is not indicated but metronidazole or penicillin may be prescribed if the patient is pyrexial. Tobacco smoking should be forbidden and the patient advised to eat a well-balanced soft diet and to obtain as much rest and sleep as is possible.

Once the acute phase of the disease has resolved, minor periodontal surgery may be required to correct cratering of the interdental soft tissues which increases plaque retention (*Fig.* 14.16).

To summarize, periodontal health is dependent upon the regular and effective removal of plaque from the teeth by the patient. Destructive periodontal disease can be halted if plaque is removed and the damaged tissues are allowed to heal.

As treatment of the damaged tissues involves the root planing of affected tooth roots it is fortunate that most root surfaces are accessible to instrumentation via the periodontal pocket. In areas in which access is restricted periodontal surgery may be employed to provide a clear view of the affected area. Various surgical procedures can be utilized to remedy gingival problems of different types and in various locations. This may involve either resection, replacement or repositioning of the gingiva or a combination of them. Periodontal surgery may also be utilized to increase the width of gingiva, to cover exposed root surfaces or to remove periodontally involved tooth roots (*Figs.* 14.12, 14.13, 14.14).

Regular routine maintenance visits involving plaque control and root planing are essential if periodontal health is to be maintained regardless of which method of periodontal treatment is employed.

SUGGESTED READING

Ahrens D., Shapira Y. and Kuftinec M. (1981) An approach to rotational relapse. *Am. J. Orthodont.* **80**, 83–91.

Bain M. (1980) Chlorhexidine in dentistry. *N. Z. Dent. J.* **76**, 49–54.

Erpenstein H. (1983) A 3-year study of hemisectioned molars. *J. Clin. Periodontol.* **10**, 1–10.

Hall W. (1981) The current status of mucogingival problems and their therapy. *J. Periodontol.* **52**, 569–75.

Kieser B. (1974) An approach to periodontal pocket elimination. *Br. J. Oral Surg.* **12**, 177–95.

Knowles J., Burgett F., Morrison E. et al. (1980) Comparison of results following three modalities of periodontal therapy related to tooth type and initial pocket depth. *J. Clin. Periodontol.* **7**, 32–47.

Lang N. and Hill R. (1977) Radiographs in periodontics. *J. Clin. Periodontol.* **4**, 16–28.

Lindhe J. (1983) *Textbook of Clinical Periodontology*. Copenhagen, Munksgaard.

Lindhe J., Westfelt E., Nyman S. et al. (1984) Long term effect of surgical/nonsurgical treatment of periodontal disease. *J. Clin. Periodontol.* **11**, 448–58.

Matter J. (1982) Free gingival grafts for the treatment of gingival recession. *J. Clin. Periodontol.* **9**, 103–14.

Newell D. (1981) Current status of the management of teeth with furcation invasion. *J. Periodontol.* **52**, 559–68.

Pihlstrom B., McHugh R., Oliphant T. et al. (1983) Comparison of surgical and non-surgical treatment of periodontal diseases. A review of current studies and additional results after 6½ years. *J. Clin. Periodontol.* **10**, 524–41.

Schluger S., Youdelis R. and Page R. (1977) *Periodontal Disease*. Philadelphia, Lea & Febiger.

Shick R. (1981) Maintenance phase of periodontal therapy. *J. Periodontol.* **52**, 576–83.

Chapter 15
Some complications of oral surgery

The possible complications of oral surgery are many and varied, and some of them may occur even when the utmost care is exercised. However, many of these mishaps can be avoided if the operator anticipates the possibility of their occurrence, takes sensible precautions and employs a plan of campaign designed to deal with the difficulties which have been diagnosed during a careful pre-operative assessment. Ill effects resulting from complications can often be either minimized or avoided by prompt treatment. For these reasons it has been thought wise to place emphasis upon the art of preoperative assessment and treatment planning throughout this text, and so it has been necessary to discuss possible complications in every chapter. There remain, however, a number of important complications which have not been discussed in detail and it is these topics that form the subject of this chapter.

SYNCOPE

A patient, or even at times a person accompanying a patient, may collapse in the dental surgery, the waiting room or elsewhere on the practice premises. Such emergencies occur most frequently in patients seated in the dental chair either at the beginning or at the end of treatment. Collapse may occur suddenly and may or may not be accompanied by loss of consciousness. In most instances these episodes are vasovagal attacks or 'faints' due to a sudden fall in the blood supply to the brain causing cerebral hypoxia and spontaneous recovery is usual. However, patients with a known history of either cardiac ischaemia or hypertension are especially at risk for a fall in blood pressure is accompanied by a reduction in cardiac output and relative myocardial ischaemia which may compromise a heart which is already abnormal. The patient often complains of feeling dizzy, weak, and nauseated, and the skin is seen to be pale, cold, and sweating.

Syncope due to a vasovagal attack is usually characterized by profound bradycardia and so the presence of a weak slow pulse is helpful in differential diagnosis.

First-aid treatment should be instituted at once and at no time should such a patient be left unattended. The first priorities are to clear and preserve the airway and to maintain respiration and circulation, thus preventing hypoxic or ischaemic injury. The ABC of treatment is thus Airway, Breathing and Circulation, and time should not be wasted at this juncture in making sophisticated diagnoses or instituting drug therapy. The vast majority of patients treated according to these principles recover quickly without further sequelae. The head should be lowered by quickly adjusting the back of the dental chair to the 10° Trendelenburg head-down position. More extreme degrees of head-down tilt interfere with cerebral venous drainage and reduce the perfusion of blood in the brain. With some designs of chair, the use of this method may entail considerable delay and in these circumstances the patient's head should be put between his knees after his collar has been loosened. Care should be taken to maintain the airway and to ensure that the patient cannot fall out of the chair. No fluids must be given by mouth until the patient is fully conscious. If sufficient help is available the patient may be lifted from the chair and laid flat on the floor. Swabs, packs, dental fragments and instruments should be removed from the mouth, using the fingers and blood aspirated with suction apparatus. If there is any indication that the patient is likely to vomit he should be turned laterally, preferably on to his left side (*Fig.* 15.1).

A woman in late pregnancy should never be placed in the supine position, for if she is, the gravid uterus may press on the inferior vena cava and produce the 'caval compression' or 'supine hypotensive syndrome' which may result in a precipitous fall in cardiac output and so delay her recovery. When such a patient faints she should be laid on her side, care being taken to maintain the airway.

The respiration and pulse rate and amplitude of all such patients should be monitored constantly if possible. Patients exhibiting acute respiratory distress, such as occurs in bronchial asthma or pulmonary oedema, should never be laid flat but should sit forward with their arms supported at table level.

When consciousness returns a glucose drink may be given if the patient has missed a meal and is being treated under local anaesthesia. Alternatively, sp. ammon. aromat. BPC (sal volatile) 1 drachm (3·6 ml or approximately 1 tea-spoonful) in at least one-third of a tumblerful of water may be administered.

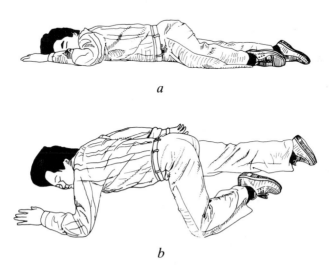

a

b

Fig. 15.1. Patient lying in the lateral position. *a*, Viewed from the side. *b*, Seen from above.

Spontaneous recovery within 15 min is usual and it is often possible to complete the surgery at the same visit if treatment is undertaken with the patient in the supine position. If the operation has not been started and is not urgent it is wise to defer it and to consider the use of premedication prior to the next appointment. In either case the patient should not be sent home for at least an hour and should preferably be accompanied during the journey.

If recovery does not occur within a few minutes of first-aid measures being instituted, the collapse is probably not of vasovagal origin and oxygen should be administered and medical aid summoned. Careful note should be taken of both the type and rate of respirations, and the rate, volume, and character of the pulse. If circumstances permit, the blood pressure should be recorded at intervals and an intravenous injection of 250 mg of aminophylline injection BP may be given slowly.

RESPIRATORY ARREST

If respiration ceases the skeletal muscles become flaccid and the pupils are widely dilated. The patient should be laid flat on the floor and his airway should be cleared by the removal of any appliances or foreign bodies and by pulling the mandible upwards and forwards to extend the head fully (*Fig.* 15.2*a*). The management of aspirated foreign bodies is described on p. 381. The airway can be secured by using the so-called neck-lift head-tilt manoeuvre. Place the clenched fist under the patient's neck and hyperextend the head by exerting downward counter-pressure on the forehead (*Fig.* 15.2*a*); if the jaw sags down then convert to jaw-lift by transferring the fist under the neck to grasp the lower jaw with the finger tips and thumbs under the angles of the mandible (*Fig.* 15.2*b*). These manoeuvres usually secure an airway but in the rare case in which such measures fail to do so, as in the very muscular or very obese patient or those having a convulsion in whom the muscles are tensed and the teeth tightly clenched a nasopharyngeal airway should be inserted. In desperate situations the obstruction to the airway must be relieved by cricothyrotomy as described on p. 384 (*Fig.* 15.10). The patient's nostrils should be compressed between the operator's finger and thumb, and mouth-to-mouth resuscitation should be performed so that

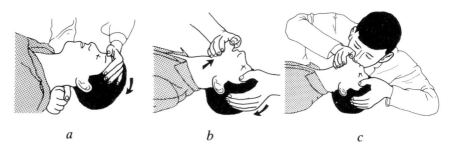

a   *b*   *c*

Fig. 15.2. Mouth-to-mouth resuscitation. *a, b,* Extending the head to clear the airway. *c,* Technique of artificial respiration. If the external nares cannot be covered by the operator's mouth they must be compressed between his finger and thumb (*see Fig.* 15.4*a*).

the chest is seen to rise every 3 or 4 sec (*Fig.* 15.2*c*). The efficiency of this form of resuscitation is greatly enhanced if a Brook airway (*Fig.* 15.3) is available and can be inserted over the tongue and the operator takes the deepest possible breath through his nose and delivers four quick deep breaths. The rise and fall of the patient's chest must be observed out of the corner of the eye of the operator who should endeavour to ensure that full expiration from the patient's lungs does not occur as this manoeuvre helps to expand them (*Fig.* 15.4). Whilst he is attempting to remedy respiratory arrest the dental surgeon must check the carotid pulse and apex beat at regular intervals, for cessation of breathing may be quickly followed by cardiac arrest, which is a more sinister emergency.

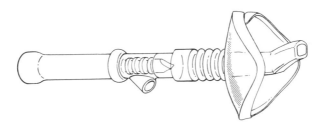

Fig. 15.3. The Brook airway.

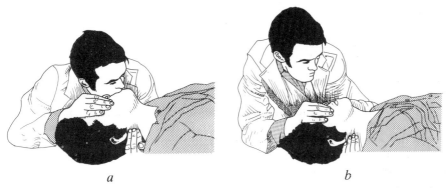

a   *b*

Fig. 15.4. Chest movements must be observed *a*, during mouth-to-mouth respiration, and *b*, following it.

CARDIAC ARREST

Unless the circulation can be restored and maintained within 3 min of cardiac arrest occurring, irreversible brain damage may occur due to cerebral anoxia or ischaemia. The patient exhibits a deathly pallor and greyness with blotches of cyanosis, and his skin is covered with a cold sweat. The carotid pulse and apex beat cannot be felt and the heart sounds cannot be heard. If the patient is a child, the heart will often start beating again if the sternum is tapped sharply. When an adult is being treated the patient should be laid flat on his back on the floor. The dental surgeon kneels at one side of his trunk and places the heel of his left hand on the lower third of the patient's sternum. If the fingers of this hand point towards the

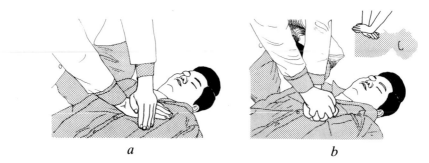

a   *b*

Fig. 15.5. External cardiac massage (*see* text for explanation).

shoulder the heel of the hand will be sited correctly and the risk of undue pressure on internal organs will be reduced (*Fig.* 15.5*a*). The operator then places his right hand on the back of the heel of his left hand and interlocks the fingers of the two hands (*Fig.* 15.5*b*). Then keeping his arms straight he utilizes his body weight to compress the chest by 2½–4 cm (1–1½ in) squeezing the heart between the sternum and the vertebral column at a rate of 60–90 compressions per minute. The compression to relaxation ratio should be equal and this can be achieved by counting 'one two' regularly like a metronome. Firm sustained pressure during compression is much more effective than jerky jabbing movements and at the end of each compression full recoil and expansion of the chest should be allowed. This is the moment at which normal ventilation of the lungs is most effective and if an assistant is available efforts should be made to achieve synchronization.

In children under the age of about 10 years a more gentle approach is necessary and adequate compression of the sternum of 3–4 cm may be achieved with one hand. Artificial ventilation of the lungs should also be less vigorous in children than in adults.

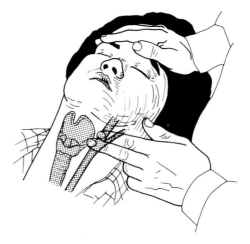

Fig. 15.6. Palpating the carotid pulse.

The circulation should be reassessed at regular intervals by feeling for the carotid pulse and noting the colour of the patient (*Fig*. 15.6). If an assistant is present she should simultaneously treat the respiratory arrest in the manner described above. When no assistance is available the dental surgeon should perform respiratory and cardiac resuscitation alternately for periods of 20 sec.

Prolonged resuscitation is an exhausting business and although theoretically it should be continued until the patient's colour improves, his pupils contract, and respiration and heart beats are restored, an unassisted operator can only maintain resuscitation for a limited period. This period can be greatly prolonged if assistance is available and the individuals participating in the resuscitation of the patient take turns at mouth-to-mouth respiration and cardiac massage alternately. In desperate situations in which it is not possible to obtain specialist help, some authorities advise the injection of 5 ml of 10% calcium chloride solution directly into the heart. The technique is as follows: The junction between the manubrium sterni and the body of sternum is easily palpable even in obese persons. This readily located landmark lies at the level of the second costal cartilage and can be used to identify the fourth costal cartilage and the intercostal space below it. A No. 1 needle is inserted into this space 3·8 cm (1½ in) from the lateral border of the sternum. After aspirating blood to check that the point of the needle is in the heart, the injection is made.

Once the vital signs have been restored and stabilized the patient should be transferred to hospital. Close surveillance must be maintained throughout the journey and artificial respiration and external cardiac massage either continued or reinstituted if necessary. Cardiac arrest not infrequently recurs in such circumstances.

FOREIGN BODIES

Foreign bodies including teeth, roots and detached fillings may be either swallowed or inhaled. A sharp foreign body, such as a fragment of a broken denture may, if swallowed, produce a pharyngo-oesophageal injury which may be complicated by mediastinitis. Such patients usually complain of dysphagia and should be referred to hospital for investigation and treatment without delay.

Patients under general anaesthesia are more likely to inhale either blood, saliva or a foreign body than conscious patients in whom a cough reflex is present. Adequate packing of the throat and the use of a cuffed endotracheal tube and suction minimize the risk of such a complication occurring.

The inhaled non-obstructing foreign body may produce dyspnoea, coughing paroxysms or stridor. Oxygen should be administered and the patient should be transferred under continuous surveillance to hospital without further delay.

The inhaled foreign body which obstructs the larynx causes a rapidly developing cyanosis and exaggeration of respiratory effort. Such a patient may clutch at his throat as he struggles for breath and immediate steps must be taken to restore the patency of the airway.

If the patient is seated he should sit forward with his head between his knees and be encouraged to cough. If this manoeuvre fails to dislodge the foreign body the operator should quickly deliver four very firm blows to the patient's back high up between the shoulder blades (*Fig*. 15.7). If this measure fails to achieve the

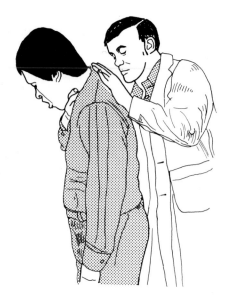

Fig. 15.7. Dislodging an inhaled foreign body.

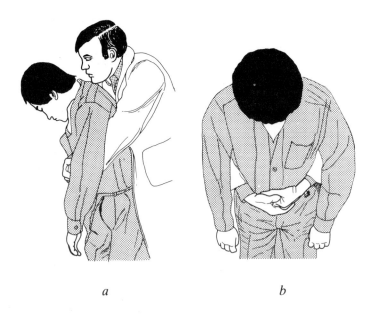

a   b

Fig. 15.8. The Heimlich manoeuvre (*see* text for explanation).

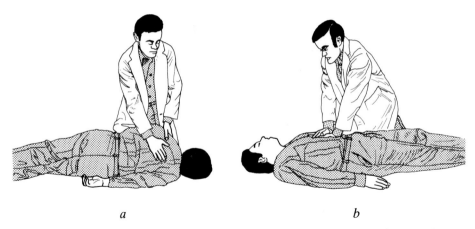

a   *b*

Fig. 15.9. The Heimlich manoeuvre performed on the supine patient (*see* text for explanation).

desired result the Heimlich manoeuvre, which mimics the action of a cough, should be undertaken without delay. The manoeuvre is performed as follows:

The operator sits or stands behind the patient and circling his or her waist with his arms places a clenched fist in the patient's epigastrium and grasps it with his other hand (*Fig*. 15.8*a*). The clenched fist is then pulled upwards sharply into the patient's epigastrium four times (*Fig*. 15.8*b*).

If this does not succeed in dislodging the inhaled foreign body the patient should be laid on his or her side and struck four times on the back in the manner described above (*Fig*. 15.9*a*). If this fails he should be rolled into the supine position and the abdominal thrust manoeuvre performed as follows:

The operator places the heel of his hand in the patient's epigastrium and thrusts sharply upwards below the xiphisternum four times (*Fig*. 15.9*b*). If this fails the patient is turned on to his or her side and the four sharp blows to the back are repeated (*Fig*. 15.9*a*).

The Heimlich manoeuvre should not be employed to treat women in the advanced stages of pregnancy or in small children in whom it is relatively easy to damage the liver.

In the unlikely event that these measures do not succeed the obstruction must be by-passed by cricothyrotomy (*see over* and *Fig*. 15.10). Oxygen must then be administered until the patient's cyanosis disappears and transfer to hospital under careful surveillance is practicable.

ANAESTHETIC EMERGENCIES

Syncope, respiratory obstruction and arrest, and cardiac arrest may complicate general anaesthesia, despite every care being taken, and both the anaesthetist and the operator must always be on the alert for warning signs. The pulse should be continuously monitored throughout the anaesthetic by either palpation of the carotid pulse or the use of a finger pulse plethysmograph with a display and pre-set alarm. If collapse occurs the administration of the anaesthetic must be stopped immediately and the airway should be cleared, all packs, apparatus and debris being removed from the mouth. The mandible and tongue should be pulled forward, the neck extended, and the head either held downwards and forwards if the patient cannot be lifted from the chair, or upwards if he can be laid on the floor. Oxygen should be given if there is excessive contraction of the accessory muscles of respiration. If the obstruction to respiration is not relieved, either endotracheal intubation or cricothyrotomy cannulation (laryngotomy) must be performed. Should either respiratory or cardiac arrest occur it should be treated in the manner outlined above.

CRICOTHYROTOMY

The establishment of an airway via the cricothyroid membrane is considered to be a safe, quick and simple procedure and the technique of choice in a number of emergency situations.

Fig. 15.10 shows the relative positions of the hyoid bone and the thyroid and cricoid cartilages as they lie just below the mandible in the midline of the neck. On the front of the thyroid cartilage the laryngeal prominence or Adam's apple is easily palpable as a notched structure except in infants and very obese patients. Above the notch lies the body of the hyoid bone whilst 2–3 cm directly below it lies the cricothyroid membrane. This membrane is approximately 22 mm wide and 10 mm high in the adult and can be palpated as an indentation. Directly below the membrane lies the cricoid cartilage which is the only complete tracheal ring and the narrowest segment of the trachea. The vocal cords lie about 1·5–2 cm above the cricothyroid membrane, the superior aspect of which is traversed by the cricothyroid vessels. The jugular and carotid vessels lie on either side of the membrane, the highly vascular thyroid isthmus and the anterior thyroid veins lie below it and the oesophagus is separated from its posterior surface by the airway. The proximity of these vulnerable and important structures makes it essential to site the incision through the cricothyroid membrane very accurately and the technique of cricothyrotomy is performed in the following manner.

Whenever possible an assistant holds the head in the midline, with the neck extended. The operator identifies the hyoid bone, the thyroid and cricoid cartilages and the cricothyroid membrane by palpation. If the patient is conscious and circumstances permit, the membrane and the skin overlying it are infiltrated with local anaesthetic solution. For example, an elective cricothyrotomy is sometimes performed on a conscious patient in whom a rapidly spreading haematoma of the neck threatens the patency of the airway. In most instances the condition of the patient is such as to render this step unnecessary. The operator places the little finger of his left hand on the hyoid bone, the two middle fingers on the thyroid cartilage immediately below the laryngeal prominence (Adam's apple) and the index finger on the cricoid cartilage (*Fig.* 15.10). Horizontal incisions 1–1½ cm in length are then made through the skin and the cricothyroid membrane just above the upper side of the left index finger. The scalpel blade should be guarded with the finger and inserted in a 30–40° caudal direction towards the posterior part of the cricoid cartilage in order to ensure that the oesophagus is not endangered. In children a large bore intravenous cannula (size 10 or 12) should be used instead of

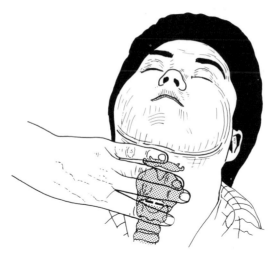

Fig. 15.10. Cricothyrotomy. The dotted line indicates the site of incision.

a scalpel, as the cricothyroid membrane is quite small. Some operators prefer to either use a cannula in all cases or to first insert a large bore cannula in adults as a guide for the incision with a scalpel.

Blunt ended scissors are then used to spread the incision horizontally and either a dilator or artery forceps used to spread it vertically to permit the placement of either an endotracheal or a tracheostomy tube. The tube may be any size from 4 to 8 but should have an outer diameter of less than 9 mm. It is advanced caudally into the trachea and tied securely in place. Experience reveals that the healing of the cricothyrotomy stoma is complete in about 2 months after removal of the tube without suture.

PRECAUTIONARY MEASURES

It is the duty of the dental surgeon to make every endeavour to avoid complications and to prevent emergencies arising. Although it is not possible to prevent them occurring completely, both their incidence and their effects can be reduced by the exercise of care and skill. Complications can only be diagnosed as soon as they occur and dealt with promptly and effectively if the possibility of their occurring has been anticipated. All too often practitioners only start thinking about emergencies and planning how to cope with them after one has arisen and exposed their inadequacies. Whilst an emergency may be a good learning experience it is an extremely bad situation in which to experience learning.

As fainting occurs more frequently when the temperature and relative humidity are high, the surgery premises should be kept cool and well ventilated. The waiting room should be light and airy and an efficient appointments system should be utilized to minimize waiting. It has been shown that dental patients, especially men under 35 years of age, with a history of fainting in the dental surgery on previous occasions, are more likel to faint than others. A firm but reassuring manner should be adopted when dealing with such patients. If the procedure has been performed with the patient in the supine position, care should be taken to raise the patient gradually from the supine to the sitting position and then to the standing position. This is particularly important when the treatment has been prolonged and especially so if the patient is either elderly and/or hypertensive. He must be carefully observed and at the first sign of pallor or sweating he should be laid flat, for in this position he is less likely to lose consciousness.

The dental surgeon should use a dental chair the design of which permits the patient to be quickly placed upon his back with his legs higher than his head (10° Trendelenburg position) in an emergency. Otherwise an unconscious patient will have to be lifted out of the chair and on to the floor. Little purpose will be served by this exhausting manoeuvre if there is insufficient free space available for the patient to be laid down and resuscitated. As it may be necessary to remove blood, mucus, or vomit from the air-passages, an efficient aspiration apparatus should be kept readily available in the surgery. A supply of oxygen and either a modern anaesthetic machine or an inflating bellows (e.g., Ambu, Porten) with which a patient's lungs can be inflated with oxygen should also be near at hand. It is as useless to have oxygen available for use when the tubing is too short to allow the mask to be applied to the face of a supine patient, as to know which drug should be given if it and the apparatus and expertise required to administer it are not readily available. Similarly it is important to ensure that all equipment is regularly inspected and properly maintained and serviced so that it is in good working order when needed.

Times of stress and crisis are ill-suited for either the acquisition of new clinical skills or the institution of a search in the telephone directory for the numbers of doctors or hospitals. For these reasons every dental surgeon should try to foresee possible emergencies and prepare for them. He should instruct each new member of his staff in the role that he or she will play when a crisis occurs and should hold regular practices and checks on his emergency and communication equipment and arrangements. Every member of staff should be trained to care for the unconscious patient, to use airways, oxygen equipment and suction apparatus and to undertake both mouth-to-mouth respiration and external chest compression in a competent fashion. Training is facilitated by the production of written protocols for equipment inspection and maintenance, preventive measures and treatment plans and communication practices. If only one emergency occurs during a lifetime of practice and the life of the patient concerned is preserved as a result of his precautionary measures, the wisdom and foresight of the dentist will have been amply rewarded.

HYPERVENTILATION

Abnormally prolonged and deep breathing is an hysterical manifestation of fear and may produce altered consciousness. Such a patient is seen to be hyperventilating, panting and pale, and may complain of tingling in the fingers or lips. The volume, rhythm and rate of the pulse are normal. If untreated the condition may be complicated by tetany with carpopedal and jaw spasm.

Once the condition is recognized treatment is simple. The patient is made to rebreathe in and out of a bag such as a waste paper basket liner until recovery occurs.

HAEMORRHAGE AT OPERATION

Sometimes a constant oozing of blood during an operation obscures vision and makes surgery difficult. A wide-bore sucker end should be used during procedures in which bone has either to be cut or removed, and to be of value the apparatus, which should produce a pressure of 0·14 kg/sq cm (20 lb/sq in), must be handled by an assistant trained in its correct use. More severe bleeding can be controlled by pressure on a hot (49 °C) normal saline pack held in position for a timed 2 min. The sucker should be used to remove excess saline from the pack. During more extensive oral surgical procedures bleeding sometimes occurs from a larger vessel and in these circumstances the vessel should be picked up, clamped with a haemostat, and tied with either 000 linen or catgut. Bleeding may be troublesome when surgery is performed on patients under general anaesthesia if oxygenation is insufficient. The vasoconstrictor present in local anaesthetic solutions usually ensures a dry operative field and thus facilitates surgery. The anaesthetist's consent must be obtained if it is planned to employ vasoconstrictors on patients under general anaesthesia as their use may predispose to cardiac complications in certain circumstances.

When the operation is completed the patient should be allowed to rinse his mouth with a bland mouthwash once. A firm gauze roll should then be placed upon the wound and the patient instructed to bite upon it for a few minutes. If the haemorrhage is not controlled within 5 min the dental surgeon should either insert further sutures or a Whitehead's varnish on ribbon-gauze pressure pack to control the bleeding.

POSTOPERATIVE HAEMORRHAGE

Following surgery the patient should be instructed to avoid violent exercise, stimulants, or very hot food or drink for the rest of the day to minimize the risk of postoperative haemorrhage. If bleeding occurs the patient should apply a clean folded handkerchief to the wound and bite on it firmly for a timed 5 min. The site of operation should be cleansed by rinsing the mouth with warm saline immediately before going to bed on the day of operation. Healing will be aided by the use of hot saline mouth-baths frequently on the following 2 or 3 days (see p. 86), and the patient should be instructed to return for consultation should anything untoward complicate the healing period.

Most patients who return complaining of postoperative haemorrhage are accompanied by anxious relatives or friends and it is essential to separate the patient from these well-intentioned, but unhelpful, companions. Until the patient has been taken to the dental surgery and the persons accompanying him asked to remain in the waiting room, it will be quite impossible to either reassure or treat him satisfactorily. After seating the patient comfortably in the dental chair and covering his clothes with a protective waterproof apron, the dental surgeon should examine the mouth in order to determine the site and amount of haemorrhage. Almost invariably an excess of blood clot will be seen in the bleeding area and this should be grasped in a piece of gauze and removed. A firm gauze pack should then be placed upon the site of the haemorrhage and the patient instructed to bite upon it. If tannic acid powder is placed upon the portion of the pack related to the bleeding tissues, it will help to arrest the haemorrhage.

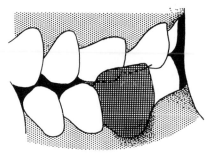

Fig. 15.11. The use of a composition block for haemostasis.

If a tear is present in the gingiva and in many other instances, it will be advisable to insert some sutures into the soft tissues, under local anaesthesia, to control the haemorrhage. When the haemorrhage is coming from the gingiva surrounding a tooth socket, interrupted horizontal mattress sutures are best suited to this purpose and should be inserted across the socket as soon as possible (*see Fig.* 3.36). The object of this form of suturing is not to close the socket by approximating the soft tissues over it, but to tense the mucoperiosteum over the underlying bone so that it becomes ischaemic. In the vast majority of cases, the bleeding arises not in the bony socket but from the soft tissues surrounding it and is stopped by the procedure described above. In the rare case in which bleeding is coming from the bone, haemorrhage can usually be arrested by crushing the bony channel containing the involved vessel by applying pressure on a blunt instrument. The patient should be instructed to bite upon a gauze pack for 5 min following the insertion of a suture. Should these measures fail to control the haemorrhage, either gelatin or fibrin foam may be tucked into the wound under the sutures and a composition block moulded over the area. After the block has been placed in situ (*Fig.* 15.11) and an extra-oral support provided, the patient should be referred to the nearest hospital for further treatment.

In most cases the haemorrhage will have been arrested by simple measures and it is prudent to re-examine the patient after he has walked about before discharging him. The mouth tastes unpleasant after an oral haemorrhage, but repeated rinsing promotes bleeding and should be avoided. The oral cavity should be cleaned carefully with gauze soaked in cold water, special attention being paid to the tongue. This simple procedure adds greatly to the patient's comfort.

BLOOD LOSS

The loss of blood which complicates multiple dental extractions and other forms of oral surgery is often either forgotten or disregarded. It is not unusual for patients who are known to be anaemic to be advised that neither the extraction of their teeth nor other oral surgical procedures need be delayed until they have responded to medical treatment. *Table* 15.1 summarizes the results of some investigations into blood loss complicating multiple extractions and reveals that

Table 15.1. Summary of the Results of some Published Studies of Blood Loss during Multiple Extractions

Author	Number of patients	Largest loss (ml)	Comments
Gores, Royer and Mann (1955)	50 (21 with local anaesthetic agents)	771	8 lost over 400 ml (no local anaesthetic agents) 2 lost over 400 ml (with local anaesthetic agents)
Johnson (1956)	175	919	Average loss 223 ml
Connors (1959)	10	700	Average loss 316 ml
Spengos (1963)	21	912	Mean value 536 ml (extractions and alveoplasty)
Meyer and Allen (1968)	35	1283	Mean value 351 ml (vasoconstrictors of limited value in controlling operative blood loss as distinct from postoperative)
Werner, Moss and Ruetz (1968)	17	1445	Mean value 363·4 ml

often between one-half to one and three-quarters of a pint of blood may be lost when a dental clearance is performed. The workers quoted claim that the average loss exceeds that sustained in simple mastectomy, inguinal herniorrhaphy, and haemorrhoidectomy, and that the maximum loss is greater than that which complicates hysterectomy, nephrectomy, cholecystectomy, and thyroidectomy, and may even equal the blood loss which accompanies gastric resection.

The amount of blood lost is directly correlated to the operating time and can be reduced by performing surgery in easy stages, the use of vasoconstrictors injected locally, and careful attention to postoperative haemostasis. This degree of blood loss is probably of little significance in fit young adults, many of whom can donate a pint of blood for transfusion purposes without suffering any ill effect. However, most dental clearances and many other oral surgery procedures are performed upon older patients, in whom haemopoiesis is less active and not infrequently some degree of anaemia exists preoperatively. Anaemia should be diagnosed and treated before oral surgical procedures are undertaken, for not only does it predispose to postoperative haemorrhage but it also makes the effects of blood loss more severe.

POSTOPERATIVE PAIN

When the patient is discharged after an oral surgical operation he should be supplied with some analgesic tablets, for use if required to control any post-operative pain (*see* p. 84).

The patient should be given a further appointment and instructed to return to the dentist if anything untoward occurs during the period of healing. Pain which varies in degree, character, and duration may complicate the healing period and may be due to a variety of causes.

SOME AVOIDABLE CAUSES OF POSTOPERATIVE PAIN

Failure to handle the soft tissues carefully during a surgical procedure may cause an oedematous swelling, soreness and delayed healing. The use of blunt instruments, the excessive retraction of badly designed flaps, or burs becoming entangled in the soft tissues are typical errors of technique which produce these avoidable sequelae. If sutures are tied too tightly, *postoperative swelling* due to oedema or haematoma formation may cause sloughing of the soft tissues and breakdown of the suture line. Usually such conditions regress if the patient uses hot saline mouth-baths frequently for 2 or 3 days (*see* p. 86).

A more serious cause of postoperative swelling is infection of the wound. No effort should be spared to prevent the introduction of pathogenic micro-organisms into the tissues. If the infection is mild, it will often respond to the application of heat intra-orally by the use of frequent hot saline mouth-baths. The patient should be cautioned against applying heat extra-orally, because this tends to increase the size of the facial swelling. A hot-water bottle applied to the cheek in an effort to relieve pain is a common cause of gross swelling of the face. If fluctuation is present, the pus should be evacuated prior to the institution of antibiotic therapy (*see* p. 234). Any patient with a postoperative infection severe enough to warrant antibiotic therapy is best treated at a hospital with oral surgery facilities, especially if the swelling involves the submaxillary and sublingual tissues.

Trismus or inability to open the mouth due to muscle spasm may complicate oral surgical procedures, particularly difficult dental extractions. It may be caused by postoperative oedema, haematoma formation, or inflammation of the soft tissues. Patients with traumatic arthritis of the temporomandibular joints exhibit painful limitation of mandibular movement. An inferior dental block injection may be followed by trismus, even when administered for reasons other than extraction, owing to either haematoma formation or the introduction of infection. The treatment of trismus varies with the underlying cause. Although the application of intra-oral heat by means of short-wave diathermy or the use of hot saline mouth-baths gives relief in mild cases, other patients may require the administration of antibiotics or specialist treatment to relieve their symptoms.

Postoperative pain may be caused by avoidable trauma during oral surgical procedures. Bone may be bruised by clumsy instrumentation or damaged by overheated burs during bone removal. Careful avoidance of these errors of technique combined with meticulous attention to the smoothing of sharp bone edges and socket toilet eliminate this cause of after-pain.

'DRY SOCKET'

This well-recognized but ill-understood complication of tooth extraction is familiar to all experienced dental surgeons and is usually regarded as a localized osteitis, involving either the whole or a part of the condensed bone lining a tooth socket, the so-called 'lamina dura'. The condition is characterized by an acutely painful tooth socket containing bare bone and broken-down blood clot (*Fig.* 15.12, and *see Table* 1.2). It is said to complicate 3% of all dental extractions and between 14–37% of lower third molar removals. The incidence is significantly higher after the removal of a single tooth than after multiple extractions. The aetiology is obscure, but many predisposing causes have been noted. Infection of

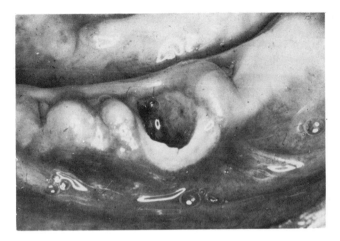

Fig. 15.12. 'Dry socket' with exposed bare bone.

the socket occurring either before, during, or after the extraction may be an exciting factor, and yet many periodontically affected, abscessed and infected teeth are extracted without a 'dry socket' occurring. Whilst it is true that the condition may follow the use of excessive force during an extraction, this is not always the case and the complication may occur after very easy extractions.

Many authorities feel that the vasoconstrictor in local anaesthetic solutions may predispose to 'dry socket' by interfering with the blood supply of the bone, and they point out that the condition occurs more frequently under local than general anaesthesia. Nevertheless, 'dry sockets' may follow extractions performed under general anaesthesia, especially if they are performed inexpertly. The incidence may be influenced by the fact that many dental surgeons perform their more difficult extractions under local anaesthesia. There is evidence that 'dry sockets' occur more frequently in wounds which display poor filling with blood clot in the immediate postoperative period. Thus the use of vasoconstrictors cannot be the basic cause of the lesion but may well be a contributory factor. Mandibular extractions are complicated by the development of a 'dry socket' more often than maxillary extractions. The mandible has much more dense bone and is less vascular than the maxilla. However, anatomical studies have revealed that the blood supply to the alveolus in the lower molar region is no poorer than that of other regions of the jaws. Lower teeth are usually more difficult to extract than upper teeth and gravity ensures that mandibular sockets become contaminated with food debris.

Some patients appear to have a predisposition to dry sockets and experience this unpleasant complication of tooth extraction on more than one occasion. This has led some authorities to postulate the existence of a systemic aetiological factor. To date there is little evidence to support this concept, although an increased titre of fibrinolytic substances has been demonstrated in the alveolar bone of patients afflicted with 'dry socket'. A number of bacteria are known to possess fibrinolytic activity and it has recently been postulated that *Treponema denticolum* may have an aetiological role in the genesis of dry sockets.

Pregnant women and those taking oral contraceptives appear to be more susceptible than others to 'dry socket'. Except for these groups the sexes display no predilection for the condition.

Whilst it is probable that a combination of two or more of these predisposing factors makes the occurrence of a 'dry socket' more likely, it is impossible to forecast preoperatively which extractions will be followed by this complication and so the following measures aimed at prevention should be employed wherever possible. The teeth should be scaled and any gingival inflammation treated prior to the extraction of teeth. Only the minimum amount of local anaesthetic solution necessary to produce analgesia should be administered and the teeth should be removed in the least traumatic manner possible.

Many procedures have been claimed to reduce the incidence of 'dry socket' most of which involve the insertion into the socket of either antibiotics or steroids or a combination of both at the time of extraction. Neither they nor the prophylactic use of antibiotics administered systemically have found widespread favour. However, the prophylactic administration of Metronidazole Tablets BP (Flagyl) in a dosage of 200 mg 8-hourly for 3 days starting on the day of extraction appears to reduce significantly the incidence of dry sockets and to be worthy of trial. It has also been shown that the same antibacterial drug provides prompt relief from pain once the complication has occurred if given in the larger dosage of 400 mg t.d.s. for 5 days. Patients should be warned to avoid drinking alcohol whilst metronidazole is being taken and for 3 days after completing the course of treatment if the unpleasant side effects of nausea and vomiting are to be avoided.

When a 'dry socket' occurs, the aims of treatment should be the relief of pain and the speeding of resolution. The socket should be irrigated with warm normal saline and all degenerating blood clot removed (*Fig.* 15.13). Sharp bony spurs should be either excised with rongeur forceps or smoothed with a wheel stone. A loose dressing, composed of zinc oxide and oil-of-cloves on cotton-wool, is tucked into the socket (*Fig.* 15.14). It must not be packed tightly or it may set hard and be very difficult to remove. Analgesic tablets (p. 84) and hot saline mouth-baths (p. 86) are prescribed and arrangements made to see the patient again in 3 days.

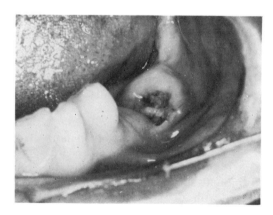

Fig. 15.13. 'Dry socket' containing degenerating blood clot.

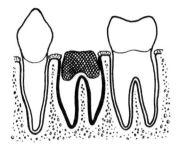

Fig. 15.14.   A sedative dressing tucked into a 'dry socket'.

Most patients treated in this manner report relief of pain, but some require a further dressing or even chemical cauterization of the exposed bare painful bone to control the symptoms. This can be performed, after isolating and drying the 'dry socket', by applying a small quantity of carbolized resin to the bare bony walls of the socket with a pair of College tweezers. A zinc oxide/oil-of-cloves cotton-wool dressing is then inserted to cover the caustic and left in situ for 3 days.

Whilst zinc oxide and oil-of-cloves dressings relieve pain they undoubtedly delay healing. Though a pack, composed of Whitehead's varnish (pigmentum iodoform compositum BPC) on ribbon gauze, is not quite so effective in controlling pain, it can be left in situ for 2 or 3 weeks and the socket will be found to be granulating when the dressing is removed (*see* p. 78).

ACUTE OSTEOMYELITIS OF THE MANDIBLE

Sometimes it may be difficult to differentiate between a patient afflicted with a severe 'dry socket' and a patient suffering from acute osteomyelitis of the mandible. The latter condition usually causes much more general prostration and toxicity. There is a marked pyrexia and pain is very severe. Often the mandible is exquisitely tender on extra-oral palpation, whilst the onset of impairment of labial sensation some hours or even days after the extraction is a characteristic feature of acute osteomyelitis of the mandible. A patient suffering from this condition should be admitted, as an emergency, to a hospital where facilities for its effective treatment exist. Traumatic extraction of a lower molar under local anaesthesia in the presence of acute gingival inflammation (e.g., pericoronitis or acute ulcerative gingivitis) predisposes to acute osteomyelitis of the mandible (*see* p. 245).

DISLOCATION OF THE TEMPOROMANDIBULAR JOINT

Complete or partial dislocation of the temporomandibular joint occurs readily in some patients and a history of recurrent dislocation should never be disregarded. Either this mishap or postoperative traumatic arthritis of the temporomandibular joint may complicate difficult extractions, or prolonged oral surgical procedures if the lower jaw is not supported throughout the procedure.

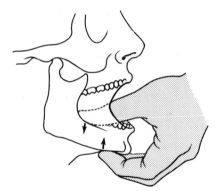

Fig. 15.15. The reduction of a dislocation of the mandible (*see* text for explanation).

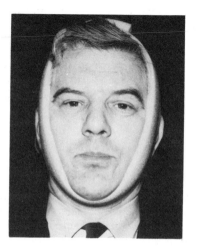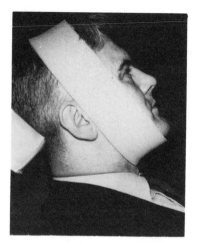

Fig. 15.16. Plastic-foam chin support (6·4 cm (2½ in) wide and 76·2 cm (30 in) long).

The support given to the jaw by the left hand of the operator should be supplemented by that given by the anaesthetist or an assistant pressing upwards, with both hands, beneath the angles of the mandible.

Dislocation may also be caused by the injudicious use of mouth gags. If dislocation occurs it should be reduced immediately. The operator stands in front of the patient and places his thumbs intra-orally on the external oblique ridges in the mandibular molar regions and his fingers extra-orally under the lower border of the mandible (*Fig.* 15.15). Downward pressure with the thumbs and upward pressure with the fingers reduce the dislocation. Many dental surgeons wrap their thumbs in thick gauze when reducing dislocations of the temporomandibular joint in order to prevent them being damaged as the mandible goes into place. If the thumbs are placed on the external oblique ridges alongside the molar teeth the risk of this mishap occurring is minimized. If treatment is delayed, muscle spasm may render reduction impossible except under general anaesthesia. The patient should be warned not to open his mouth too widely or to yawn for a few days postoperatively, and an extra-oral support for the joint should be applied (*Fig.* 15.16) and worn until tenderness in the affected joint subsides.

FRACTURE OF THE MANDIBLE

Fracture of the mandible may complicate oral surgical procedures performed upon atrophic mandibles unless great care is exercised (*see* p. 108). Excessive force should never be used to extract teeth. If a tooth does not yield to moderate pressure the reason should be sought and remedied.

The mandible may be weakened by senile osteoporosis and atrophy, osteo-myelitis, previous therapeutic irradiation, or such osteodystrophies as osteitis deformans, fibrous dysplasia, or fragilitas ossium. Unerupted teeth, cysts, hyper-parathyroidism, or tumours may also predispose to fracture. In the presence of one of these conditions, surgery should be undertaken only after careful clinical and radiographic assessment and the construction of splints preoperatively. The patient should be informed before operation of the possibility of mandibular fracture and, should this complication occur, treatment must be instituted at once. For these reasons these cases are best dealt with in specialist oral surgery centres. If a fracture of the mandible occurs in the dental surgery an extra-oral support (*see Fig.* 15.16) should be applied and the patient referred immediately to a hospital where facilities for definitive treatment exist (*see* Chapter 16).

POSTOPERATIVE IMPAIRMENT OF SENSATION

Postoperative impairment of labial sensation may complicate the removal of large mandibular cysts and the extraction of mandibular cheek teeth or roots, which are in close relationship to the inferior dental and mental nerves. The techniques employed to minimize the risk of nerve damage during the removal of roots from the edentulous mandible are discussed on p. 106 and during the extraction of impacted lower third molars on p.129. Unerupted or partially erupted second premolars may also be grooved, notched, or perforated by the contents of the inferior dental canal, and this can be diagnosed radiographically using the criteria described in relation to third molars (*see Fig.* 3.28). Fractures of the body of the mandible, acute osteomyelitis of the mandible, and acute infections in the tissues related to the mental nerve may also cause impairment of labial sensation. Abscesses situated in the buccal sulcus in the mandibular premolar region should be opened using Hilton's method in order to minimize the risk of damaging the mental nerve (*see* p. 234, *Fig.* 9.9).

The lingual nerve may be damaged either during a traumatic extraction of a lower molar in which the lingual soft tissues are trapped in the forceps, or by being caught up with the bur during the removal of bone. A metal retractor should be used to protect adjacent soft tissues from harm whenever a bur is in use.

The unpleasant symptoms of labial anaesthesia and paraesthesia may be of varying severity and may persist for periods lasting from a few hours to many months, depending upon the amount of damage sustained by the involved nerves.

Although anaesthesia may be tolerated with equanimity, paraesthesia is often the cause of considerable distress. All such patients should be seen at regular intervals until sensation has returned to normal. The dental surgeon should elicit and carefully record the nature and extent of sensory loss present at each visit so that the rate of recovery may be determined and any necessary supportive treatment provided. It is wise to seek a second opinion in such cases.

FAILURE TO COMPLETE THE OPERATION

The dental surgeon may not be able to complete the operation due to inadequacy of anaesthesia, lack of co-operation from the patient, or a lack of either the facilities or skill which is required. The experienced practitioner avoids these pitfalls by making a thorough preoperative assessment and a careful treatment plan.

Failure to secure anaesthesia is usually due to either faulty technique or insufficient dosage of the anaesthetic agent. It is impossible to perform surgery well unless both the operator and the patient have complete confidence in the anaesthesia under which the operation is performed. The employment of a skilled anaesthetist will ensure this when a general anaesthetic is administered, but when local anaesthesia is employed its efficacy should be tested with a sharp probe before the operation is commenced. If nothing is felt by the patient, anaesthesia has been secured. If he feels pressure but not pain, analgesia has been obtained, whilst pain indicates that a further injection of local anaesthetic solution is required.

Nervous patients are often helped by premedication and all patients find it easier to relax and co-operate with a dental surgeon who has a calm, courteous, and confident manner and who encourages them as he works in a methodical and unhurried fashion.

SUGGESTED READING

Allwright W. C. and Cheong E. (1964) Cardiac resuscitation in the dental surgery. *Br. Dent. J.* **116**, 260–2.
Banks P. (1981) *Killey's Fractures of the Middle Third of the Facial Skeleton*, 4th ed. Bristol, Wright.
Banks P. (1983) *Killey's Fractures of the Mandible*, 3rd ed. Bristol, Wright.
Birn H. (1966) The vascular supply of the periodontal membrane. *J. Periodont. Res.* **1**, 51–68.
Birn H. (1970) Fibrinolytic activity in 'dry socket'. *Acta Odontol. Scand.* **28**, 37–58.
Bourne J. G. (1980) The common fainting attack. *Br. Dent. J.* **149**, 101–4.
Brown A. S. (1961) Complications in the office practice of minor oral surgery. *J. Canad. Dent. Assoc.* **27**, 514–20.
Connors J. J. (1959) Blood loss in the surgical removal of teeth. *Ann. Dent.* **18**, 74–6.
Gores R. J., Royer R. Q. and Mann F. D. (1955) Blood loss during operation for multiple extraction with alveoplasty and other surgical procedures. *J. Oral Surg.*, **13**, 299–306.
Hannington-Kiff J. G. (1969) Fainting and collapse in dental practice. *Dent. Pract.* **20**, 2–7.
Harvey W. (1964) Notes on the management of emergencies. *Dent. Mag.* **81**, 167–70.
Heimlich H. J. (1975) A life-saving maneuver to prevent food choking. *JAMA* **234**, 398–401.
Howe G. L. (1962) Some complications of tooth extraction. *Ann. R. Coll. Surg.* **30**, 309–23.
Johnson R. L. (1956) Blood loss in oral surgery. *J. Dent. Res.* **35**, 175–84.
Kay L. W. (1961) A review of the aetiology, diagnosis and treatment of cardiac arrest. *Br. Dent. J.* **111**, 201–9.

Kouwenhoven W. B., Jude J. R. and Knickerbocker G. C. (1960) Closed chest cardiac massage. *JAMA* **173**, 1064–7.

Krekmanov L. (1981) Alveolitis after operative removal of third molars in the mandible. *Int. J. Oral Surg.* **10**, 173–9.

Kress T. D. and Balasubramanian S. (1982) Cricothyroidotomy. *Ann. Emerg. Med.* **11**, 197–201.

MacGregor A. J. (1968) Aetiology of dry socket: a clinical investigation. *Br. J. Oral Surg.* **6**, 49–58.

Meyer R. and Allen G. D. (1968) Blood volume studies in oral surgery. *J. Oral Surg.* **26**, 721–6.

Nitzan D. W. (1983) On the genesis of 'dry socket'. *J. Oral Maxillofac. Surg.* **41**, 706–10.

Rood J. P. and Murgatroyd J. (1980) Metronidazole in the prevention of dry socket. *Br. J. Oral Surg.* **17**, 62–70.

Rood J. P. and Danforth M. (1981) Metronidazole in treatment of dry socket. *Int. J. Oral Surg.* **10**, 345–7.

Spengos M. N. (1963) Determination of blood loss during full mouth extraction and alveoplasty by plasma volume studies with I^{131}-tagged human albumin. *Oral Surg.* **16**, 276–83.

Werner P., Moss R. W. and Ruetz P. P. (1968) Determination of total blood loss after oral surgical procedures. *J. Oral Surg.* **26**, 794–9.

Chapter 16
Reference of patients to a specialist

As knowledge advances and new techniques are developed it becomes increasingly difficult for the dental surgeon to keep up to date with progress in his field. These difficulties are particularly marked when he is engaged wholly in general practice. The good practitioner does his best to solve this problem by attending post-graduate courses, lectures and dental society meetings whenever possible, in addition to reading selected dental periodicals. Comparatively few general dental practitioners are afforded the opportunity of working in a hospital or clinic for a few hours each week. This is a great pity, for although it usually entails both inconvenience and some personal sacrifice, there is no better way of increasing one's knowledge and improving one's skill.

However hard he tries, the dental surgeon will find it impossible to provide both expert opinion upon and treatment for a number of patients presenting in his practice. In such cases it is his duty to enlist the aid of those of his colleagues who have either more experience or better facilities to cope with the particular problem. A good general practitioner never loses respect by referring a patient for specialist opinion and treatment. In many instances he gains in stature, for the intelligent patient appreciates his desire to maintain the highest standards of practice. If the practitioner's diagnosis is correct an able specialist will tell the patient so and institute treatment promptly, whilst if it is incorrect any worthwhile specialist will not make any adverse comment upon the matter but will discreetly either alter any existing treatment or institute the treatment required. Most patients have more respect for and confidence in those dental surgeons who ensure that they receive the best treatment available for any oral problem which may be encountered.

Whilst no specialist would refuse to help a practitioner with a genuinely difficult case, he is more likely to assist those colleagues who accord him both the courtesy and consideration which he merits, by reason of his professional experience and responsibilities. Patients should never be sent to a specialist without an appointment or without a letter signed personally by the dental surgeon seeking his aid. In genuine cases of emergency the arrangements may be made by telephone, but the patient should still be given a letter. Simple cases which are merely either inconvenient or unremunerative for the practitioner to treat himself should not be sent to specialist colleagues, all of whom base their opinions about both the ethical standards and professional competence of general dental practitioners upon their professional dealings with them. If a dental surgeon makes a genuine attempt to assist with or co-operate in the treatment plan, thus helping his patient, it is always noted with appreciation. Note is also taken of those practitioners who prefer to shelve all their responsibilities once the patient has received specialist advice about a particular problem.

A case history should be taken in each instance and a summary of it included in the letter of reference. Except in genuine cases of emergency, it is usually preferable if all routine dental treatment is completed before the patient is referred for specialist opinion and treatment. Prior scaling of the teeth facilitates clinical examination, whilst a knowledge of both the status and prognosis of individual teeth may be of assistance to the specialist during both diagnosis and treatment planning. Thus, if there is a treated pulpal exposure in a second mandibular molar, he may decide to extract this tooth rather than the third molar adjacent to it. In other cases prior scaling and polishing of the teeth and the resultant improvement in the periodontal condition of the teeth may aid him in making an accurate assessment of the prognosis of the patient's remaining natural teeth.

Copies of all correspondence relating to a patient should be carefully filed with the case history. Many dental surgeons treat every case they refer to a specialist as a miniature postgraduate course and try to learn something from it. This is an excellent and rewarding practice.

Most general practitioners refer their patients when necessary to specialist colleagues whom they know and whose opinions and ability they trust and respect. Many hospitals issue lists of names of the consultants employed in their institution, together with details of the timings of clinics and the relevant administrative arrangements, to medical and dental practitioners on request. Whenever possible, it is best to write a letter requesting that an appointment be sent to the patient rather than just arranging one by telephoning an appointments clerk or bureau. Prior warning enables the specialist to arrange to see the patient at a time convenient to himself and under optimum conditions.

If the correct name and status of the specialist is known the letter should be addressed to him in person, but if these details are not known it should be addressed to the Head of the appropriate department. The dental surgeon will find that it facilitates the reference of patients if he builds up a list of the addresses, qualifications, and other details of those specialists who consult and treat patients whom he is either not equipped to treat or feels unable to treat himself. A dental surgeon should take care not to commit a specialist to any particular form of treatment. It is unfortunate that some general practitioners sometimes promise patients, whom they refer for specialist advice, that an operation will be performed under intravenous anaesthesia. This practice may create difficulties in patient management if a specialist anaesthetist decides that this form of anaesthesia is not indicated. Letters of reference, wherever practicable, should be posted separately and not handed to the patient for him to read *en route* to the hospital. This is especially important when confidential reports, opinions, or information are contained within the letter. The handwriting of both medical and dental practitioners is notorious for its illegibility. Typewritten letters are always legible and should be used whenever possible. Where handwritten letters are employed, legibility is of prime importance.

The letter of reference should contain the following details.

1. The name, address and age of the patient, together with details of previous hospital attendances and the hospital number, if known.

2. An indication whether the patient is receiving, or wishes to receive,

J. BLOGGS, B.D.S.
DENTAL SURGEON
—

TELEPHONE: ANYTOWN 1234

18 LITTLE GRANGE,

ANYTOWN,

WESSEX.

29th February, 1985

Dear Mr. Sawyer,

re: John Nobody, Aged 25 years
25, Hawthorn Avenue,
Anytown.

I would be grateful if you would send an out-patient appointment to this patient whom I am treating under the National Health Service.

<u>Exam</u>ination revealed the presence of caries in several teeth including 8 7/. I have removed the caries from both these teeth and inserted sedative dressings. Although both cavities were <u>deep</u> there is no evidence of pulpal involvement in either tooth. As 8/ is mesio-angularly impacted and unopposed I felt that it should be removed and I would value your opinion about this. Should you agree that extraction of the tooth is indicated, I would be grateful if you would undertake it as the enclosed radiograph shows the tooth to have an unfavourable root pattern. You might like to know that I extracted his /6 with some difficulty eighteen months ago and had to insert a suture to control the bleeding post-operatively. I would be happy to remove any sutures or provide any other post-operative treatment required if you would like me to do so. When he has been discharged from your department I will complete his routine dental treatment.

The patient would prefer his appointment with you to be on either a Wednesday or a Saturday if this is possible.

Would you please return the radiograph to me at your earliest convenience as I shall have to submit it to the Dental Estimates Board.

Yours sincerely,

S.Sawyer,Esq. M.D.S.,F.D.S.R.C.S.
Department of Oral Surgery,   (Eng),
City Hospital,
Anytown,
Wessex.

James Bloggs

(James Bloggs)

Fig. 16.1. Specimen letter referring a patient to a specialist.

treatment as a private patient or as a patient under the terms of the National Health Service.

3. A concise case history, a clear account of any clinical findings, and an honest statement, including dates, of any unsuccessful treatment which has been given (e.g., attempted tooth extractions, retained or misplaced roots, etc.).

4. All relevant information which the patient is either unable or unlikely to supply. This should include details of drug therapy already given, the development of symptoms and change of signs over a period, drug sensitivities or steroid treatment, social background, and attitude of the patient to or his knowledge about the condition which has necessitated reference to the specialist.

5. A clear statement of the reason for referral or the specific problem, and the service required, e.g., opinion and advice alone or both advice and treatment. It should also be made clear what proportion of the treatment the practitioner is prepared to undertake. For example, it is quite customary for a dental surgeon to ask a specialist to undertake the surgical treatment of a localized lesion and to then refer the patient back for any remaining dental treatment of a routine nature.

6. An indication that the practitioner is prepared to participate in the treatment of the patient if so desired, by removing sutures, doing dressings, or either providing or adjusting prosthetic or orthodontic appliances.

As has already been stated, a typewritten letter should be sent whenever possible and it is courteous to ensure that all such letters are signed by the dental surgeon himself. Headed notepaper on which the practitioner's name is clearly printed should be used for letters of reference whenever this is possible. When a handwritten letter is sent, the practitioner's name should always be printed under his unreadable signature. Whenever records, models, or radiographs are enclosed, it should be clearly indicated whether they should be returned when finished with. If circumstances permit, the dental surgeon will derive the maximum benefit from referring the patient by attending the consultation with the specialist and any operation performed upon his patient.

A typical letter of reference is shown in *Fig.* 16.1.

Sound judgement and common sense must govern the decision to refer a patient for specialist advice and treatment. The dental surgeon who fails to make full use of the specialist facilities available does both himself and his patients a disservice.

Appendix A

Instruments for oral surgery

Every dental surgeon has his favourite instruments and this results in a bewildering array of patterns being available for use. It is obviously uneconomic to accumulate a large number of different implements, many of which are seldom if ever used. The beginner should endeavour to acquire proficiency in the use of a limited range of instruments in the first instance. When a practice is equipped it is better to buy several identical surgical kits each containing a limited range of oft-used instruments if delays due to sterilization are not to occur. Whilst different teachers would probably have differing views on the composition of such a kit, most of them would agree that stainless-steel instruments should be used as far as is practicable.

The standard kit employed by the author for this purpose can conveniently be divided into two parts. The forceps, elevators, gags and props are used initially and only when the technique of intra-alveolar extraction has been mastered is the student introduced to the instruments employed in trans-alveolar extraction.

The kit comprises:

Dental Extraction Forceps

For Permanent Teeth	Pattern Number
Lower root (fine)	74N
Lower root (heavy)	137
Lower full molar	73
Upper straight (fine)	29
Upper straight (heavy)	2
Upper premolar (Read)	76S
Upper premolar (fine)	147
Upper full molar (right and left)	94 and 95
Upper bayonet	101

For Deciduous Teeth	
Upper straight	163
Upper root	159
Upper full molar	157
Lower root	162
Lower full molar	160

Elevators

Warwick James' pattern (right and left)
Cryer's pattern 30/31 (right and left)
Lindo Levien's pattern (large, medium, and small)

Gags and Props

Mouth gags with Ferguson ratchet
McKesson mouth props (set of three)

Other Surgical Instruments

Cheek retractor (Kilner's pattern)
Flap retractor (Austin's pattern)
Flap retractor (Bowdler Henry's pattern)
Scalpel handle No. 3
Scalpel blades Nos. 15, 12, and 11
Mitchell's trimmer or Cumine's scaler
Waugh's mouse-toothed forceps
Gillies 6 in (15 cm) toothed dissecting forceps
Periosteal elevator (Howarth's pattern)
Ash surgical burs (Toller's pattern)
Chisels (French's pattern), 5 mm, 7 mm, 9 mm, 11 mm in width
Mallet (Weiss pattern), B178 7½ in (19 cm)
Curved artery forceps (Mosquito pattern)
Syringe (for irrigation)
Needle-holders (Kilner's pattern)
Suture needles (Lane's No. 22 half-circle cutting)
Mersilk, No. 000
Ash's No. 5 alveolotomy shears
Rongeur forceps (Ash's No. 3)
Ash's 'acrylic tools' (Nos. 6, 8, 20R)
Dental mirror, straight probe, and College tweezers
Scissors 11·4 cm (4½ in) straight
Scissors (Kilner) 10 cm (4 in)
Skin hooks (Gillies)
Bone file (Miller 52 pattern)

Difficulties have long been experienced in avoiding a break in the chain of sterility when using a bur to remove bone or to divide teeth.

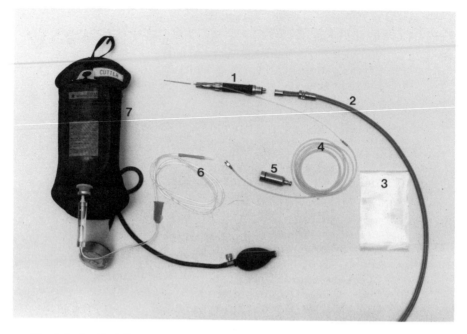

Fig. A.1. Sterile drill system for surgical use. 1, Integral straight handpiece and air motor. Fully autoclavable. 2, Standard dental unit air supply tube—Midwest 4 bore type or similar (exhaust air returned to unit, away from wound site). 3, Sterile nylon sleeve and autoclave tape. 4, Sterile silicone tubing with female Luer–Lok connector. 5, Air-operated pinch valve (connected to drill air supply in use). 6, Standard basic drip-set with male Luer–Lok connector. 7, Standard inflatable rapid transfusion pressure cuff or simple gravity drip supply of normal saline. (*Courtesy of Dr R. N. W. Clark.*)

It is now possible to achieve these objectives conveniently by using a fully autoclavable integral straight handpiece and air motor on a standard dental unit 4-bore air supply tube which ensures that the exhaust air is not directed upon the site of operation. The tubing is covered with a sterile nylon sleeve secured with autoclave tape (*Fig.* A.1).

The bur is cooled with sterile normal saline delivered via sterile silicone tubing connected to a standard basic drip set by means of male and female Luer–Lok connectors. Flow is ensured by either a simple gravity supply or by the use of a standard inflatable rapid transfusion pressure cuff and the rate of flow is controlled by an air-operated pinch valve which is connected to the drill air supply.

The items of equipment required are the following:

DynaTorq Micro Air Motor Model D × S 4100
Cutter 'Safticuff' pressure cuff
Normal saline in 500 ml plastic containers
Disposable sterile nylon sleeves
Autoclave tape

Appendix B
Instruments for periodontal surgery

Two mouth mirrors
'Michigan O' periodontal probe
Columbia curettes 13, 14
Goldman Fox curettes 2, 3, 4, 5
Gracey's curettes 13, 14
Cavitron tips P10
Two Bard Parker No. 3 scalpel handles, with Nos. 11, 12 and 15 blades
Goldman Fox knives Nos. 7, 11
Blake knife
Periosteal elevators (Ash No. 9)
Adson large tissue forceps
Goldman Fox No. 16 scissors
Crile–Wood needle holder
Ochsenbien periodontal chisels, left and right
No. 6 round bone bur
Rough diamond gingivoplasty stones
Arkansas sharpening stone
Ethicon eyeless sutures 4·0 B/B
   (with FS-2 18·7 mm needle) and 5·0 B/B
Bulb syringe (for use with normal saline)

Appendix C

Other equipment and materials required

a. For treatment purposes
Whitehead's varnish
Thrombin
Gelfoam
Phytomenadione (Konakion) 10–20 mg
Prilocaine 3% with felypressin
Iodine solution (for periodontal use)
Neb. Ephedrine 1% in normal saline
Tinct. Benzoin Co. inhalations
Karvol inhalant capsules
Carbolized resin
Pom-poms
Tannic acid powder
Phenindamine tablets BP
Plastic foam chin supports
Trichloracetic acid
Glycerine
Capillary tubes containing lead shot

b. To facilitate investigations
Capillary tubes containing a lead shot
Filter paper
Acetest and Clinitest tablets
Sickledex testing kit
Browne's tubes
Autoclave tape
Bacteriology swabs
West nasopharyngeal swabs
Intra-oral adhesive bandage
Microscope slides
Wooden spatulas
Cytospray, Spraycyte; solution of equal parts ether/95% ethyl alcohol
Sterile disposable syringes (2·5 ml and 10 ml side-nozzle)
Sterile No. 1 needles
Ellis biopsy drill
10% formol-saline
Specimen containers

c. For use in emergencies

Most of the emergencies which are likely to occur in the dental surgery can be dealt with effectively by the prompt application of the basic methods of resuscitation without recourse to drug therapy. Carefully planned arrangements and well designed equipment can facilitate resuscitation in the following ways:

Requirement	Achieved by
1. Patient in supine position	Use of dental chair designed to effect this quickly, and/or surgery design permitting the patient to be laid on floor with ease
2. A patent airway	Efficient suction apparatus (0·14 kg/sq cm, 20 lb/sq in) Guedel's airways Oxygen ⎫ Readily available
3. Artificial respiration	Brook airway Inflating bellows (Ambu, Porten) Training of all members of staff
4. External cardiac massage	Training of all members of staff

On occasions the use of the following drugs may prove to be life saving:

1. *When given intravenously:*
    50% dextrose solution 20–100 ml ampoules.
    Hydrocortisone sodium succinate injection BP 100 mg in 2 ml.
    Phentolamine methane sulphonate (Rogitine) 5 mg.

2. *When injected directly into the heart:*
    10% calcium chloride solution 5 ml.

3. *When given intramuscularly:*
    0·1% (1:1000) adrenaline solution 1 ml.
    Lorazepam 4 mg.

The *cricothyrotomy kit* should be kept sterile and ready for use in a convenient place, and comprises:
    Scalpel handle No. 3
    Scalpel blades Nos. 10 and 15
    Scissors (Kilner) 10 cm (4 in)
    Abelson cricothyrotomy cannula
    Large-bore intravenous cannula (size 10 or 12)
    Endotracheal or tracheostomy tubes (size 4–8)

Index